Surface Engineering and Technology for Biomedical Implants

Surface Engineering and Technology for Biomedical Implants

YOSHIKI OSHIDA

MOMENTUM PRESS

MOMENTUM PRESS, LLC, NEW YORK

First published by Momentum Press®, LLC
222 East 46th Street New York, NY 10017
www.momentumpress.net

ISBN-13: 978-1-60650-627-1 (hard back, case bound)
ISBN-13: 978-1-60650-628-8 (e-book)
DOI: 10.5643/9781606506288

Cover design by Jonathan Pennell
Interior design by Exeter Premedia Services Private Ltd., Chennai, India

10 9 8 7 6 5 4 3 2 1

Printed in the United States of America

To my wife
for putting up with me

&

To my parents and family members
for their love, support, and encouragement

Contents

Preface

As society is increasingly concerned with quality of life for an ever-growing elderly population and those with sports and military injuries, greater attention is being paid to managing diseases and pains, as well as treating these populations. Orthopedics and dental implants still face many challenges to facilitate the aged society, in particular, because implant receiving vital hard tissue gradually deteriorates (in the sense of reduced bone density and quality). In addition, special developments in materials, as well as treatment techniques, are urgently needed for dental/medical implant candidates who have already developed serious or lifestyle-related diseases which are contraindicative to implant treatments.

And there is much development going on. As detailed in the Prologue and Chapter 1, there are no fewer than 120 journals in the medical/dental and engineering fields related to the subject in this book. The challenges are interdisciplinary and of worldwide interest.

Chapters 2 through 4 discuss materials and compatibility requirements. Well-established treatments are discussed in Chapter 5, followed by evaluations in Chapter 6. But there are still many materials, modification methods, as well as treatment techniques, which are under R&D stage, as seen in Chapter 7. These should include an extensive application of 3D bioprinting technology toward a successful fabrication of customized implant systems, functionally gradient material/structure, biofunctionalization of newly developed materials, and so forth.

Keywords

surface, interface, surface engineering and modification, biomaterials, implantable materials, compatibilities

Acknowledgements

In closing, I admit to having a very long list of individual names to be mentioned with my memories and appreciation–from my teachers who inspired me, friends and colleagues who challenged me, and most importantly students (some of them are now my colleagues) who continue to both inspire and challenge me. To all of them, I owe my knowledge and capability to comprehend the cited articles presented in this book. These people, who were and are valuable to me and to this book, should at least include the late T. Nakayama, S. Iguchi, V. Weiss, H. W. Liu, the late J. A. Schwartz, T. Koizumi, N. Saotome, T. Nishihara, F. Farzin-Nia, G. K. Stookey, the late C. J. Andres, the late T. M. Barco, M. Kowolik, V. John, D. Brown, D. Burr, M. Siefert, R. Shew, J. A. Parr, R. Miyamoto, M. Kingsley, J. Williams, J. Levon, A. Zuccari, A. Hashem, A. Wu, M. Yapchulay, S. Isikbay, C. Kuphasuk, C-M. Lin, I. Garcia, W. Panyayong, Y-J Lim, M.Reyes, W. C. Lim, J-C. Chang, S. Al-Ali, B. Anbari, D. Bartovic, F. Hernandez, I. W. Koh, Z. H. Khabbaz, R. Xirouchaki, P. Agarwal, N. Al-Nasr, C. B. Sellers, J. Dunigan-Miler, S. Al-Johancy, C. S. Wang, E. Matsis, R. Rani, Y-C. Wu, K. Mirza, I. Katsilieri, C. N. Elias, E. B. Tuna, O. Aktören, K. Gençay, Y. Güven, L. Oshida, and JIP (Japan Implant Practice) Association members. Special thanks should also go to M. A. Dirlam for excellent professional illustrations of all figures in this book, and to the Editorial team at Momentum Press (S. Goldberg, J. Stein, and M. Treloar). Finally, but not least important, special thanks should go to J. Schulterbrandt for his comments on the text. Thank you all.

Prologue

This book is based on a review of about 1,500 carefully selected articles and presents itself as a typical example of evidence-based learning (EBL). Evidence-based literature reviews can provide foundation skills in research-oriented bibliographic inquiry, with an emphasis on such review and synthesis of applicable literature. Information is gathered by surveying a broad array of multidisciplinary research publications written by scholars and researchers.

In order for EBL to be used effectively, the content of every publication must be critically evaluated in terms of its degree of reliability. There is an established protocol for ranking the reliability of sources—this is a especially useful tool in the medical and dental fields. The ranking, from the most to least reliable evidence source, follows: (i) clinical reports using placebo and double blind studies, (ii) clinical reports not using placebo, but conducted according to well-prepared statistical test plans, (iii) study reports on time-effect on one group of patients during predetermined period of time, (iv) study/comparison reports, at one limited time, on many groups of patients, (v) case reports on a new technique or idea, or both, and (vi) retrospective reports on clinical evidence. Unfortunately, the number of published articles increases in this descending reliability order. The greatest advantage of the EBL review is that it helps identify common phenomena in a diversity of fields and literature. It is then possible to create synthetic, inclusive hypotheses that deepen and further our understanding.

As important as the diversity of source material is to the EBL review, it can pose unique challenges. The sources used in this review are mainly journal articles published in the medical/dental and engineering fields. These two groups' studies have very different analytical criteria and inherent issues.

In medical/dental journals authors typically present statistically analyzed results; this lends these studies a high degree of reliability. Though we may be confident in the conclusions drawn from statistical analysis, it can be difficult to develop generalized ideas from this literature. Some controversy exists in the medical and dental fields on the relationship between *in vitro* and *in vivo* test results. This situation is further complicated and confusing because among the various *in vivo* tests exists a wide variety of animal model species. The *in vitro* studies are also not without weakness—it is almost impossible to broadly extrapolate *in vitro* test results, since it is very rare to find articles where identical test methods were employed.

In contrast to medical/dental studies, the data presented in the engineering journals are normally not subjected to statistical analysis. The characterization of data is considered more important to interpretation results because researchers try to explain phenomena, mechanisms, and kinetics.

Discoveries in the engineering realm are vitally important to the advancement of medicine and dentistry: the materials and most of the technologies currently employed in medical and dental fields were originally developed in the engineering field. In this book, the author draws upon his unique experience in both fields to bridge the gap between medical/dental and engineering research.

At the early stages of preparing this book, the author chose appropriate journals in both medical/dental and engineering fields, which were directly and indirectly relevant to a group of key words including: surface, interface, surface engineering and modification, biomaterials, implantable materials, and compatibilities. There are about 120 journals in front of me. These are surprisingly a large number of journals. For those who might be interested in the literature survey in similar scope of this book, here is a lengthy list of journals; *Am J Orthod, Am J Dent, Angle Orthod, Advanced Material Process, American J Orthod Dentofacial Orthop, ASM Intl, Apply Sur Sci, Advances Dent Res, Amer J Orthod, Acta Biomater, Ann Biomed Eng, Appl Sur Sci, ACS Nano, Adv Orthop Surg, Biomaterials, Br Med J, Bone Joint Surg Br, Biomed Mater, Bioelectrochemistry, Biochemistry, CRC Crit Rev Biocompatibility, Cell Clin Implant Dent Relat Res, Clin Orthop, Clin Oral Implant Res, Clin Oral Investing, Clin Mater, Contact Dermatitis, Crit Rev Oral Boil Med, Corr Sci, Corrosion, Colloids Surf B Biointerfaces, Dent Mater J, Digest J Nanometer and Biostructures, Electrochem Acta, Faraday Discuss, Gen Dent, Intl Dental Jour, Int J Oral Maxillofac Implants, Int J Oral Surg, Int J Nanomed, Int J Prosthodont, Implant Dent, Int Arch Allergy Apply, Immunol, Int J Mol Sci, J Adhes, J Adhes Sci Technol, J Alloys Compound, J Am Ceram Soc, J Appl Phys, J Apply Biomater, J Assoc Ad Med Instrum, J Arthroplasty, J Bacterial J Biochem Biophys Method, J Biosci Polym Ed, Journal of Metals, J Biomech, J Biomed Mater Res A, J Biomed Mater Res B, J Bio-Med Mater Eng, J Bone Joint Surg Am, J Bone Miner Res, J Cardiovasc Technol, J Chronic Dis, J Clin Invest, J Clin Pathol, J Colloid Interface Sci, J Dent Res, J Electroceramics, J EngTribol, J Exp Med, J Invest Dermatol, J Jpn Soc Dental Mater Devices, J Less-Common Metal, J Mater Sci, J Mater Sci Let, J Mater Process Technol, J Mech Behav Biomed Mater, J Mater Sci Mater Med, J Nanosci Nanotechnol, J Prosthet Dent, J Electrochem Soc, J Oral Implants, J Oral Rehabil, J Prosthodont, J Vac Sci Technol, Jpn Inst Metals, Jpn Dent Mater, Langmuir, Metall Mater Trans A, Metall Mater Trans B, Mater Manufac Process, Mater Science Eng A, Mater Science Eng B, Mater Perform, Mater Science Forum, Mol Biology of the Cell, Med Device Technol, Med Sci Monit, Med Prog Technol, Orthopedics, Oral Microbial Immunol, Proc Royal Soc, Prog Organ Coat, Quint Intl, Quint Dent Technol, Surf Coat Technol, Surf Technol, Surf Interface Anal, Tribology Industry, Tissue Eng, Tribol Letter, The Amer Soc Metals, Trans Orthop Res Soc, Trans Soc Biomater, Trans Electrochem Soc, Thin Solid Films, Toxicology*, and *Wear*. I suspect there should be more than these.

Let's do a simple calculation, suppose each journal is published monthly (of course, some of these are published quarterly). Looking only at the last 10 years, it might be simply 120 journals × 12 months × 10 years = 14,400 individual journals. Of course, all of these articles are not equally relevant to the scope of this book; let us assume that approximately 10% of these should possess reasonable relevancy to this book. As I mentioned in the prologue, I carefully selected about 1,500 articles, which is about 10% of the aforementioned number. In other words, at least one article out of the 120 journals published monthly is somewhat related to this book. Accordingly, the contents of this book should well-represent worldwide researches.

Chapter 1

Introduction

We have a tremendous number of artificial organs or devices that help to maintain patients' quality of life (QOL); they include hydrocephalus shunts, ocular and contact lenses, orbital floors, artificial ears, cochlear implants, nasal implants, artificial chins, mandibular mesh, artificial skin, blood substitutes, artificial hearts and heart valves, pacemakers, breast prostheses, pectus implants, glucose biosensors, dialysis shunts and catheters, absorbable pins, temporary tendons, artificial kidneys, birth control implants, vascular grafts, artificial live, spinal fixations, finger joints, cartilage replacements, artificial legs, bone plates and bars (including sacroiliac joint), and Harington spinal bars. There are also a variety of dental prostheses, including dental implants, bridges and crowns, endodontic devices, orthodonticarch wires, and brackets. The development of dental and orthopedic implants (particularly, knee, and total hip replacements) is particularly important and the most challenging, because it involves the collective knowledge and synthesis of several diverse disciplines such as biomaterials science and engineering, and surface modification and technology in order to obtain its ultimate goal: That their surfaces are biologically accepted by a host's vital hard and soft tissues and function in body.

This chapter introduces the three basic requirements for placed implants to exhibit satisfactory biofunctionality: *Biological* (or in short, biocompatibility), *morphological*, and *biomechanical compatibility*. In the following chapters of this book, we will discuss implantable materials, the nature of surfaces and interfaces, some important interfacial reactions, requirements for successful implant systems, and surface modifications and its methods, characterization, and evaluations of modified surfaces. At the end, we will introduce the application of newly developed technology into dental and medical implantology.

1.1. Literature Review Results

Figure 1.1 shows the popularity of pure titanium (CpTi: commercially pure titanium) and its alloys (typically, Ti–6Al–4V and Ti–6Al–7Nb) in dental and medical fields by counting the manuscripts published in different journals, most of which will be cited in this book, and the number of publication on the term "biocompatibility" [1,2]. Referring

DOI 10.5643/9781606506288/ch1

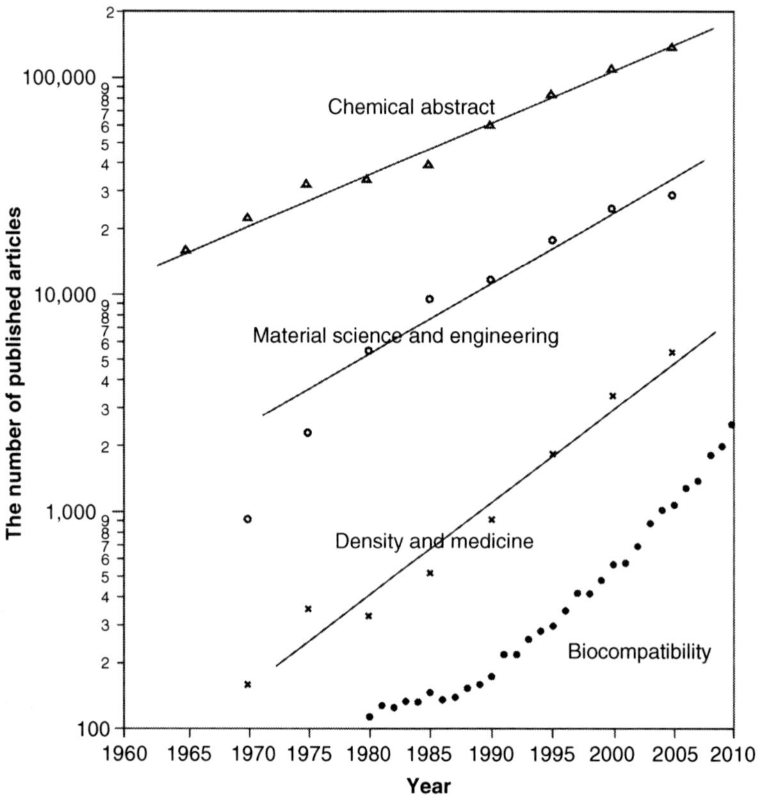

Figure 1.1. Accumulated number of published articles on titanium materials and biocompatibility.

to the figure, there are three straight lines in the semi-log plot that demonstrate the total accumulated number of published articles every 5 years. The uppermost line represents the accumulated number of all articles listed in Chemical Abstract. It represents a wide scattering of articles in many areas including refining, metallurgy, dentistry, medicine, bioengineering, engineering, industries, pure chemistry, and chemical engineering. The second straight line from the top is obtained when the search area is limited to materials science in both the engineering and medical/dentistry fields. If our search is further defined within only medicine/dentistry area, we still have an exponential increase in publications. If we search only for articles related to "biocompatibility," the number of published articles by year again appears to be increasing almost in parallel to those on titanium biomaterials in dentistry and medicine, indicating that the concept of biocompatibility is recognized as very important when biomaterials are used for both dental (intraoral) and orthopedic (extraoral) implant systems.

1.2. Acceptability and Prevalence of Implants

A questionnaire yielded interesting results about the differences in attitudes toward implant treatment among middle-aged and older Swedish subjects over a 10-year interval in 1989 and 1999 [3]. One thousand six hundred sixty-five subjects responded to both surveys. It was reported that (i) in 1989, few respondents indicated an interest in implant treatment, (ii) whereas, in 1999, 92% of those who had not indicated an interest in the earlier survey now indicated that they desired implant treatment, and (iii) changes in awareness of implant treatment, along with an expansion in the number of qualified providers, may have contributed to this increase [3]. Advances in medical science and developments in biomedical materials have led to a remarkable increase in life span and improvement of QOL. Monitoring friction and wear in the human body has played a very significant role in those improvements.

There are six major joint systems in our body: the shoulder, elbow, wrist, hip, knee, and ankle joints. Replacement surgery is commonly performed on hip and knee joints. Hip prosthesis or hip replacement surgery becomes necessary when the hip joint has been badly damaged from causes such as arthritis, congenital malformation or abnormal development, and damage from injury. A natural hip is composed of a femoral (thigh bone) with a femoral head on top of it that articulates with the acetabular cup in the acetabulum. As in all other joints, cartilage is found between the acetabular cup and the femoral head, and acts to lubricate their movement and facilitate the articulation. In an arthritic hip joint, the cartilage has been damaged, narrowed or even lost by a degenerative process or by inflammation.

Thus, several organs, joints, and critical parts of the human body wear out and may be replaced [4]. According to a report, the amount of predicted implant placements in 2002 in the United States will be as follows: total hip joint replacements: 448,000; knee joint replacements: 452,000; shoulder joint replacements: 24,000; dental implants: 854,000; coronary stents: 1,204,000; and coronary catheters: 1,328,000 [5,6]. Further, even when the implantation has been successfully performed and the prognosis has been excellent, dental and medical implants can fail due to wear, fatigue, chemical degradation, infection, and lead to osteolysis and loosening [4,7].

1.3. Overview of Implant Technology

In order to place an implantable material, the host's hard tissue has to be traumatized. Injured or diseased tissues will be removed to some extent in the process of implantation. The success of the entire operation depends on the kind and degree of tissue response (*biocompatibility*) toward the implants during the healing process. The tissue response toward the injury may vary widely according to the site, species, contamination, and so forth [5,7].

Endosseous dental implants have created a revolution in the routine approach to dental care for patients missing one or more teeth. The success of this procedure was obtained through a series of clinical and biological steps, starting with the initial primary stability provided by the amount, quality, and distribution of bone within the proposed implant site [8–10]. Following the placement of the dental implant, a series of bone modeling and remodeling steps take place. Bone adaptation or integration of an implant is characterized by a series of biological reactions that start with bone turnover at the interface: a process of localized necrosis, followed by rapid repair [11]. The long-term success of implant therapy is not just dependent on enhanced osseous stability, greater attention being given to the transmucosal dental implant or implant abutment interfaces. The mechanical and biological stability derived from the design and surfaces in this connective tissue and adjacent epithelial environment are critical to maintaining a sufficient volume of connective tissue with minimal inflammatory infiltrate [12]. In order to increase the predictability of implant therapy, significant efforts have gone into the development of implant biomaterials that hold the promise of improving clinical success. These technologies have evolved from simple modification of the oxide surface to precise nanoscale modification technologies that involve the formation of a uniform and consistent surface that leads to altered cellular response. Further, there are developing technologies that utilize changes in surface chemistry. Also, biologics are also being added to the oxide surface in order to assist in stability of both the osseous and transmucosal environment [12–16].

With regard to bone healing immediately after placing an implant(s) in traumatized bone, there are three distinct and crucial stages: (i) the first and most important healing phase, osteoconduction, relies on the recruitment and migration of osteogenic cells to the implant surface, through the residue of the peri-implant blood clot. Among the most important aspects of osteoconduction are the indirect effects generated at the implant surface, by the initiation of platelet activation, which results in directed osteogenic cell migration, (ii) the second healing phase, de novo bone formation, results in a mineralized interfacial matrix equivalent to that seen in the cement line in natural bone tissue; these two healing phases, osteoconduction and de novo bone formation, result in contact osteogenesis and, given an appropriate implant surface, bone bonding, and (iii) the third healing phase, bone remodeling, relies on slower processes [17,18].

Osseointegration, which can be defined as a direct structural and functional connection between living bone and the surface of a load-carrying implant and is recognized as a time-depending bone healing, is critical for implant stability, and is considered a prerequisite for implant loading and long-term clinical success of endosseous dental implants. The implant/tissue interface is an extremely dynamic region of interaction. This complex interaction involves not only biomaterial and biocompatibility issues but also alteration of mechanical environment. The processes of osseointegration involve an initial interlocking between alveolar bone and the implant body, and later, biological fixation through continuous bone apposition and remodeling toward the implant. The process itself is quite complex and there are many factors that influence the formation and maintenance of bone at the implant surface. Ideally, an implant's appearance can histologically resemble a functional ankylosis, with no intervention of fibrous or connective tissue between bone and implant surface [19,20]. The successful outcome of any implant procedure is mainly dependent on the interrelationship of the various factors, including biocompatibility of the implant material, macroscopic and microscopic nature of the implant surface and designs, the status of the implant in both a health and a morphology (bone quality) context, the surgical technique, the health of the patient, the undisturbed healing phase, and loading conditions [19,21].

Various modifications of the implant surface can alter the percentage of osseointegration. New types of reinforcements for implants and the use of growth factors to augment bone regeneration have been developed [17]. As mentioned before, osseointegration is a major factor influencing the success of dental implants. To achieve rapid and strong durable osseointegration, biomaterial researchers have investigated various surface treatment methods, particularly for titanium dental implants. Current dental implant research has studied the interaction between bone and implant surfaces in order to understand and improve the osseointegration process. The implant surface treatment, chemical or topographic modification, and cellular interactions can affect bone healing, promote accelerated osteogenesis, and increase bone–implant contact and bond strength.

Surface characteristics determine not only aesthetic appearance but also interaction with the environment, including mechanical interactions such as friction and wear and chemical interactions such as adherence and biocorrosion. Coatings, claddings, thin films, and other surface modifications may be categorized in many ways. One of these is principally by the form of the material deposited at any given instant on a small area of the surface. Such forms include atoms or molecules, particles, bulk, and others. Atomic deposition include electroplating, CVD (chemical vapor deposition), PVD (physical vapor deposition), ion implantation, vacuum evaporation, molecular beam epitaxy, plasma and sputter deposition, and spray pyrolysis. Particulate deposition includes thermal spray, flame spray, high velocity oxyfuel spray, impact packing, fusion coating, enameling, and electrophoresis. Bulk coating/cladding should include wetting processes such as painting and dip coating, electrostatic spraying such as spin coating, laser cladding, and high temperature synthesis. In addition to these, shot peening and laser peening can be included as mechanical modification [22,23]. Surface transformations (such as ceramization, nitrization, etc.) can be performed on metals in order to combine their load-bearing properties to the inertness and wear resistance of ceramics. In a joint prosthesis, metals are useful for their high fatigue strength and ductility, but they are more sensitive to superficial corrosion and wear than ceramics. Coating a ceramic on metal surface will improve the qualities of the metallic component [24].

References

1. Oshida, Y., 2007, *Bioscience and Bioengineering of Titanium Materials*, Elsevier, London, UK, pp.4–5.
2. Annual number of published articles in peer-review journals on "Biocompatibility" between 1970 and 2007. en.wikipedia.org/wiki/Biocompatibility.
3. Narby, B., Kronström, M., Söderfeldt, B. and Sigvard Palmqvist, S., 2008, Changes in attitudes toward desire for implant treatment: A longitudinal study of a middle -aged and older Swedish population, *Int J Prosthodont* 21:481–485.
4. Shtansky, D.V. and Roy, M., 2013, Surface engineering for biotribological application, In: M. Roy ed., *Surface Engineering for Enhanced Performance against Wear*, Springer, New York, NY, pp. 277–310.
5. Black, J. and Hastings, G. ed., 1998, *Handbook of Biomaterial Properties*, Chapman & Hall, Thomson Science, UK.
6. Zivić, F., Babić, M., Grujović, N. and Mitrović, S., 2010, Tribometry of materials for bioengineering applications, *Tribol Industry* 32:25–32.
7. Helsen, J.A. and Missirlis, Y., 2010, *Biomaterials, Biological and Medical Physics, Biomedical Engineering,* Springer-Verlag, Berlin/Heidelberg, Germany.

8. Roos, J., Sennerby, L. and Albrektsson, T., 1997, An update on the clinical documentation on currently used bone anchored endosseous oral implants, *Dent Update* 24:194–200.
9. De Freest, C.F. and Savett, D.A., 1996, Longevity of osseointegrated dental implants, In L. L.Hence and J. Wilson ed., *Clinical Performance of Skeletal Prostheses*, Springer, New York, NY, pp. 237–254.
10. Schliephake, H. and D. Scharnweber, D., 2008, Chemical and biological functionalization of titanium for dental implants, *J Mater Chem* 18:2404–2414. doi: http://dx.doi.org/10.1039/B715355B.
11. Stanford, C.M. and Brand, R.A., 1999, Toward an understanding of implant occlusion and strain adaptive bone modeling and remodeling, J Prosthet Dent 81:553–561.
12. Salvi, G.E. and Lang, N.P., 2001, Changing paradigms in implant dentistry, *Crit Rev Oral Biol Med* 12:262–272.
13. Berglundh, T., Persson, L. and Klinge, B., 2002, A systematic review of the incidence of biological and technical complications in implant dentistry reported in prospective longitudinal studies of at least 5 years, *J Clin Periodontol* 29:197–212. doi: http://dx.doi.org/10.1034/j.1600-051X.29.s3.12.x.
14. Renvert, S., Roos-Jansaker, A-M., Lindahl, C., Renvert, H. and Persson, G.R., 2007, Infection at titanium implants with or without a clinical diagnosis of inflammation, Clin Oral Implant Res 18:509–516. doi: http://dx.doi.org/10.1111/j.1600-0501.2007.01378.x.
15. Roos-Jansaker, A-M., Renvert, H., Lindahl, C. and Renvert, S., 2006, Nine- to fourteen-year follow-up of implant treatment. Part III: Factors associated with peri-implant lesions, *J Clin Periodontol* 33:296–301.
16. Stanford, C.M., 2010, Surface modification of biomedical and dental implants and the processes of inflammation, wound healing and bone formation, Int J Mol Sci 11:354–369.
17. Davies, J.E., 2003, Understanding peri-implant endosseous healing, *J Dent Educ* 67:932-949. doi: http://dx.doi.org/10.3390/ijms11010354.
18. Fritz, M.E., 1999, Two-stage implant systems, *Adv Dent Res* 13:162–169. doi: http://dx.doi.org/10.1177/08959374990130010601
19. Parithimarkalaignan, S. and Padmanabhan, T.V., 2013, Osseointegration: An update, *J Ind Prosthodon Soc* 13:2–6. doi: http://dx.doi.org/ 10.1007/s13191-013-0252-z.
20. Abjanich, J.H. and Orenstein, I.H., 2002, Prosthodontic considerations in dental implant restoration, In: A.M. Greenberg and J. Prein ed., Craniomaxillofacial Reconstructive and Corrective Bone Surgery*: Principles of Internal Fixation Using the AO/ASIF Technique*, Springer, New York, NY, pp. 232–261.
21. Oshida, Y., 2007, *Bioscience and Bioengineering of Titanium Materials*, Elsevier, London, UK, pp. 180–182.
22. Tucker, R.C., 2002, Surface engineering, *JOM* 160:1–3.
23. Oshida, Y., 2007, *Bioscience and Bioengineering of Titanium Materials*, Elsevier, London, UK, pp. 317–319.
24. Rieu, J., 1993, Ceramic formation on metallic surfaces (ceramization) for medical applications, *Clin Mater* 12:227–235.

Chapter 2

Implantable Materials

Each of the joints in the six major components in the body, that is, the shoulder, elbow, wrist, hip, knee, and ankle, possesses a unique biomechanistic function. Orthopedic implant material for these joints requires distinct mechanical properties of ductility, rigidity, and strength to the respective joints. In addition, biological parameters should not be ignored for orthopedic implant material selections, because it will become a crucial issue if there were a problem of wear debris toxicity involved. As to dental implants, although each of the 32 teeth has different biofunctions, we can roughly divide them into anterior teeth portion versus posterior teeth portion and maxilla teeth portion versus mandibular teeth portion. These quadrants show distinct force and moment during the masticatory activity. Accordingly, appropriate dental implant systems should be selected and certain types of surface modification (modification for material's case zone) should be applied to the properly selected implantable material(s). In this chapter, basic properties of the three major materials (as material's core zone) along with composite materials will be reviewed.

2.1. Introduction

The oral environment, in which saliva and bacteria are found, is corrosive to dental restoration materials. Implanted material should be tested for various biochemical reactions within the body. This includes (i) nearly inert materials, with minimal chemical reactivity; (ii) totally resorbable materials, with possible dissolution into metabolic constituents; and (iii) materials with controlled-activity surfaces. These biomaterials can be found in the metallic materials group, polymeric materials group, ceramic materials group, and composite materials group. Over the last 15–20 years, tests and standards have been developed to assess and categorize the chemical and biological suitability of these materials; they now serve as the basis for the recommendation of any dental restoration material. Until a few years ago, almost all national and international dental standards and testing programs focused entirely on the physical and chemical properties of a material. However, today dental material standards require biological testing as well. The science of dental materials now encompasses a broad knowledge and appreciation of the biological restraints

DOI 10.5643/9781606506288/ch2

associated with the selection and use of materials designed for use in the oral cavity. According to the existing standards, all dental materials should pass primary tests (screening to indicate cellular response), secondary tests (evaluating tissue responses), and usage tests in animals before being evaluated clinically in humans. Testing programs for dental materials are based on specifications or standards established by national or international standards organizations, such as the American National Standards Institute (ANSI) and the International Standards Organization. The oldest and largest of these programs has been operated continuously by the American Dental Association (ADA) since the late 1920s. Evaluation of dental products for safety and efficacy has historically been the scope of both the ADA and the Food and Drug Administration (FDA). In accordance with these regulations (US Medical Device Amendments, 1976), all dental materials are reviewed for safety and effectiveness and classified by the FDA as Class I, II, or III. Class I materials are considered to be of low risk in causing adverse reactions. Materials in Class II must satisfy the requirements outlined in the current ANSI/ADA specifications. The most extensive testing is required for Class III materials, which includes full safety and efficacy assessments prior to marketing [1,2].

This chapter describes all the materials that have been evaluated as implantable. Within this assortment of biomaterials, titanium and Co–Cr–Mo alloys are almost exclusively used for metallic implants. Of these, the titanium alloy seems best suited for orthopedic and dental uses due to its superior biocompatibility, light weight, low stiffness, and cost. However, its relatively poor abrasion resistance can be improved by a hard coating, such as TiN, so that Ti-based alloys can be used for the artificial hip or knee joint replacement. Aluminum alloys and stainless steels are used in medical instruments. Aluminum is used where low weight and low cost are important and great strength and abrasion resistance are not needed. Surgical class stainless steels behave differently; the 300 series stainless steel is used where good corrosion resistance and strength are important but not abrasion resistance, whereas the 400 series steels are used where abrasion resistance is important such as in cutting tools and guides and some corrosion resistance can be sacrificed. The precipitation hardening steels are used where improved corrosion resistance is needed but at the sacrifice of hardness and strength, in comparison to the 400 series. Ultra-high-molecular-weight polyethylene (UHMWPE) is exclusively used for implant bearings with a highly cross-linked version commonly used for the hip replacement bearings due to its greatly apparent, improved wear resistance. However, the increased stiffness and brittleness makes the use of such materials in incongruent knee devices questionable. Acetal and other engineering plastics are used for many instrument applications [3].

2.2. Metallic Biomaterials

Metallic biomaterials continue to be used extensively for the fabrication of surgical implants primarily for the same reason that led to their initial selection of these devices many decades ago: high strength and fracture and corrosion resistance. These qualities make them suitable and reliable for long-term implant performance in major load-bearing situations. This, coupled with a relative ease of fabrication of both simple and complex shapes using well-established and widely available fabrication techniques (e.g., casting, forging, machining, and advanced manufacturing technologies such as superplastic forming or laser forming), has promoted the use of metallic biomaterials primarily in the fields of orthopedics and dentistry, the two disciplines in which highly loaded devices are most common. It is noteworthy to add that similar reasons have led to their widening use in cardiovascular devices (e.g., artificial heart valves, blood conduits, and other components of heart assist devices, vascular stents) and neurovascular implants (aneurysm clips) [4–6]. In addition, the electrical conductivity of metals favors their use as neuromuscular stimulation devices, the most common example being cardiac pacemakers. These favorable properties (good fracture resistance, electrical conductivity, and formability) are related to the metallic interatomic bonding that characterizes this class of material. An understanding of material properties and the fabrication processes of metallic components is critical for ensuring the desired performance of implants in service. While mechanical failure is unacceptable for most engineered structures, it is particularly so for surgical implants where failure can cause pain in patients and, in certain cases, death (e.g., heart valve component fracture), or the need for complicated and life-threatening revision surgery [4].

Titanium materials (including CpTi and Ti-based alloys) are extensively used in both dental and medical fields—particularly in dental implantology and orthopedics. CpTi possesses four grades: I, II, III, and IV. Ti-based alloys include TiNi, Ti–6Al–4V, and Ti–6Al–7Nb. TiNi's superelastic (SE) nature and shape memory effect (SME) property have been effectively used for orthopedic implants, devices, and tools in endodontic dentistry and orthodontic mechanotherapy [7–9]. The bulk material forms of Ti and its alloys have been widely used in orthopedic implants due to their good biocompatibility, high strength-to-weight ratio (i.e., high specific strength), relative low elastic modulus (or low stiffness), high fatigue strength, and excellent corrosion resistance, as compared to the widely used biomedical Co–Cr alloys and stainless steels. Nevertheless, porous implant components manufactured from biocompatible metallic materials are known to promote interactions between bone and the surrounding tissue. Pores facilitate bone tissue formation by allowing the migration and proliferation of osteoblasts and mesenchymal cells into the implant [10,11]. In addition, a porous surface provides mechanical interlocking between the implant and the surrounding bone, enhancing mechanical stability at the interface. The minimum pore size suitable for bone replacement was reported to be larger than 100 μm, while the tendency of fibrous tissue formation increased above a pore size of 1 mm [10].

A major goal of endosseous dental implant use is to achieve osseointegration or biointegration of the bone with the implant. Although a wide variety of materials have been used for such implants, only a few promote or achieve osseointegration and biointegration; these are CpTi- and Ti-based alloys. The surface oxide of titanium appears to be central to the ability of this material to osseointegrate. The oxide limits the dissolution of elements and promotes the deposition of biological molecules that allow bone to exist as close as 30 Å to the surface of the implant. The epithelial interface between the gingiva and titanium appears to contain many of the structural characteristics of the native tooth–gingiva interface, but details are still vague. The connective tissue interface with the titanium appears to be one of tightly fitting tissues rather than adhesion. Ceramic coatings appear to improve the ingrowth of bone and to promote chemical integration of the implant with the bone. While the complex characteristics of these coatings affect the ossification response, the mechanisms remain obscure. Progress in dental implantology is likely to continue as the interface between the material and bone is more clearly understood, and biological molecules and artificial tissues are developed [11]. Stainless steel (316L) and Co–Cr alloys have been widely used as materials in orthopedic implants because of their biocompatibility, physical properties, and manufacturing ease [12]. In general, these alloys have excellent corrosion resistance and are not believed to cause any local or systemic responses. However, fretting corrosion of metallic implants is sometimes observed in biological systems and leads to the release of metallic ions from the implants [13,14]. These ions, such as Ni, Co, and Cr, are known to cause adverse tissue and allergic reactions [15–18].

Although Ti and its alloys are currently considered the most attractive metallic materials for orthopedic and dental surgeries, the mechanical/tensile strength of CpTi is insufficient for its use as an artificial hip joint, pin, or screws [19,20], and its wear resistance is also inferior to that of stainless steels and Co–Cr alloys [20]. The appearance of increased wear debris from Ti has been associated with inflammation, bone resorption, and pain [21–25]. To improve mechanical strength and wear resistance, various elements have been added to create new Ti alloys.

Ti–6Al–4V is a high-strength Ti alloy, but its biocompatibility is considered lower than that of CpTi. The wear and corrosion resistances of Ti–6Al–4V are inferior to those of Ti; further, Ti–6Al–4V releases compounds and wear debris containing V or V ions, both of which are toxic [21]. At present, it is difficult to avoid the wear or fretting of implanted alloys, or both, in a living body, resulting in the release of elements contained in the alloy and the formation of wear debris. Therefore, it is preferable not to use highly toxic elements in alloys. This gives a basic reason for developing new, V-free Ti alloys with strengths equivalent to Ti–6Al–4V. Accordingly, Ti–6Al–7Nb and Ti–5Al–2.5Fe [7] have been developed and used in service.

Recently, Ti–13Nb–13Zr [26] (elastic modulus of 40–80 GPa) and Ti–29Nb–13Ta–4.6Zr [27] have been developed for orthopedic applications in order to avoid the "stress shielding" effect caused by the modulus mismatch between the implant and the bone. The Ti–Zr binary alloy has better corrosion resistance and mechanical properties than CpTi. Ikarashi et al. [28] placed Ti–Zr samples in a subcutaneous position in rats for 8 months. It was reported that all Ti–Zr samples showed similar mitogen-induced blastogenesis as was observed in Ti, Zr, and Cr samples, suggesting that the implantation of Ti–Zr alloy did not cause systemic toxicity or a decrease in immune activity. It is interesting to note that (i) the fibrous capsule membranes around the Ti and Ti–Zr alloy implants were thinner than those around the Cr implants; (ii) the number of macrophages, inflammatory cells, and other cells involved in immune responses in and around the fibrous capsules of the Cr- and Ti-implant groups were higher than those of the Ti–Zr alloy- and Zr-implant groups; and (iii) the Ti–Zr alloy had the lowest total score of tissue responses among the materials tested. None of the animals from the Ti-, Zr-, and Ti–Zr alloy-implant groups exhibited a skin reaction after exposure to Ti or Zr salt solutions, indicating that Ti–Zr alloy has better biocompatibility than Ti for use as an artificial surgical implant [14]. Similar evaluations on Ti–Zr alloy as dental implant materials are reported [29,30].

Due to the specific properties of its SME or SE effects, or both, NiTi intermetallic alloy has been widely utilized in both the dental field (as an implant material, endodontic file and reamers, orthodontic archwires, etc.) and the medical field (as stents, Harrington spiral plate, etc.). NiTi alloys can be solid or porous, like a foam metal [31,32]. The porous NiTi, whose porosity was controlled by self-propagating high-temperature synthesis, provided appropriately sized and interconnected (open) pores, thus creating implant morphologies similar to bone. A porous implant structure allows ingrowth of mineralized tissue, establishing a biological fixation of the implant. It has been shown that 50% porous NiTi provides greater initial bone ingrowth than 30% porous hydroxyapatite (HA), primarily due to the greater exposed surface area [32].

After the invention of stainless steel in the 1920s, metallic implants have experienced a renaissance. The ASTM (American Society for Testing and Materials) Committee F04 on Medical and Surgical Materials and Devices, formed in 1962, has played an important role in metallic implant development, practice, and standardization. A great variety of corrosion-resistant metals have been developed and used for medical implants including the class of 316L (Fe–18Cr–12Ni–3Mo with low carbon content) stainless steels, Co–27Cr–2Mo alloys, and Ti biomaterials [7,8,33].

The new generation of metallic biomaterials has been made nickel free via novel processing including nanoprocessing and amorphization. Other developments have raised the concept of biodegradable rather than inert metals where temporary medical implants, which function only during specific period and then degrade, are targeted [33]. Due to the excellent biocompatibility of Ta (tantalum) [34], several studies have focused on the dental and medical applications of Ta materials. The use of pure, porous Ta for total hip arthroplasty [35–37] and Ta oxide nanotube for various medical usages [38] have been investigated and support prior studies of tantalum's outstanding biocompatibility. NiTi alloys [39] or dental implants [40] were coated with Ta in order to improve biocompatibility. Ta was also demonstrated as an effective alloying element to Ti. Villa et al. [41] investigated the biocompatibility of Ti–Ta (containing in a range of 40–50 wt.%) alloys. It was reported that methylthiazoletetrazolium assay tests indicated a higher degree of proliferation on Ti–Ta alloys, suggesting that the newly developed Ti–Ta binary alloys are biocompatible.

Implants can be used either to replace diseased tissue or to assist in the healing process. The former type of implant should remain in the body permanently, while the latter is temporary. An example of a temporary implant application is stenting, where remodeling of the arterial wall is expected to take place and a continuous presence of the stent becomes unnecessary [42]. Thus, in situations where a permanent implant is used for a short-term application, additional surgeries are required to remove these devices once the healing process is complete. This removal process increases the cost of health care and patient mobility. In contrast, biodegradable materials dissolve after the healing process is complete; no additional surgeries are required for the removal of these implants. Biodegradable implants also eliminate the complications associated with the long-term presence of implants in the body. Lastly, once these materials degrade within the body, it is important that the degradation products are able to be metabolized by the body. Therefore, implants should be bioabsorbable [43]. Since traditional metallic biomaterials (like surgical stainless steels, Co–Cr alloys, and Ti biomaterials) are typically biocompatible but not biodegradable, the potential for magnesium-based alloys in biomedical applications has gained more interest [43]. In recent years, research on magnesium (Mg) alloys had increased significantly for hard tissue replacement and stent application due to their outstanding advantages. There are several remarkable reasons why Mg alloys are so important: (i) Mg alloys have mechanical properties similar to bone, which avoids stress shielding; (ii) they are essentially biocompatible with the human metabolism because the main degradation product, Mg, is an essential trace element for human enzymes; and (iii) the most important reason is that they are perfectly biodegradable in the body fluid [42–44].

Though these metallic implantable materials show excellent corrosion resistance, biocorrosion or biodegradation, or both, may occur [45,46]. In later chapters, various surface treatments to stabilize the surface oxide film as well as surface modifications to further improve biocorrosion resistance will be discussed.

2.3. Polymeric Biomaterials

Polymeric biomaterials have been extensively used in medicinal applications [47]. Commonly used synthetic polymers include poly(lactic acid) and poly(lactic-co-glycolic acid) [48–50], poly(ethylene glycol) [51,52], 2-hydroxyethyl methacrylate [53] and poly(vinyl alcohol) [53–55], polytetrafluoroethylene, polyethylene terephthalate, polymethyl methacrylate (PMMA), polyethylene (PE), polypropylene, polysulfone, silicone rubber, polyoxymethylene [56], and benzocyclobutene [57]. However, in terms of protein adsorption, cell adhesion, cytotoxicity, blood compatibility, and tissue compatibility, the factors that determine their biocompatibility are still not very clear [58]. Indirectly related to biocompatibility, potential wear debris toxicity of polymers remains an unexplored issue. UHMWPE, with its superior wear resistance and low-friction surface properties, has been applied successfully as a key material in artificial knee and hip joint replacement. However, the wear debris generated during the joint motions can cause osteolysis and loosening of the implant, thereby contributing to the main cause for joint revision. Many attempts have been made to improve the wear resistance of PE materials in order to elongate their service life. It was reported that various nanofillers, including carbon nanofibers, carbon nanotubes, nano-alumina, and nano-montmorillonite, have been applied as ideal reinforcing components to modify the tribological properties of PE [58].

The interdisciplinary field of biomaterials and tissue engineering has been one of the most dynamic and rapidly expanding disciplines during the past two decades. Polymers are especially useful in this area mainly because of their flexibility in chemical structure engineering and physical property design. Many noncytotoxic and biodegradable polymers can be fabricated into medical devices for numerous applications, including tissue replacement, drug delivery, cancer therapy, and nonviral gene therapy [59]. In recent years, there has been a great demand for polymers designed with better functions that include blood and tissue compatibility (biocompatibility) and an antimicrobial activity. The surface modification of existing polymers is one of the most attractive ways to accomplish this. Treatment with plasma, gamma ray, or electron beams leads to a sufficient level of activation of polymers, so that specific monomers may be grafted. The extent of modification, that is, the degree of grafting, may be easily controlled by the careful manipulation of the radiation exposure and reaction conditions. Graft modification may be carried out almost on all polymers, thus yielding the ability to create a desired functional chemistry both on the surface and in the bulk matrix. The grafting is applicable to almost all polymer–monomer combinations, with enormous possibilities, in regard to physicochemical and biological characteristics, to attain goal-driven antimicrobial activity and biocompatibility [60].

There is a technology developed in the field of engineering that can be applied to the manufacture of medical polymers, which is electrospinning. It has been recognized as a versatile method for the fabrication of continuous ultrafine fibers using electrical forces. Various natural and synthetic polymers have been successfully electrospun into nonwoven mats or oriented fibrous bundles with high porosity and large surface areas. Despite the numerous reports on the production of electrospun fibers, these fiber mats did not gain much interest for use in the biomedical field until the past decade. This review summarizes the research and development related to the electrospinning of some common biocompatible polymers and gives an overview of their potential in many biomedical applications such as tissue engineering, wound dressing, carriers for drug delivery or controlled release, and enzyme immobilization [61].

2.4. Ceramic Biomaterials

Ceramics used for the repair and reconstruction of diseased or damaged parts of the musculoskeletal system, termed bioceramics, may be bioinert (e.g., titania, alumina, and zirconia), resorbable (e.g., tricalcium phosphate), bioactive (e.g., HA, bioactive glasses, and glass ceramics), or porous (e.g., HA coated metals) for tissue ingrowth [62 71]. Applications include replacements for hips, knees, teeth, tendons, and ligaments and repair for periodontal disease, maxillofacial reconstruction, augmentation and stabilization of the jaw bone, spinal fusion, and bone repair after tumor surgery. Pyrolytic carbon coatings are thromboresistant and are used for prosthetic heart valves. The mechanisms of tissue bonding to bioactive ceramics have resulted in the molecular design and development of bioceramics for interfacial bonding with hard and soft tissue. Bioactive composites are being developed with high toughness and an elastic modulus that matches bone. Therapeutic treatment of cancer has been achieved by localized delivery of radioactive isotopes via glass beads. Clinical success of bioceramics has led to a remarkable advance in the quality of life for millions of people [72–74].

Zirconia ceramics are showing themselves to be another important tool to both medical and dental fields. Currently, zirconia (ZrO_2) ceramics are being extensively investigated for medical applications, and the results demonstrate excellent levels of osseointegration [75–86]. Further, ZrO_2 ceramics have been widely used in implant dentistry. When ZrO_2 was used as a blasting media on titanium substrates, it was reported that (i) the blasting media and the blasted titanium surface showed superior reduction of bacterial adhesion, especially after coating with saliva pellicle, and (ii) modifying titanium with ZrO_2 endows the same surface properties of pure ZrO_2—namely, reducing bacterial adhesion [87].

Ceramics, glasses, and glass–ceramics are increasingly being tested for use in the human body. These materials often have excellent chemical properties for biomedical use, but they are brittle and show fatigue. Careful analysis of their mechanical properties is needed to determine appropriate applications. HA is emerging as the most promising bioceramics because it shows no foreign body reactions and bonds strongly to bone. If properly made without pores or second phases, it has excellent fatigue resistance. Glass–ceramics containing HA crystals also show good promise for many applications. Different forms of these materials, such as dense, granular, mixed granular with plaster of Paris, and coatings on metals are being tested and have very good potential as bioceramics [88–90].

2.5. Composites

There are several types of hybrid or composite implantable materials. A fiber-reinforced composite was prepared from PMMA and E-glass to enhance the bone bonding properties of the material [91]. Chitosan-clay-based bio-nanocomposites were developed as advanced functional materials [92]. The adhesion of proteins involved in osteoblast cells was examined on composite polyurethane/$CaCO_3$surfaces with promising results [93]. Bond coats based on bioinert ceramic materials such as titania and ZrO_2 were developed to increase the adhesion strength of the coating system HA-bond coat to Ti–6Al–4V alloy surfaces used for hip endoprostheses and dental root implants. It was reported that the bond coats improved the adhesion strength, as measured by a modified ASTM D 3167-76 peel test, by up to 100%. Further, the resorption resistance, as determined by *in vitro* leaching in simulated protein-free body fluid, endured for up to 28 days [94].

A glass in the SiO_2–Al_2O_3–CaO–CaF_2–K_2O–B_2O_3–La_2O_3 system was prepared. It was found that miserite [$KCa_5(Si_2O_7)(Si_6O_{15})(OH)F$] was the main crystalline phase. The composite possesses a modulus of elasticity of 96 ± 3 GPa and a fracture toughness, K_{IC}, of 4.77 ± 0.27 $MPam^{0.5}$. The attachment and proliferation of MC3T3-E1 osteoblastic cells were evaluated, and it was found that MC3T3-E1 cells exhibited attachment, spreading, and proliferation on composite glass surfaces, thus demonstrating excellent biocompatibility [95].

The carbon fiber-reinforced polyetheretherketone (PEEK) was evaluated for dental implants. It was reported that although PEEK could represent a viable alternative material for dental implants, further experimental studies on the chemical modulation of PEEK seem to be necessary, mainly to increase the bone–implant contact ratio and to minimize the stress distribution to the peri-implant bone [96].

We have discussed implantable materials in metallic, polymeric, ceramic, and composite forms. There are other implantable materials that ordinarily are not good implant candidates, yet become viable alternatives when their surfaces have been modified through a variety of methods. The latter types of implantable materials will be extensively discussed in the following chapters. Overall, there is a spectrum of implant materials at our disposal. Many factors contribute to the choice and suitability of an implant material—biocompatibility, corrosion and wear resistance, longevity, strength, and toxicity are but a few examples. Promising new research continues to add to our knowledge base and to the set of materials at our disposal.

References

1. Anusavice, K.J., 2003, *Phillips' Science of Dental Materials,* Saunders: An Imprint of Elsevier Science., St. Louis, MO, pp. 185–196.
2. Moore, B.K. and Oshida, Y., 1995, Materials science and technology in dentistry, In: D.L. Wise ed., *Encyclopedic Handbook of Biomaterials and Bioengineering*, Marcel Dekker, Co., New York, NY, pp. 1325–1430.
3. Buechel, F.F. and Pappas, M.J., 2012, Properties of materials used in orthopaedic implant systems, In: F.F. Buechel and M.J. Pappas ed., *Principles of Human Joint Replacement—Design and Clinical Application*, Springer, Berlin/Heidelberg, Germany, pp. 1–35.
4. Pilliar, R.M., 2009, Metallic biomaterials, In: R. Narayan, ed., *Biomedical Materials*, Springer Science+Business Media, New York, NY, pp. 41–42.
5. Lemons, J.E., 2004, Biomaterials, biomechanics, tissue healing, and immediate-function dental implants, *J Oral Implantol* 30:318–324. doi: http://dx.doi.org/10.1563/0712.1.
6. Drago, C. and Howell, K., 2012, Concepts for designing and fabricating metal implant frameworks for hybrid implant prostheses, *J Prosthodon* 21:413–424. doi: http://dx.doi.org/10.1111/j.1532-849X.2012.00835.x.
7. Oshida, Y., 2007, *Bioscience and Bioengineering of Titanium Materials*, Elsevier, London, UK, pp. 269–271.
8. Lemons, J.E. and Dietsh-Misch, F., 1999, Biomaterials for dental implants, In: C.E. Misch ed., *Contemporary Implant Dentistry*, St. Louis, MO, pp. 271–286.
9. Hanawa, T., 1999, In vivo metallic biomaterials and surface modification, *Mater Sci Eng* 267:260–266. doi: http://dx.doi.org/10.1177/0885328206055998.
10. Dizlek, M.E., Guden, M., Turkan, U. and Tasdemirci, A., 2009, Processing and compression testing of Ti6AL4V foams for biomedical applications, *J Mater Sci* 44:1512–1519. doi: http://dx.doi.org/10.1007/s10853-008-3038-7.
11. Wataha, J.C., 1996, Materials for endosseous dental implants, *J Oral Rehab* 23:79–90. doi: http://dx.doi.org/10.1111/j.1365-2842.1996.tb01214.x.
12. Jacobs, J.J., Gilbert, J.L. and Urban, R.M., 1998, Corrosion of metal orthopaedic implants, *J Bone Joint Surg Am* 80:268–282.
13. Tsuchiya, T., Ikarashi, Y., Uchima, T., Doi, H., Nakamura, A., Ohshima, Y., Fujimaki, M., Toyoda, K., Kobayashi, E., Yoneyama, T. and Hamanaka, H., 2002, A method to monitor corrosion of chromium–iron alloys by monitoring the chromium ion concentration in urine, *Mater Trans* 43:3058–3064. doi: http://dx.doi.org/10.2320/matertrans.43.3058.
14. Savarino, L., Granchi, D., Ciapetti, G., Cenni, E., Greco, M., Rotini, R., Veronesi, C.A., Baldini, N. and Giunti, A., 2003, Ion release in stable hip arthroplasties using metal-on-metal articulating surfaces: A comparison between short- and medium-term results, *J Biomed Mater Res A* 66A:450–456. doi: http://dx.doi.org/10.1002/jbm.a.10595.
15. Ryhänen, J., Kallioinen, M., Tuukkanen, J., Junila, J., Niemelä, E., Sandvik, P. and Serlo. W., 1998, In vivo biocompatibility evaluation of nickel-titanium shape memory alloy: Muscle and perineural tissue responses and encapsule membrane thickness, *J Biomed Mater Res* 41:481–488.

16. Uo, M., Watari, F., Yokoyama, A. Matsuno, H. and Kawasaki. T., 2001, Tissue reaction around metal implants observed by X-ray scanning analytical microscopy, *Biomaterials* 22:677–685. doi: http://dx.doi.org/10.1016/S0142-9612(00)00230-1.
17. Kanerva, L., Sipilainen-Malm, T., Estlander, T., Zitting, A., Jolanki, R. and K. Tarvainen, K., 1994, Nickel release from metals, and a case of allergic contact dermatitis from stainless steel, *Contact Dermatitis* 31:304–307.
18. Kanerva. L. and Forstrom, L., 2001, Allergic nickel and chromate hand dermatitis induced by orthopaedic metal implant, *Contact Dermatitis* 44:103–104. doi: http://dx.doi.org/10.1034/j.1600-0536.2001.4402096.x.
19. Kobayashi, E., Matsumoto, S., Doi, H., Yoneyama, T. and Hamanaka, H., 1995, Mechanical properties of the binary titanium-zirconiumalloys and their potential for biomedical materials, *J Biomed Mater Res* 29:943–950. doi: http://dx.doi.org/10.1002/jbm.820290805.
20. Oshida, Y., 2007, *Bioscience and Bioengineering of Titanium Materials*, Elsevier, London, UK, pp. 217–281.
21. Long, M. and H. J. Rack, H.J., 1998, Titanium alloys in total joint replacement—A materials science perspective, *Biomaterials* 19:1621–1639. doi: http://dx.doi.org/10.1016/S0142-9612(97)00146-4.
22. Galante, J.O., Lemons, J.E., Spector, M., Wilson, Jr., P.D. and Wright, T.M., 1991, The biologic effects of implant materials, *J Orthop Res* 9:760–775. doi: http://dx.doi.org/10.1002/jor.1100090516.
23. Katou, F., Andoh, N., Motegi, K. and Nagura, H., 1996, Immuno-inflammatory responses in the tissue adjacent to titanium miniplates used in the treatment of mandibular fractures, *J Craniomaxillofac Surg* 24:155–162. doi: http://dx.doi.org/10.1016/S1010-5182(96)80049-7.
24. Williams, D.F., 1994, Titanium: Epitome of biocompatibility or cause for concern, *J Bone Joint Surg Br* 76B:348–349.
25. Rogers, S.D., Howie, D.W., Graves, S.E., Pearcy, M.J. and Haynes, D.R., 1997, In vitro human monocyte response to wear particles of titanium alloy containing vanadium or niobium, *J Bone Joint Surg Br* 79B:311–315. doi: http://dx.doi.org/10.1302/0301-620X.79B2.7192.
26. Henriques, V.A.R., Galvani, E.T., Petroni, S.I.G., Paula, M.S.M. and Lemos, T.G., 2010, Production of Ti–13Nb–13Zr alloy for surgical implants by powder metallurgy, *J Mater Sci* 45:5844–5850. doi: http://dx.doi.org/10.1007/s10853-010-4660-8.
27. Niinomi, M., 2008, Metallic biomaterials, *J Artif Organs* 11:105–110. doi: http://dx.doi.org/10.1007/s10047-008-0422-7.
28. Ikarashi, Y., Toyoda, K., Kobayashi, E., Doi, H., Yoneyama, T., Hamanaka, H. and Tsuchiya, T., 2005, Improved biocompatibility of titanium-zirconium (Ti-Zr) alloy: Tissue reaction and sensitization to Ti-Zr alloy compared with pure Ti and Zr in rat implantation study, *Mater Trans* 46:2260–2267.
29. Berner, S., Dard, M., Gottlow, J., Molenberg, A. and Wieland, M., 2009, Titanium-Zirconium: A novel material for dental implants, *Euro Cell Mater* 17:S1–S16.
30. Grandin, H.M., Berner, S. and Dard, M., 2012, A review of Titanium–Zirconium (TiZr) alloys for use in endosseous dental implants, *Materials* 5:1348–1360. doi: http://dx.doi.org/10.3390/ma5081348.
31. Ayers, R.A., Bateman, T.A. and Simske, S.J., 2000, Porous NiTi as a material for bone engineering, In: L. Yahia ed., *Shape Memory Implants*, Springer-Verlag, Berlin, Germany, pp. 73–88.
32. Bansiddhi, A., Sargeant, T.D., Stupp, S.I. and Dunand, D.C., 2008, Porous NiTi for bone implants: A review, *Acta Biomaterialia* 4:773–782. doi: http://dx.doi.org/ 10.1016/j.actbio.2008.02.009.

33. Hermawan, H., 2012, Introduction to metallic biomaterials, In: *Springer Briefs in Materials*, Springer, Berlin, Germany, pp. 1–11.
34. Matsuno, H.,Yokoyama, A., Watani, F., Uo, M. and Kawasaki, T., Biocompatibility and osteogenesis of refractory metal implants, titanium, hafnium, niobium, tantalum and rhenium, *Biomaterials* 22:1253–1262. doi: http://dx.doi.org/10.1016/S0142-9612(00)00275-1.
35. Levine, B., Della Valle, C.J. and Jacobs, J.J.J., 2006, Applications of porous tantalum in total hip arthroplasty, *J Am Acad Orthop Surg* 14:646–655.
36. Siegmeth, A., Duncan, C.P., Masri, B.A., Kim, W.Y. and Garbuz, D.S., 2009, Modular tantalum augments for acetabular defects in revision hip arthroplasty, *Clin Orthop Relat Res* 467:199–205. doi: http://dx.doi.org/10.1007/s11999-008-0549-0.
37. Kim, W.Y., Greidanus, N.V., Duncan, C.P., Masri, B.A. and Garbuz, D.S., 2008, Porous tantalum uncemented acetabular shells in revision total hip replacement: Two to four year clinical and radiographic results, *Hip Int* 18:17–22.
38. Wang, N., Li, H., Wang, J., Chen, S., Ma, Y. and Zhang, Z., 2012, Study on the anticorrosion, biocompatibility, and osteoinductivity of tantalum (186 GPA as MOE) decorated with tantalum oxide nanotube array films, *ACS Appl Mater Interf 26:*4516–4523.
39. Cheng, Y., Cai, W., Li, H.T. and Zheng, Y.F., 2006, Surface modification of NiTi alloy with tantalum to improve its biocompatibility and radiopacity, *J Mater Sci* 41:4961–4964. doi: http://dx.doi.org/10.1007/s10853-006-0096-6.
40. Fathi, M.H. and Vajihesadat, M., 2007, Tantalum, niobium and titanium coatings for biocompatibility improvement of dental implants, *Dent Res J* 4:74–82.
41. Villa, R., Ortiz, C.R., Tapia, S., Ganzalez, G., Trillo, E., Garza, K.M., Stafford, S.W. and Murr, L.E., 2002, In vitro biocompatibility of fibroblast cells on Ti–Ta alloys, *Maters Trans* 43:2991–2994.
42. Virtanen, S., 2012, Biodegradable Mg alloys: Corrosion, surface modification, and biocompatibility, *Mod Aspect Electroc* 55:101–125. doi: http://dx.doi.org/10.1007/978-1-4614-3125-1_3.
43. Brar, H.S., Platt, M.O., Sarntinoranont, M., Martin, P.I. and Manuel, M.V., 2011, Magnesium as a biodegradable and bioabsorbable material for medical implants, *JOM* 61:31–34. doi: http://dx.doi.org/10.1007/s11837-009-0129-0.
44. Yang, J., Cui, F. and Lee, I.S., 2011, Surface modifications of magnesium alloys for biomedical applications, *Ann Biomed Eng* 39:1857–1871. doi: http://dx.doi.org/10.1007/s10439-011-0300-y.
45. Kamachimudali, U., Sridhar, T.M. and Baldev Raj, B., 2003, Corrosion of bio implants, *Sadhana* 28:601–637. doi: http://dx.doi.org/10.1007/BF02706450.
46. Singh, R. and Dahotre, N.B.J., 2007, Corrosion degradation and prevention by surface modification of biometallic materials, *J Mater Sci Mater Med* 18:725–751. doi: http://dx.doi.org/10.1007/s10856-006-0016-y.
47. Plastics used in some medical devices break down in a previously unrecognized way, ACS News Service Weekly Press Pac., December 5, 2012.
48. Lunsford, L., McKeever, U., Eckstein, V. and Hedley, M.L., 2000, Tissue distribution and persistence in mice of plasmid DNA encapsulated in a PLGA-based microsphere delivery vehicle, *J Drug Target* 8:39–50. doi: http://dx.doi.org/10.3109/10611860009009208.
49. Ronneberger, B., Kissel, T. and Anderson, J.M., 1997, Biocompatibility of ABA triblock copolymer microparticles consisting of poly(L-lacticco-glycolic-acid) A-blocks attached to central poly(oxyethylene) B-blocks in rats after intramuscular injection, *Eur J Pharm Biopharm* 43:19–28. doi: http://dx.doi.org/10.1016/S0939-6411(96)00006-9.
50. Royals, M.A., Fujita, S.M., Yewey, G.L., Rodriguez, J., Schultheiss, P.C. and Dunn, R.L., 1999, Biocompatibility of a biodegradable in situ forming implant system in rhesus

monkeys, *J Biomed Mater Res* 45:231–239. doi: http://dx.doi.org/10.1002/(SICI)1097-4636(19990605)45:3<231::AID-JBM11>3.0.CO;2-H.

51. Dalsin J.L., Hu, B.H., Lee, B.P., Messersmith, P.B., 2003, Mussel adhesive protein mimetic polymers for the preparation of nonfouling surfaces. *J Am Chem Soc* 125:4253–4258. doi: http://dx.doi.org/10.1021/ja0284963.
52. Tsai, W.B., Grunkemeier, J.M., McFarland, C.D. and Horbett, T.A., 2002, Platelet adhesion to polystyrene-based surfaces preadsorbed with plasmas selectively depleted in fibrinogen, fibronectin, vitronectin, or von Willebrand's factor, *J Biomed Mater Res* 60:348–359. doi: http://dx.doi.org/10.1002/jbm.10048.
53. Paradossi, G., Cavalieri, F., Chiessi, E., Spagnoli, C. and Cowman, M.K., 2003, Poly(vinyl alcohol) as versatile biomaterial for potential biomedical applications, *J Mater Sci Mater Med* 14:687–691. doi: http://dx.doi.org/10.1023/A:1024907615244.
54. Oka, M., Ushio, K., Kumar, P., Ikeuchi, K., Hyon, S.H., Nakamura, T. and Fujita, H., 2000, Development of artificial articular cartilage, *Proc Inst Mech Eng H* 214:59–68. doi: http://dx.doi.org/10.1016/0267-6605(90)90053-X.
55. Maruoka, S., Matsuura, T., Kawasaki, K., Okamoto, M., Yoshiaki, H., Kodama, M., Sugiyama, M. and Annaka, M., 2006, Biocompatibility of polyvinylalcohol gel as a vitreous substitute, *Curr Eye Res* 31:599–606. doi: http://dx.doi.org/10.1080/02713680600813854.
56. Xu, S. and Tangpong, X.W., 2013, Review: Tribological behavior of polyethylene-based nanocomposites, *J Mater Sci* 48:578–597. doi: http://dx.doi.org/10.1007/s10853-012-6844-x.
57. Lee, K., Massia, S. and He, J., 2005, Biocompatible benzocyclobutene-based intracortical neural implant with surface modification, *J Micromech Microeng* 15:2149–2155. doi: http://dx.doi.org/10.1088/0960-1317/15/11/022.
58. Wang, Y.X., Robertson, J.L., Spillman, W.B. Jr. and Claus, R.O., 2004, Effects of the chemical structure and the surface properties of polymeric biomaterials on their biocompatibility, *Pharm Res* 21:1362–1373. doi: http://dx.doi.org/10.1023/B:PHAM.0000036909.41843.18.
59. Wang, S., Lu, L., Wang, C., Gao, C. and Wang, X., 2010, Polymeric biomaterials for tissue engineering applications, *Int J Polymer Sci* 2010. doi: http://dx.doi.org/10.1155/2010/148513.
60. Shintani, H., 2005, Bulk and/or surface modification of medical polymers to attain antimicrobial activity and/or biocompatibility, *Biocontrol Sci* 10:13–19. doi: http://dx.doi.org/10.4265/bio.10.13.
61. Supaphol, P., Suwantong, O., Sangsanoh, P., Srinivasan, S., Jayakumar, R. and Nair, S.V., 2012, Electrospinning of biocompatible polymers and their potentials in biomedical applications, *Adv Polym Sci* 213–239. doi: http://dx.doi.org/10.1007/12_2011_143.
62. Andreiotelli, M., Wenz, H.J. and Ralf-Joachim Kohal, R-J., 2009, Are ceramic implants a viable alternative to titanium implants? A systematic literature review, *Clin Oral Implants Res* 20:S32–S47. doi: http://dx.doi.org/10.1111/j.1600-0501.2009.01785.x.
63. Treccani, L., Maiwald, M., Z□llmer, V., Busse, M., Grathwohl, G. and Rezwan, K., 2009, Antibacterial and abrasion-resistant alumina micropatterns, *Adv Eng Mater* 11:B61–B66. doi: http://dx.doi.org/ 10.1002/adem.200800372.
64. Lin, Y-S. and Burggraaf, A.J., 1991, Preparation and characterization of high-temperature thermally stable alumina composite membrane, *J Am Ceram Soc* 74:219–224. doi: http://dx.doi.org/10.1111/j.1151-2916.1991.tb07320.x.
65. Liu, Y., Chen, O.Y., Wei, C.C. and Li, K., 2006, Preparation of yttria-stabilised zirconia (YSZ) hollow fibre membranes, *Desalination* 199:360–362.
66. Wenz, H.J., Bartsch, J., Wolfart, S. and Kern, M., 2008, Osseointegration and clinical success of zirconia dental implants: A systematic review, *Int J Prosthodont* 21:27–36.
67. Femández-Fairén, M., Sala, P. and Gil, F.J., Failures of yttria-stabilised tetragonal zirconia: 52 retrieved ceramic femoral heads of total hip prostheses, *Biomed Mater Eng* 16:415–422.

68. Schincaglia, G.P., Marzola, R., Scapoli, C. and Scotti, R., 2007, Immediate loading of dental implants supporting fixed partial dentures in the posterior mandible: A randomized controlled split-mouth study: Machined versus titanium oxide implant surfaces, *Int J Oral Maxillofac Implants* 22:35–46.
69. Domanski, M., Winnubst, L., Luttge, R., Lamers, E., Walboomers, X.F., Jansen, J. and Gardeniers, H., 2012, Production and characterization of micro- and nano-features in biomedical alumina and zirconia ceramics using a tape casting route, *J Mater Sci Mater Med* 23:637–1644. doi: http://dx.doi.org/10.1007/s10856-012-4635-1.
70. Rahaman, M.N., Yao, A., Bal, B.S., Garino, J.P. and Ries, M.D., 2007, Ceramics for prosthetic hip and knee joint replacement, *J Am Ceram Soc* 90:1965–1988. doi: http://dx.doi.org/10.1111/j.1551-2916.2007.01725.x.
71. Xie, C., Lu, H., Li, W., Chen, F.M. and Zhao, Y.M.J., 2011, The use of calcium phosphate-based biomaterials in implant dentistry, *J Mater Sci Mater Med* 23:853–862. doi: http://dx.doi.org/10.1007/s10856-011-4535-9.
72. Hench, L.L., 1998, Bioceramics, *J Am Ceram Soc* 81:1705–1728. doi: http://dx.doi.org/10.1111/j.1151-2916.1998.tb02540.x.
73. Hench, L.L., 1991, Bioceramics: From concept to clinic, *J Am Ceram Soc* 74:1487–1510. doi: http://dx.doi.org/10.1111/j.1151-2916.1991.tb07132.x.
74. Heimke, G. and Griss, P., 1980, Ceramic implant materials, *Med Biolog Eng Computing* 18:503–510. doi: http://dx.doi.org/10.1007/978-0-387-37880-0_6.
75. Salem, N.A., Taleb, A.L.A. and Aboushelib, M.N., 2013, Biomechanical and histomorphometric evaluation of osseointegration of fusion-sputtered zirconia implants, *J Prosthodon* 22:261–267.
76. Egawa, M., Miura, T., Kato, T., Saito, A. and Yoshinari, M., 2013, In vitro adherence of periodontopathic bacteria to zirconia and titanium surfaces, *Dent Mater J* 32.101–106. doi: http://dx.doi.org/10.4012/dmj.2012-156.
77. Özkurt, Z. and Kazazoğlu, E., 2011, Zirconia dental implants: A literature review, *J Oral Implantol* 37:367–376. doi: http://dx.doi.org/10.1563/AAID-JOI-D-09-00079.
78. Bankoğlu, M., Aydin, C., Yilmaz, H. and Gül, E.B., 2012, An overview of zirconia dental implants: Basic properties and clinical application of three cases, *J Oral Implantol* 2012. doi: http://dx.doi.org/10.1563/AAID-JOI-D-12-00109.1, 2012.
79. Baldassarri, M., Zhang, Y., Thompson, V.P., Rekow, E.D. and Stappert, C.F.J., 2011, Reliability and failure modes of implant-supported zirconium-oxide fixed dental prostheses related to veneering techniques, *J Dent* 39:489–498. doi: http://dx.doi.org/10.1016/j.jdent.2011.04.006.
80. Hisbergues, M., Vendeville, S. and Vendeville, P., 2009, Zirconia: Established facts and perspectives for a biomaterial in dental implantology, *J Biomed Mater Res Part B* 88B:519–529. doi: http://dx.doi.org/10.1002/jbm.b.31147.
81. Koch, F.P., Weng, D., Krämer, S., Biesterfeld, S., Jahn-Eimermacher, A. and Wagner, W., 2010, Osseointegration of one-piece zirconia implants compared with a titanium implant of identical design: A histomorphometric study in the dog, *Clin Oral Implants Res* 21:350–356. doi: http://dx.doi.org/10.1111/j.1600-0501.2009.01832.x.
82. Shin, D., Blanchard, S.B., Ito, M. and Chu, T-M.G., 2011, Peripheral quantitative computer tomographic, histomorphometric, and removal torque analyses of two different non-coated implants in a rabbit model, *Clin Oral Implants Res* 22:242–250. doi: http://dx.doi.org/10.1111/j.1600-0501.2010.01980.x.
83. Bormann, K-H., Gellrich, N-C., Kniha, H., Dard, M., Wieland, M. and Gahlert, M., 2012, Biomechanical evaluation of a microstructured zirconia implant by a removal torque comparison with a standard Ti-SLA implant, *Clin Oral Implants Res* 23:1210–1216. doi: http://dx.doi.org/10.1111/j.1600-0501.2011.02291.x.

84. Gahlert, M., Roehling, S., Sprecher, C.M., Kniha, H., Milz, S. and Bormann, K., 2012, In vivo performance of zirconia and titanium implants: A histomorphometric study in mini pig maxillae, *Clin Oral Implants Res* 23:281–286.doi: http://dx.doi.org/10.1111/j.1600-0501.2011.02157.x.
85. Nakamura, K., Kanno, T., Milleding, P. and Örtengren, U., 2010, Zirconia as a dental implant abutment material: A systematic review, *Int J Prosthodont* 23:299–309.
86. Gremillard, L., Meille, S., Chevalier, J., Zhao, J., Fridrici, V., Kapsa, P., Geringer, J. and Uribe, J., 2012, Degradation of bioceramics, In: N. Eliaz ed., *Degradation of Implant Materials,* Springer Science, New York, NY, pp. 195–252.
87. Al-Radha, A.S.D., Dymock, D., Younes, C. and O'Sullivan, D., 2012, Surface properties of titanium and zirconia dental implant materials and their effect on bacterial adhesion, *J Dent* **40:**146–153. doi: http://dx.doi.org/10.1016/j.jdent.2011.12.006.
88. Doremus, R.H., 1992, Review: Bioceramics, *J Mater Sci* 27:285–297. doi: http://dx.doi.org/10.1007/BF00543915.
89. Coelho, P.G., de Assis, S.L., Costa. I. and Thompson, V.P., 2009, Corrosion resistance evaluation of a Ca- and P-based bioceramic thin coating in Ti-6Al-4V, *J Mater Sci Mater Med* 21:215–222. doi: http://dx.doi.org/10.1007/s10856-008-3562-7.
90. Huhtinen, R., Sandeman, S., Rose, S., Fok, E., Howell, C., Fröberg, L., Moritz, N., Hupa, L. and Lloyd, A., 2013, Examining porous bio-active glass as a potential osteo-odonto-keratoprosthetic skirt material, *J Mater Sci Mater Med* 24:1217–1227. doi: http://dx.doi.org/10.1007/s10856-013-4881-x.
91. Hautamäki, M.P., Puska, M., Aho, A.J., Kopperud, H.M. and Vallittu, P.K., 2013, Surface modification of fiber reinforced polymer composites and their attachment to bone simulating material, *J Mater Sci Mater Med* 24:1145–1152. doi: http://dx.doi.org/10.1007/s10856-013-4890-9.
92. Darder, M., Aranda, P. and Ruiz-Hitzky, E., 2012, Chitosan-clay bio-nanocomposites, In: L. Avérous and E. Pollet ed., *Environmental Silicate Nano-Biocomposites; Green Energy and Technology*, Springer-Verlag, London, UK, pp. 365–391.
93. Dulińska-Molak, I., Lekka, M. and Kurzydłowski, K.J., 2013, Surface properties of polyurethane composites for biomedical applications, *Appl Surf Sci* 270:553–560. doi: http://dx.doi.org/10.1016/j.apsusc.2013.01.085.
94. Heimann, R.B., 1999, Design of novel plasma sprayed hydroxyapatite-bond coat bioceramic systems, *J Thermal Spray Technol* 8:597–603. doi: http://dx.doi.org/10.1361/105996399770350304.
95. Saadaldin, S.A., Dixon, S.J., Costa, D.O. and Rizkalla, A.S., 2013, Synthesis of bioactive and machinable miserite glass-ceramics for dental implant applications, *Dent Mater* 29:645–655. doi: http://dx.doi.org/10.1016/j.dental.2013.03.013.
96. Schwitalla, A.D. and Müller, W-D., 2011, PEEK dental implants: A review of the literature, *J Oral Implantol* 39: 743–749. doi:http://dx.doi.org/10.1563/AAID-JOI-D-11-00002.

Chapter 3

Interfacial Reactions Between Vital Tissue and Nonvital Implant Surfaces

In some cases, once a certain type of implantable core material is chosen, the material is almost ready for implantation due to the acceptable biocompatibility. In most cases, the surface itself is not good enough to achieve successful implant performance. The surface needs to be altered accordingly to accommodate/facilitate the actual biological activities upon placement of the implants. It is, therefore, essential to review interfacial reactions between placed nonvital implant surfaces (either surface treated or untreated) and receiving vital hard/soft tissues.

3.1. Introduction

Any material applicable for surgical implantation gives rise to a wide spectrum of biochemical reactions within the body. This spectrum can be roughly divided into three categories: (i) almost inert materials, with minimal chemical reactivity, (ii) totally resorbable materials, with possible dissolution into metabolic constituents, and (iii) materials with controlled-activity surfaces. Titanium materials that are exposed to biological environments, and their behaviors in such environments, are needed to be known. This chapter will discuss biological reactions, and reactions in biomechanical environment in general and particularly emphasizing on the discrete stress field under strain continuum situation since this concept should be essential for designing and material selection for dental and orthopedic implants.

Dental implants are an ideal option for people in good general oral health who have lost a tooth (or teeth) due to periodontal disease, an injury, or some other reason. Dental implants (as an artificial tooth root and usually made from titanium materials) are biocompatible metal anchors surgically positioned in the jaw bone underneath the gums to support an artificial crown where natural teeth are missing. There are main three different types of dental implants: (i) root form implants, (ii) plate form

DOI 10.5643/9781606506288/ch3

implants, and (iii) subperiosteal implants. Using the *root form implants (*the closest in shape and size to the natural tooth root), the healing period usually varies from as few as three months to six or more. During this time osteointegration occurs. The bone grows in and around the implant creating a strong structural support. Plate (or blade) form implants are usually used when the bone is so narrow that it may not be suitable for the root form implant, and the area is not suitable for bone grafting. Like root form implants, there is usually a healing period for osteointegration, although some plate form implants are designed for immediate restoration (or immediate loading). With very advanced jawbone resorption there may not be enough bone width or height for the root form or plate form implant, and the subperiosteal implant may be prescribed. The subperiosteal implant is custom made and designed to sit on top of the bone, but under the gums.

Generally, any edentulous (toothless) area having enough bone support can be an indication for restoring a missing tooth with an implant. A decision has to be made on case-by-case bases whether it is a good idea based on the patient's requirements and expectations. Even though there are practically no absolute contraindications for placement of implants, there are few factors that can put it in a high-risk situation. The followings are normally believed as contraindicative factors: (i) endocrine disorders, such as uncontrolled diabetes mellitus, pituitary and adrenal insufficiency, and hypothyroidism can cause considerable healing problems, (ii) uncontrolled granulomatous diseases, such as tuberculosis and sarcoidosis, may also lead to a poor healing response to surgical procedures, (iii) patients with cardiovascular diseases, taking blood thinning drugs and patients with uncontrolled hematological disorders, such as generalized anemia, hemophilia (Factor VIII deficiency), Factor IX, X, and XII deficiencies, and any other acquired coagulation disorders are contraindicated to surgical procedures due to poor hemorrhage control, (iv) patients with bone diseases, such as histiocytosis X, Paget's disease, and fibrous dysplasia, may not be good candidates for implants, because there is a higher chance for the implant to fail due to poor osteointegration, (v) cigarette smoking, and (vi) patients receiving radio and chemotherapy should not have implants within the 6 months period of therapy [1].

For most patients, the placement of dental implants involves two surgical procedures. First (surgical stage), implants are placed within the jawbone. For the first 3 to 6 months following surgery, the implants integrate with the jawbone—osteointegration (due to successful growing of osteoblasts on and into the rough surfaces of the implant, forming a structural and functional connection between the hard tissue and placed implant). After some months the implant is uncovered and a healing abutment and temporary crown is placed onto the implant. This encourages the gum to grow in the right scalloped shape to approximate a natural tooth's gums and allows assessment of the final aesthetics of the restored tooth. After the implant has integrated/bonded to the jawbone, the second (prosthetic) phase begins. The placed implants are uncovered and small posts are attached which will act as anchors for the artificial teeth. These posts protrude through the gums. When the artificial teeth (or permanent crowns) are placed, these posts will not be seen. The entire procedure usually takes four to eight months.

There are four major factors influencing the success rates of placed implants. They include (i) correct indication and favorable anatomic conditions (bone and mucosa), (ii) good operative technique, (iii) patient cooperation (oral hygiene), and

(iv) adequate superstructure design and fabrication. Failure of a dental implant is usually related to failure to osteointegrate correctly. A dental implant is considered to be a failure if it is lost, mobile, or shows peri-implant bone loss of greater than 1 mm in the first year after postimplanting and greater than 0.2 mm a year after that. Dental implants are not susceptible to dental caries but they can develop a periodontitis condition called peri-implantitis where correct oral hygiene routines have not been followed. Unfortunately, it is true that many times a patient who was evaluated as a good implant patient candidate has a bad history of dental hygiene practice. Failure in dental implants is found to be increased in the anterior mandible where bone quality is not as dense. More rarely, an implant may fail because of poor positioning at the time of surgery, or may be overloaded initially causing failure to integrate. Implant surgery is believed to exhibit its success rate of more than 90% of the time. Occasionally, an implant fails to bond with the surrounding bone. This is usually discovered at the second stage surgery when the implant is uncovered and the surgeon finds it is loose. In this case, the "failed" implant has to be removed, and another implant can be placed either immediately or later. Potential reasons for implants failing to integrate with surrounding bone include: surgical trauma, infection around the implant, smoking (this appears to decrease blood flow to the healing gums and bone, which could interfere with the bonding process), lack of healthy bone (if there is not enough bone for the implant to remain stable, the implant may move around within the bone and bonding will not occur), titanium allergies (these are extremely rare) [2,3]. Problems can also develop years after implants are placed. For example, just like natural teeth and gums, the gums around implants can become infected by bacteria, leading to a form of periodontal disease called peri-implantitis. If that situation is left untreated, this condition can cause bone loss, which could cause the implant to become loose and have to be removed. Generally, this situation can be treated using procedures that are very similar to those used to treat periodontal disease affecting natural teeth. Another type of complication that can happen over time is the implant-supported restoration (crown, bridge, or denture) can break, or the implant itself can fracture. This usually happens if the occlusion is not aligned properly. If the occlusion is off, too much force (in most cases, torsional or shear force) might be placed on the restoration or implant. Broken restorations often can be repaired, but a fractured implant has to be removed. A broken implant or an implant that fails because of an infection can be replaced with a new implant [1].

On the other hand, orthopedic implants are used to replace damaged or troubled joints. Each implant procedure involves removal of the damaged joint and an artificial prosthesis replacement, including hip, knee, finger, elbow, shoulder, ankle, and trauma products. Orthopedic implants are mainly constructed of titanium alloys for strength and lined with plastic to act as artificial cartilage. Some are cemented into place and others (i.e., cementless) are pressed to fit and allow the patient's bone to grow into the implant for strength. The advantages of orthopedic implants should include an increased mobility, reduced pain, and a higher quality of life (QOL). The disadvantages can include a strict postsurgery recovery plan (rehabilitation), infection, and possible malfunction. Each implant is designed to withstand the movement and stress associated with each individual joint and to provide increased mobility and decreased pain. The primary need for orthopedic implants is the result of osteoarthritis, also called degenerative joint disease. When cartilage is worn down, painful bone to bone contact occurs, or cartilage might break down as a result of excess body weight and or the lack of joint movement. Historically for the domain of the elderly, orthopedic implants are now increasingly used to replace arthritic or damaged joints, or both. For hip implants, the form characteristics of the femoral cup and head are critical to its load-bearing capability. Typically, however, the main cause of failure in hip joints is due to wear, and in particular the particles that are generated, resulting in wear debris toxicity. For example, the most common cause of femoral bone loss is due to osteolysis. Although the total cause is not known, it has been attributed to a variety of factors including foreign body reaction to particulate debris, in particular to polymeric debris. As such, the avoidance of wear in hip joints is critical [4,5].

Today, titanium and some of its alloys are considered to be among the most biocompatible materials. The fact that titanium is being used preferentially in many of the more recent applications in maxillofacial, oral, neuro-surgery, and cardiovascular-surgery, as well as gaining increasing preference in orthopedics, indicates superiority. Moreover, commercially they have been successfully used for orthopedic and dental implants. Several studies show that when titanium is inserted into human bone it forms an intimate contact with the bone in a process called osteointegration [6–8], due to good biocompatibility which is greatly relied on formation of stable passive oxide film in a biological system including chemical and mechanical environments. However, the presence of the passive film is only part of the answer when we consider the complex interfacial phenomena to be found between titanium and a biological system.

3.2. Toxicity

Toxicity can be measured by the effects on the target (organism, organ, or tissue). Because individuals typically have different levels of response to the same dose of a toxin, a population-level measure of toxicity is often used which relates the probability of an outcome for a given individual in a population. One such measure is the LD50 (LD stands for lethal dose), which is a concentration measure for a toxin at which 50% of the members of an exposed population die from exposure [9]. When such data does not exist, estimates are made by comparison to known similar toxic things, or to similar exposures in similar organisms. Then the safety factors must be built in to protect against the uncertainties of such comparisons, in order to improve protection against these unknowns. Toxicity can refer to the effect on a whole organism (such as a human, a bacterium, or a plant), or to a substructure (such as the liver, kidney, and spleen). In the science of toxicology, the subject of such study is the effect of an external substance or condition and its deleterious effects on living things: organisms, organ systems, individual organs, tissues, cells, and subcellular units. Toxicity of a substance can be affected by many different factors, such as the route of administration, the time of exposure, the number of exposures, physical form of the toxin (solid, liquid, and gaseous), the genetic makeup of an individual, an individual's overall health, and many others.

There are generally three types of toxic entities: chemical, biological, and physical.

3.2.1. Chemical Toxicity

Chemicals include both inorganic substances, such as lead, hydrofluoric acid, and chlorine gas, as well as organic compounds such as ethyl alcohol, most medications, and poisons from living things.

Chemicals (which can be toxic) should include corrosion product such as oxides, chlorides, or sulfides as well as dissolved metallic ions through the anodic reaction. The toxicity is related to primary biodegradation products (simple and complex cations and anions), particularly those of higher atomic weight metals. Factors to be considered include (i) the amount dissolved by biodegradation per time unit, (ii) the amount of material removed by metabolic activity in the same time unit, and (iii) quantities of solid particles and ions deposited in the tissue and any associated transfers to the systemic system. Hence, the extent of toxicity is indirectly related to corrosion rate [10–13]. An *in vivo* corrosion experiment can always be followed up by a tissue examination. This type of tissue reaction is observed for both corrosion-resistant materials (Mo-containing stainless steel and Co–Cr–Mo alloys) and for the strongly corroding metals Fe, Mo, and Al. It must be assumed that the unwanted corrosion product itself is the determining factor. Elements like Fe, Mo, and Al (as nontoxic metals) do not trigger an extreme tissue reaction despite high corrosion rates (about 300 times higher than that of stainless steel). On the other hand, the very low corrosion rates of stainless steel and Co–Cr alloys, comparable to that of Ti, Nb, and Zr, release sufficient quantities of the highly toxic elements nickel and cobalt, to trigger a noticeable tissue reaction. It should be mentioned at this point that no limiting concentration is commonly admitted for an allergic reaction. Gold and silver are also to be found in this middle group, as these noble metals can also corrode in a living tissue. As demonstrated above, a low corrosion rate alone is not sufficient to guarantee compatibility, nor is the elemental dose the only determining factor. It would appear that the intrinsic toxicity of the element and its ability to bind to macromolecules are equally important. Chemical data for Ti, Zr, Nb, and Ta show that organic complexes of this type are unlikely, and it is also known that organo-metallic compounds of these elements, as far as they exist, are unstable [14].

There are certain types of elements which are essential for living organism and types of elements that are different between kinds of living substances. For plants, there are macronutrients including N, P, S, Ca, Mg, and Fe, and micronutrients such as Mn, Zn, Cu, Mo, B, and Cl [15,16]. On the other hand, essential trace elements for living organisms (particularly, the higher animals) include Fe, F, Si, Zn, Sr, Pb, Mn, Cu, Sn, Se, I, Mo, Ni, B, Cr, As, Co, and V. Among these elements, the following nine elements are considered as the most important bioelements, since they are able to exist as a constituting element for metalloproteins, metalloenzymes, or even vitamins: Fe, Zn, Mn, Cu, Se, Mo, Ni, Co, and V [16,17].

Despite reports associating tissue necrosis with implant failure, the degree to which processes, such as metal toxicity, negatively impact implant performance is unknown. Hallab et al. [18] evaluated representative human peri-implant cells (i.e., osteoblasts, fibroblasts, and lymphocytes) when challenged by Al^{+3}, Co^{+2}, Cr^{+3}, Fe^{+3}, Mo^{+5}, Ni^{+2}, and V^{+3} chloride solutions (and Na^{+2} as a control) over a wide range of concentrations (0.01–10.0 mM). It was reported that (i) differential effects were found to be less a function of the cell type than of the composition and concentration of metal challenge, (ii) no preferential immuno-suppression was demonstrated, and (iii) soluble Co released from the Co–Cr alloy and V released from the Ti–6Al–4V alloy could be implicated as the most likely to mediate cell toxicity in the peri-prosthetic milieu [18].

Maurer et al. [19], using diluted concentration of vanadate and titanium tetrachloride as salts, investigated the cellular uptake of titanium and vanadium. It was found that (i) titanium was not observed to be toxic to the cells, but (ii) vanadium was toxic at levels greater than 10 μg/ml. The percentage of cellular association of titanium was shown to be about 10 times that of vanadium. The percentage of cellular association of either element was greater from fretting corrosion than from the addition of salts. It was also mentioned that (i) the presence of vanadium did not affect the cellular uptake of titanium, but (ii) the presence of titanium decreased the cell association of vanadium [19].

Corrosion resistance is one of the most important properties which can determine the biocompatibility of metallic biomaterials. The high corrosion resistance of metallic materials is attributed to a passive film on their surfaces. However, the passive film on these metals may be continuously damaged by wear when these materials are used as bone plates and screws, artificial joints, or dental restorations. The wear on metallic biomaterials can generate debris and accelerate metal ion release. Powders of the Co–Cr–Mo alloy were produced by grinding larger particles for 8 h in water, serum, or joint fluid and were administered in low doses (0.05–0.5 mg/ml) for 1–6 days to human dermal fibroblasts *in vitro*. Particles were ground in a biological fluid in order to simulate conditions in an artificial hip joint. It was found that (i) such particles adhered to, or were phagocytosed, by the cells far less than those ground in water, and (ii) the toxicity of the alloy was linked with a failure of test cells to grow as quickly as the controls—particles ground in water were the most toxic [20].

3.2.2. Biological Toxicity

Biological toxicity can be more complicated to measure. In a host with an intact immune system the inherent toxicity of the organism is balanced by the host's ability to fight back; the effective toxicity is then a combination of both parts of the relationship. A similar situation is also present with other types of toxic agents. In particular, toxicity of cancer-causing agents is problematic, since for many such substances it is not certain if there is a minimal effective dose or whether the risk is just too small to see. Here, too, the possibility exists that a single cell transformed into a cancer cell is all it takes to develop the full effect. Yang et al. [21] demonstrated an increase in levels of elemental Ti in the blood and lung of rats with a Ti alloy implant. Rats were implanted with Ti alloy disks for 4 weeks. The levels of elemental Ti in the blood and lung were especially increased compared with other tissues. The Ti alloy implant enhanced lung injury related to endotoxin from gram-negative bacteria (lipopolysaccharide [LPS]), which was characterized by lung edema and other histological changes such as recruitment of neutrophils, interstitial edema, and alveolar hemorrhage in the lung. In the presence of endotoxin, an increase of nitrite production was shown in the plasma and bronchoalveolar lavage fluid of rats implanted with a Ti alloy. Moreover, the Ti alloy implant further enhanced the induction of inducible nitric oxide (NO) synthase (iNOS) protein expression induced by LPS in the lung. These endotoxin-related responses in the presence or absence of the Ti alloy implant could be inhibited by aminoguanidine (an iNOS inhibitor). It was first indicated that circulating Ti released from Ti alloy implants had an ability to affect pulmonary iNOS protein expression and enhance the pathogenesis of acute lung injury during endotoxemia [21].

3.2.3. Physical Toxicity

Physically toxic entities include things not usually thought of as such by the lay person: direct blows, concussion, sound and vibration, heat and cold, nonionizing electromagnetic radiation such as infrared and visible light, ionizing nonparticulate radiation, such as X-rays and gamma rays, and particulate radiation, such as alpha rays, beta rays, and cosmic rays [22]. Besides these, particulate macrophages should be included here; even species per se are not toxic, but because of size, they will exhibit physical toxicity. Particulate wear-debris is detected in histiocyte/macrophages of granulomatous tissues adjacent to loosen joint prostheses. Such cell–particle interactions have been simulated *in vitro* by challenging macrophages with particles dosed according to weight percent, volume percent, and number of particles. Each of these dosage methods has inherent shortcomings due to varying size and density of challenging particles of different compositions. In studies done by Shanbhag et al. [23], P388D1 macrophages with titania (TiO_2) and polystyrene particles (<2 μm), with dosage based on the ratio of the cells, were challenged. The effect of size and composition on the bone reabsorbing activity and fibroblast proliferation was studied. It was reported that (i) macrophage response to particulate debris appears to be dependent on particle size, composition, and dose as given by the surface area ratio, and (ii) macrophages stimulated by wear particles are expected to synthesize numerous factors affecting events in the bone–implant interface [23].

Recently, Takeda et al. [24] discussed on health effects of nanomaterials on next generation. For discussing the health effects of nanomaterials, people cannot disregard the research on the health effect of air-borne particles which could be any types of nanosize of biomaterials (including fine powder of titanium dioxide [TiO_2]). The results of not only animal experiments but many epidemiologic surveys and volunteer intervention experiments in humans are reported on the health effects of particles. Although the health effects of the particles matter particle sizes below 10 μm were investigated in the initial studies, recently even smaller particle has come to be regarded as questionable and research of the health effects of the minute particulate matter below 2.5 μm has been done. The health effects of various types of intentionally produced nanomaterials such as carbon black, carbon nanotube (which is recently becoming very popular material in the advanced tissue engineering field), and TiO_2 were examined on their influence on next generation. Regardless of the dosage and administration method, such as inhalation, endotracheal administration, nasal drip, and subcutaneous administration, once nanomaterials enter the bloodstream of another pregnant mouse, they move to the offspring and have effects on them. The effects may appear as various symptoms in the process of growth after birth and can sometimes lead to the onset and aggravation of serious diseases [24].

During the orthodontic mechano-therapy, there is complex stress situations developed. Such stress might accelerate the potential corrosion reaction. Removable osseointegrated titanium mini-implants were successfully used as anchorage devices in orthodontics. The early load is necessary to simplify the mini-implant methodology, but can lead to failure during osseointegration. The Ti–6Al–4V alloy was used instead of commercially pure Ti due to its superior strength. However, the corrosion resistance is low, allowing for metal ion release. Morais et al. [25] analyzed the immediately loaded mini-implant fixation and to gauge the vanadium ion release during the healing process. Titanium alloy mini-implants were inserted in the tibiae of rabbits. After 1, 4, and 12 weeks, they were submitted to removal torque testing and the kidney, liver, and lung were also extracted and analyzed by atomic absorption spectrometry. A stress analysis indicated that CpTi and Ti–6Al–4V deformed plastically and the shear strength of the interface, suggesting that the removal torques for CpTi dangerously approach the yield stress. It was also reported that the detected concentration of vanadium did not reach toxic levels in the animal model [25].

3.3. Allergic Reaction

Allergy is the opposite of acquired immune deficiency syndrome (AIDS). Allergy symptoms are the result of too much immunity. The immune system produces antibodies to fight infections. If one has AIDS, he has too little immunity to defend himself against getting sick. AIDS is too little immunity, and allergy is too much. Metal sensitivity is thought to be a very important factor in the overall biocompatibility of implants. Although titanium has not been found to show sensitivity, other materials such as nickel from stainless steel, other high nickel alloys such as NiTi, and cobalt from cobalt-based alloys have been shown to be sensitizers in skin dermatitis and might, therefore, show an allergic response upon implantation [26]. Allergic contact dermatitis to metals is a common skin disease in many countries of the world. Ni allergy is most frequent, and the prevalence is reported to be 10% in females and 1% in men [27]. The incidence of Ni allergy has increased especially in the young female generation, where the cause is probably due to the increased habit of ear piercing in females in recent years [28,29]. Cr is another well-known metal allergen. Especially in men, occupational chromium dermatitis occurs among cement workers, Cr platers, and workers dealing with leather tanning [30]. Sensitization to orthopedic implant materials is an unpredictable event that might affect implant performance. Candidate materials for hip or knee joint prosthesis implantation were subjected to evaluate preoperative assessments for identifying patients with metal sensitivity, to determine the percentage of patients who developed metal sensitivity at 1 year after prosthesis implantation, and to examine the clinical relevance of patch tests and lymphocyte transformation tests (LTT-MELISA®) for the evaluation of metal sensitization. Based on the result that the percentage of patients who tested positive for metal sensitivity 1 year postimplantation suggests the possibility of prosthesis-induced sensitization, it is strongly suggested that that the objective determination of metal sensitivity at preoperative assessment should be considered in planning arthroplasty intervention, as it would help the surgeon in selecting the most appropriate prosthesis for the patient and could benefit implant performance [31].

Ti is considered as a nonsensitizing or less sensitizing metal, and the application of Ti materials is increasing rapidly in a variety of products such as glasses' rims, wrist watches, eyeglass frames, and dental and medical devices and equipment. However, there are some reports of contact dermatitis due to Ti [32,33]. Titanium allergy is barely recognized in mainstream medicine—yet it was reported that as many as one in ten people can be affected by it. For those afflicted with titanium allergy, the symptoms can be multiple and bewildering. These can range from simple skin rashes to muscle pain and fatigue. From foodstuff to medicine, titanium is now an everyday metal. Several brands of candy, such as Skittles and M&M, have TiO_2 in the coating—often described by its E-number: E171. Like all metals, titanium releases particles through normal corrosion. These metals become ions in the body and then bind to body proteins. For those who react, the body will try to attack this structure. This starts a chain reaction which can lead to many symptoms including Chronic Fatigue Syndrome (CFS) or, in the most severe cases, Multiple Sclerosis (MS). The MELISA® test is the only scientifically-proven test which can diagnose titanium allergy and measure its severity. Those who test positive should avoid exposure or remove the titanium from their body to stop the internal reaction. This can be simple, like changing brand of toothpaste. Or it may be more complex, such as replacing titanium implants [34].

Identification of the causative chemical of contact dermatitis, comparison of the sensitization potency of chemicals and the finding of cross-reactivity among these chemicals are important to develop a safe material for the metal-sensitized patients. For this purpose, reproducible animal models are useful. Cr sensitization is easily induced in animals by using potassium dichromate ($K_2Cr_2O_7$), which is recognized as a strong sensitizer [35–39]. Although the sensitization rate to Ni in humans is the highest among various allergens, the sensitization potential of Ni salts was reported to be weak to mild in the animal studies [35,36,40–43]. On the other hand, there is little knowledge about the sensitization potential of zirconium and titanium salts by animal assays using these salts. Ikarashi et al. [44] evaluated contact sensitization capacity of four metal salts, nickel sulfate ($NiSO_4$), $K_2Cr_2O_7$, titanium chloride ($TiCl_4$) and zirconium chloride ($ZrCl_4$), using guinea-pigs and mice. In the guinea-pig sensitization tests, an injection concentration to 1% for all chemicals was set up, and the challenge concentration was changed. Guipea-pigs were sensitized with $NiSO_4$, $K_2Cr_2O_7$, and $TiCl_4$. It was found that (i) among the test metal salts, $K_2Cr_2O_7$ showed the highest sensitization rate and strongest skin reactions, (ii) $ZrCl_4$ did not cause any sensitization responses under our experimental conditions, (iii) minimal challenge concentration to cause a skin response was <0.25% for $K_2Cr_2O_7$, 0.5% for $NiSO_4$, 2% for $TiCl_4$, and (iv) in the sensitive mouse lymph node assay, $TiCl_4$ as well as $ZrCl_4$ caused mild lymph node responses, but was classified as a nonsensitizer. Based on these findings, it was concluded that the order of sensitization potential was $K_2Cr_2O_7 > NiSO_4 > TiCl_4 > ZrCl_4$ [44].

Titanium brackets are used in orthodontic patients with an allergy to nickel and other specific substances. Harzer et al. [45] studied the corrosive properties of fluoride-containing toothpastes with different pH values on titanium brackets. Molar bands were placed on 18 orthodontic patients. In the same patients, titanium brackets were bonded on the left quadrants and stainless steel brackets on the right quadrants of the upper and lower arches. Fifteen patients used Gel Kam containing soluble tin fluoride (pH 3.2), whereas three used fluoride-free toothpaste. The brackets were removed for evaluation by light microscopy and scanning microscopy 5.5–7.0 months and 7.5–17 months after bonding. It was observed that (i) the matte gray color of titanium brackets dominating over the silver gleam of the steel brackets was noticed, (ii) the plaque accumulation on titanium brackets was high, and (iii) pitting corrosion and crevices were observed in only three of the 165 brackets tested. It was concluded that the *in vivo* study confirms the results of *in vitro* studies, but the changes are so minor that titanium brackets can safely be used for up to 18 months [45].

Although no cytotoxic effect caused by the NiTi alloy has been reported [46], information concerning the biological side effects of Ni is available in the literature [47–50]. Ni is capable of eliciting toxic and allergic responses [47]. Ni can produce more allergic reactions than all other metal elements [48]. In the *in vivo* study, NiTi alloys show cytotoxic reactions [49]. Cases also show the conversion of Ni-nonsensitive subjects into Ni-sensitive subjects following the use of NiTi wires [50].

It is well documented that some metals are known to produce inflammatory responses (e.g., Cr, Co, Cu, Ni, Pd, Ti, Zr, and their based alloys) *in vitro* [51–53] and allergic reactions (e.g., Cr, Co, Ni, Ti, and NiTi) *in vivo* [2,54]. Several studies highlight that elements can diffuse from appliances and accumulate in tissues [55,56]. Ti–6Al–4V is the most frequently employed as an orthopedic implant material as well as device. However, it was reported that Al is an element involved in severe neurological, for example, metabolic-bone disease and osteomalacia [57] and Alzheimer's disease [56]. Bone remodeling will produce further Al release, even after the appliances no longer leach out Al, perpetrating the dangerous side-effect of this element [57,58]. Takemoto et al. [59] studied CpTi plates, Ti–6Al–4V screws, and surrounding tissues to evaluate the release and accumulation of ions. Optical microscopy, scanning electron microscopy (SEM) and X-ray microanalysis were carried out to evaluate the plates and screws removed from patients presenting inflammation and biopsies. It was reported that (i) ions released from metallic appliances or leaching from granules toward soft tissues was observed, (ii) an accumulation of Al but not Ti was found in soft tissues, and (iii) a peculiar accumulation of Al in the dense lamella of newly formed bone was recorded, indicating that biological perturbations may be related to Al release from the tested biomaterials [59].

3.4. Compatibility

In the field of dental or orthopedic implantology, or both, there are many compatibilities which essentially determine acceptance, rejection, and long-term survival. These compatibilities should include biological compatibility, biomechanical compatibility, morphological compatibility, hemocompatibility, cyctocompatibility, MRI compatibility, and so forth. In this chapter we will review two important combatibilities against blood (hemocompatibility) and cell (cytocompatibility), since these molecules need to be adhered, proliferated and differentiated properly right after placing implants. These compatibilities, especially the surface energy condition, are controlling factors, and certain types of surface modifications can change the surface energy, as discussed in Chapter 5.

Biological, Biomechanical, and Morphological Compatibilities will be discussed in Chapter 4, since these are essential for successful implantology.

3.4.1. Hemocompatibility

Blood-contacting materials for long-term implantation in the body, such as artificial hearts, artificial valves, and stents, are required to have good blood compatibility. Hemocompatibility is a key property of biomaterials that come in contact with blood. Surface modification has shown great potential for improving the hemocompatibility of biomedical materials and devices. The hemocompatibility of the titanium oxide films was characterized in terms of clotting, time, blood platelet adhesion and activation, thrombin time, and thrombinogen time. Huang et al. [60] studied the behavior of protein adsorption by irradiation labeling with ^{125}I. Ti–O thin films were prepared by plasma immersion ion implantation (PI^3 or PIII) and deposition, and by sputtering. Systematic evaluation of hemocompatibility, including *in vitro* clotting time, thrombin time, prethrombin time, blood platelet adhesion, and *in vivo* implantation into a dog's ventral aorta or right auricle from 17 to 90 days, proved that Ti–O films have excellent hemocompatibility. It is, hence, suggested that the significantly lower interface tension between Ti-O films, blood and plasma proteins, and the semiconducting nature of Ti–O films give them their improved hemocompatibility [60].

Already widely used in the orthopedic field as biomaterials, Ti–6Al–4V could be selected as the construction material for blood-contacting devices, such as the left ventricular assist device [61]. Several authors have discussed the biocompatibility and hemocompatibility of pure titanium [61–65]. Protein adsorption studies on titanium oxide TiO_2 have been reported [66,67]. The Ti–6Al–4V alloy behavior toward bovine serum albumin (BSA) and bovine gamma-globulin has been studied using an enzyme-linked immunosorbent assay, and has demonstrated a greater protein binding for the Ti–6Al–4V alloy than for stainless steel [68]. These results indicate that the Ti–6Al–4V alloy is well tolerated by blood [62]. It was also suggested that the Ti–6Al–4V alloy is well tolerated by the blood and, therefore, is a promising biocompatible material for the construction of biomedical devices, either in the orthopedic field or in the cardiovascular one [62].

Muramatsu et al. [69] evaluated the fibrin deposition and blood platelet adhesion onto alkali- and heat-treated CpTi, alkali- and water-treated CpTi, and alkali- and heat-treated CpTi formed with apatite in simulated body fluid (SBF). They were evaluated by exposure to anticoagulated blood or washed platelet suspension under static conditions and subsequent observation with SEM. It was reported that (i) thrombus formation on alkali-treated CpTi surfaces, which were exposed to heparinized whole blood for 1 h, was significantly less than that on untreated control CpTi, on which pronounced depositions of fibrin-erythrocytes and lymphocytes were observed, (ii) no thrombus was observed on the apatite-like formed CpTi surface, and (iii) the apatite-like formed CpTi surface exhibits stronger antithrombogenic characteristics than CpTi and other materials examined in heparinized blood [69].

Suska et al. [70] mentioned that the role of apoptosis/cell death in the inflammatory response at the implanted materials is unexplored. Two surfaces with different cytotoxic potential and *in vivo* outcomes, titanium (Ti) and copper (Cu), were incubated *in vitro* with human monocytes and studied using a method to discriminate apoptotic and necrotic cells. It was found that Ti surfaces displayed enhanced monocyte survival and production of IL(interleukin)-10 and TNF(tumor necrosis factor)-α. Cu adherent cells exhibited apoptotic signs as early as 1 hour after incubation, but (ii) in contrast to Ti, after 48 hours the predominance of apoptotic cells switched to apoptotic/necrotic cells on Cu surfaces, and (iii) material properties rapidly influence the onset of human monocyte apoptosis and progression to late apoptosis/necrosis, concluding that early detection of apoptosis and cell death may be important for the understanding of the biological response to implanted materials [70].

Ion implantation onto NiTi has been used to decrease the surface nickel concentration of this alloy and produce a titanium oxide layer [61]. Nothing is known yet about the blood compatibility of this surface and the suitability for implants in the blood vessels, like vascular stents. Maitz et al. [71] treated superelastic NiTi by oxygen or helium plasma-immersion ion implantation to deplete surface Ni, leading to the formation of a nickel-poor titanium-oxide surface with a nanoporous structure. Fibrinogen adsorption and conformation changes, blood platelet adhesion, and contact activation of the blood clotting cascade have been checked as *in vitro* parameters of blood compatibility; metabolic activity and release of cytokines IL-6 and IL-8 from cultured endothelial cells on these surfaces give information about the reaction of the blood vessel wall. It was found that (i) the oxygen-ion-implanted NiTi surface adsorbed less fibrinogen on its surface and activated the contact system less than the untreated nitinol surface, but (ii) conformation changes of fibrinogen were higher on the oxygen-implanted nitinol, (iii) no difference between initial and oxygen-implanted NiTi was found for the platelet adherence, endothelial cell activity, or cytokine release, and (iv) oxygen-ion implantation is seen as a useful method to decrease the nickel concentration in the surface of nitinol for cardiovascular applications [71].

Untreated Ti–6Al–4V and glow-discharge treated Ti–6Al–4V samples were tested on human peripheral blood mononuclear cells. It was found that (i) apoptosis, undetectable after 24 hours contact of peripheral blood mononuclear cells with the two sample types, is induced after 48 hours by treated samples, and, after 48 hours, but in the presence of 1.5 μg/ml PHA, by both sample types, and (ii) although the plasma-treated titanium alloy shows a better biocompatibility in comparison with the untreated one, attention must be paid to the careful control of the first signs of inflammation [72]. Thor et al. [73] investigated the thrombogenic responses of whole blood, platelet-rich plasma and platelet-poor plasma in contact with a highly thrombogenic surface as titanium. The thrombogenic responses of clinically used surfaces as hydroxyapatite (HA), machined titanium, titania-blasted titanium, and fluoride ion-modified grit-blasted titanium were also investigated. It was concluded that (i) whole blood is necessary for sufficient thrombin generation and platelet activation during placement of implants, and (ii) a fluoride ion modification seems to segment the thromgoneic properties of titanium [73].

3.4.2. Cytocompatibility

Although it is commonly accepted that titanium and the titanium alloying, and elements of tantalum, niobium, zirconium, molybdenum, tin, and silicon are biocompatible, some newly developed titanium alloys containing molybdenum, niobium, and silicon produced by powder metallurgy show a certain degree of cytotoxicity. Li et al.[74] had hypothesized that the cytotoxicity is linked to the ion release from the metals. The cytotoxicity of titanium and titanium alloying elements in both forms of powder and bulk was assessed, using osteoblast-like $SaOS_2$ cells. Results indicated that the metal powders of titanium, niobium, molybdenum, and silicon are cytotoxic, and the bulk metals of silicon and molybdenum also showed cytotoxicity [74].

Over the years, many metal and polymer implants have been developed for internal fracture fixation. However, there are some problems associated with their application, such as implant loosening or infection. Cytotoxicity of soluble and particulate Ti, V, and Ni by biochemical functional analysis and by microscopic morphology with elemental analysis *in vitro* using human neutrophils as probes and *in vivo* in animals was compared. It was concluded that (i) the biochemical analysis of LDH (lactate dehydrogenase), superoxide anion, inflammatory mediator TNF-α, and SEM showed that Ni in solution destroys the cell membranes of neutrophils, whereas Ti and V in solution stimulate neutrophils and increase the quantity of released superoxide anions, (ii) fine Ti particles (1–3 μm), which are smaller than neutrophils (about 5 μm), were phagocytized by the cells, and the results were similar *in vivo*, and (iii) these results showed that the cytotoxic effect of Ti particles is size dependent, and that they must be smaller than that of cells [75].

Harris et al. [76] studied the morphology and adhesion of both fibroblasts and osteoblasts to manufactured commercially pure, medical implant-quality anodized titanium surfaces, and five modified titanium surfaces, and examined their relative cytocompatibility to assess which modified surface could potentially be used *in vivo*. It was reported that (i) small variations were observed both qualitatively and quantitatively in the spreading and adhesion of fibroblasts and osteoblasts to the studied surfaces, but (ii) noticeable fibroblast and osteoblast spreading and adhesion were found on the anodized surfaces, and (iii) coating medical implant-quality anodized titanium surfaces could probably improve soft tissue adhesion or osseointegration of bone, or both, *in vivo* [76].

The cytotoxicity and mutagenicity of metal salts were systematically evaluated by Yamamoto et al. [77–79]. Metal ions released from the wear debris of Ti alloys [80], and the cytotoxicity of ceramic particles (mainly metal oxides) [81] were investigated, and it was confirmed that active oxygen species generated by macrophages phagocytosing high density polyethylene particles induced metal ion release from Ti [82].

Manceur et al. [83] reported on the biocompatibility of NiTi single crystals, since certain orientations of single crystals present several advantages over the polycrystalline form in terms of maximal strain, fatigue resistance, and temperature range of superelasticity (which is one of two uniquenesses associated with NiTi material; the other one is SME—shape memory effect). The *in vitro* biocompatibility evaluation of 50.8 wt% Ni–Ti single crystals in the orientation ⟨0 0 1⟩ was conducted after four different heat treatments in a helium atmosphere followed by mechanical polishing. The study was performed on the material extracts after immersion of the specimens in cell culture medium (DMEM) for 7 days at 37 °C. Cytotoxicity studies were performed on L-929 mouse fibroblasts using the MTT (3-[4,5-dimethylthaiazol-2-yl]-2,5 diphenyl tetrazolium bromide) assay. The J-774 macrophages were used to assess the potential inflammatory effect of the extracts by IL1-β and TNF-α dosage (sandwich ELISA method). It was found that (i) exposure of L-929 to material extracts did not affect cell viability, and (ii) IL1-β and TNF-α secretion were not stimulated after incubation with NiTi extracts compared to the negative controls, concluding that TiNi single crystals did not trigger a cytotoxic reaction [83].

Titanium alloys have been proven to behave poorly in friction due to detection of wear particles in tissues and organs associated with titanium implants. Bordji et al. [84] investigated three surface treatments in order to improve the wear resistance and the hardness of Ti–6Al–4V and Ti–5Al–2.5Fe: (i) glow discharge nitrogen implantation (10–17 atoms/cm^2), (ii) plasma nitriding by plasma diffusion treatment (PDT), and (iii) deposition of the TiN layer by plasma-assisted chemical vapor deposition (PACVD) additionally to PDT. A cell culture model using human cells was chosen to study the effect of such treatments on the cytocompatibility of these materials. The results showed that (i) the Ti–5Al–2.5Fe alloy was as cytocompatible as the Ti–6Al–4V alloy, and the same surface treatment led to identical biological consequences on both alloys, (ii) nitrogen implantation did not at all modify the cellular behavior observed on untreated samples, (iii) after the two nitriding treatments, cell proliferation, and viability appeared to be significantly reduced, and the SEM study revealed somewhat irregular surface states, but (iv) osteoblast phenotype expression and protein synthesis capacity were not affected. Hence, it was concluded that plasma diffusion nitriding treatment and TiN deposition by the chemical vapor process may be an interesting alternative to the physical vapor deposition technique [84]. Wever et al. carried out a dilution minimal essential medium extract cytotoxicity test, a guinea-pig sensitization test and two geneotoxicity (Salmonella reverse mutation and the chromosomal aberration) tests on NiTi. It was reported that the NiTi alloy showed no cytotoxic, allergic, nor genotoxic activity similar to the clinical reference control material AISI 316 stainless steel [85].

By the prolonged use of NiTi material in a human body, deterioration of the corrosion resistance of the materials becomes a critical issue because of the increasing possibility of deleterious ions released from the substrate to living tissues. It was proven that certain surface modifications, such as nitrogen, acetylene, and oxygen plasma immersion ion implantation (PIII or PI^3), can improve the corrosion resistance and mechanical properties of the materials. With this modification, it was reported that (i) the release of nickel is drastically reduced as compared with the untreated control, and (ii) the *in vitro* tests show that the plasma-treated surfaces are well tolerated by osteoblasts [86,87].

Although the Ti–Ni alloy has been increasingly applied to medical and dental devices such as coronary stents and orthodontic wires, the alloy contains nickel, which is known to give to cytotoxicity, metal allergy, and carcinogenicity. The corrosion resistance of the Ti–Ni alloy was studied by electrolytic treatment in lactic acid, water, and glycerol [88]. It was found that, with the electrolytic treatment, nickel concentration in the surface oxide layer decreased, and the thickness of the surface oxide layer increased.

A number of ternary NiTi–X alloys have been introduced with the aim to improve the fatigue properties and to decrease the thermal hysteresis range; well-known ternary alloying elements are Cu and Fe [19,21,89]. Particularly, Cu has been shown to dissolve in the B2 (austenitic) phase in concentrations up to 30 at%. However, NiTi-Cu solid solutions containing more than 10 at% are characterized by poor formability, so that alloys of technical interest usually contain Cu in the range from 5 to 10 at%. NiTi (57.6 wt%Ni, 42.4 wt%Ti) and NiTiCu (50.7 wt%Ni, 42.4 wt%Ti, 6.9 wt%Cu) were evaluated by the Tada method [89]. It was concluded that (i) a significant difference in the *in vivo* biocompatibility between the binary and ternary alloy was shown and (ii) the presence of the binary alloy lead to few morphological changes and a slight reduction of dehydrogenase activity of epithelial cell cultures, whereas the effect of the ternary alloy appears to be more pronounced, obviously due to the releasing of copper ions [90].

Newly developed β-type titanium alloys, Ti–29Nb–13Ta–4.6Zr, CpTi, and Ti–6Al–4V, were evaluated in terms of cytotoxicity [91]. Each plate specimen was put on zirconia (ZrO_2) balls in a vessel, and in an autoclave. The vessel with 10 ml Eagle's culture solution at a temperature of 310 K was rotated with a speed of 240 rpm, and extraction periods were 7 and 14 days. As-extracted solution and filtrated extract solution using a 0.22 μm membrane filter were prepared. In the as-extracted solution and filtrated extracted solution, the survival rate of L929 cells derived from mice was evaluated using the Neutral Red (NR) [92] and MTT [93] methods. The exposure period of L929 cells to extract the solutions was 2 days. The MTT method is a method for evaluating cell respiration by the mitochondria, while the NR method is a method for evaluating the ratio of sound cells of which cell membranes have no lesion by the amount of NR pigment. The survival rate of L929 cells indicates the cytotoxicity level of the extracts, and it was also reported that the new alloy is equivalent to that of CpTi and Ti–6Al–4V [91].

Spriano et al. [94] treated Ti–6Al–7Nb as prosthetic implant material by various methods: surfaces were (i) mechanically polished with SiC paper, (ii) passivated in 35 wt.% HNO_3 for 30 minutes, (iii) treated in alkali 5 M NaOH at 60 °C for 24 hour, (iv) heated at 600 °C for 1 hour in air, and (v) heated at 600 °C for 1 hour in vacuum. These treated surfaces were characterized in order to evaluate their surface properties and cell interaction, in order to assess if the treatments were effective in obtaining a surface presenting at the same time bone-like apatite induction ability, and low metal ion release. Wettability was examined by surface contact angle measurements. The untreated surface showed 55 degrees, which was the highest value of the surface contact angle, indicating that the untreated surface is not at the active stage. On the SiC-polished surface, it was 50°, then it follows very low values of contact angle; the in-air oxidized surface exhibits almost zero degree of the contact angle, indicating very high wettability. It was also reported that such active surface was covered with a film of a composition close to the standard Ca/P ratio bone-like apatite after the surfaces were immersed in SBF for 30 days [94].

Hou et al. [95] used the rat oral implant model to assess histological changes in the mechanical environment surrounding loaded and unloaded dental implants. The maxillary left first molar from rats was extracted, and the site was allowed to heal for 1 month. A titanium mini-screw implant was then placed into the site and allowed to heal for 21 days. The madibular left first molars in one group of rats were extracted to create an unloaded condition. In a second group of rats, the mandibular left first molars were left in occlusion with the opposing screw head to simulate loading. Radiographs were taken on the day of placement and at 7 days, 14 days, and 21 days after post-implantation and were used to estimate the bone-implant contact (BIC) ratio. It was reported that (i) areas of high shear stress adjacent to the helical threads of loaded implants were associated with ostecalcin localization and bone formation but only minimal localization of matrix metalloproteinase 13, and (ii) bone adjacent to unloded implants showed fibrous tissue and extensive matrix metalloproteinase 13 localization surrounding the apical two-thirds of each implant [95].

The antibacterial effect and cytocompatibility of a nanostructured TiO_2 (titania) film containing Cl on the CpTi surface was investigated [96]. The nanostructured TiO_2 was prepared by anodization with hydrofluoric acid, followed by secondary anodization with the NaCl solution of different concentrations (0.4 M, 1 M, and 2 M). The antibacterial effect was evaluated by the film adhesion method and cytocompatibility was tested by the viability of MG-63 cells in an MTT assay. It was found that (i) the contact angle (as a function of surface wettability) showed anodized titanium as a hydrophilic nature, and (ii) TiO_2 nanostructured film anodized in 1 M NaCl exhibited the best antibacterial effect and cell cytocompatibility [96]. The titanium dioxide layer is composed mainly of anatase and rutile. This layer is prone to break (mainly due to its britlle ceramic nature), releasing particles to the milieu. Based on previous finding that commercial anatase TiO_2 was deposited in organs with macrophagic activity, transported in the blood by phagocytic-mononuclear cells, and induced an increase in the production of reactive oxygen species, Olmedo et al. [97] further evaluated the effects of rutile TiO_2, using male Wistar rats being injected with a suspension of rutile TiO_2 powder. It was reported that (i) titanium was found in phagocytic mononuclear cells, serum, and in the parenchyma of all the organs tested, (ii) although rutile TiO_2 provoked an augmentation of reactive oxygen species, it failed to induce damage to membrane lipids, possibly due to an adaptive response, and (iii) rutile TiO_2 is less bioactive than anatase TiO_2 [97].

Normally measuring the surface contact angle is performed by placing one liquid droplet onto the target substrate, followed by measuring height (h) of the droplet, and length (d) of the droplet after wetting. Using the sphere approximation, the contact angle (θ) can be obtained by the formula $\theta = 2\tan^{-1}(2h/d)$. And it is the common practice to measure the advancing angle instead of receding angle which is much lower angle since the wetting front is travelling on already-wet area. The contact angle (if the used liquid does not show any corrosiveness against the substrate surface material), the contact angle normally spreads; hence the contact angle (θ) can be partial-differentiated with respect to time (t) as the formula $\delta\theta/\delta t = [-4h(\delta d/\delta t) + 4d(\delta h/\delta t)]/(d^2 + 4h^2)$ [98].

In terms of wettability, hydrophilicity has been gaining increasing interest as a factor that might influence the osseointegration of dental implants. Rupp et al. [99] used nine screw-type implant systems from eight manufacturers to measure dynamic water contact angles. Wettability was quantified by first advancing contact angles. It was concluded that (i) the first advancing mean contact angles of all implants ranged from 0 to 138 degrees, demonstrating statistically significant differences among implant systems, and (ii) because of kinetic hysteresis, initially hydrophobic implants became to be hydrophilicity during following immersion loops [99].

3.5. Bone Healing

Once cytocompatibility is established on the placed implant's surface, the attached cells should grow to achieve the initial stage of osseointegration. As mentioned in the previous chapter, osseointegration is a time-dependent process and success of the osseointegration is strongly related to the quality and condition of receiving hard tissue. In some clinical cases, patients need to receive bone grafting to the alveolar bone structure in dental implantology, or bone grafting for orthopedic implants. In this section, bone healing mechanisms and grafting will be reviewed.

3.5.1. Cellular Response to Biomaterials

Eriksson et al. [100] pointed out the importance of surface topography on cellular reactions. Surface plays a crucial role in biological interactions for four reasons. First, the surface of a biomaterial is the only part in contact with the bioenvironment. Second, the surface region of a biomaterial is almost always different in morphology and composition from the bulk. Differences arise from molecular rearrangement, surface reaction, and contamination. Third, for biomaterials that do not release nor leak biologically active or toxic substances, the characteristics of the surface govern the biological response. And fourth, some surface properties, such as topography, affect the mechanical stability of the implant/tissue interface [101]. Biomaterials used in a living organism may come into contact with cells in the related tissue for a long period of time. For this reason, they should naturally be harmless to the organism, and their mechanical properties should be suited to the purpose and compatible with receiving tissue surfaces. Furthermore, they should possess a biological effect capable of providing favorable circumstances for the properties and functions of the cells at the implant site. For example, materials used in the construction of an artificial heart or heart valve must provide for anti-thrombogenesis, which for a dental or bone implant must be suitable for cell attachment, because both the connective and epithelial cells (with which these materials mainly come into contact) are anchorage-dependent, and therefore need a cell attachment scaffold for cell division and cell differentiation to be conducted. It is therefore important to investigate attachability of the cells to the materials, which is one of the parameters in the evaluation of biomaterials.

It has been shown that methods of implant surface preparation can significantly affect the resultant properties of the surface and subsequently the biological responses that occur at the surface [102–104]. Recent efforts have shown that the success or failure of dental implants can be related not only to the chemical properties of the implant surface, but also to its micromorphologic nature [105–107]. From an *in vitro* standpoint, the response of cells and tissues at implant interfaces can be affected by surface topography or geometry on a macroscopic basis [105,106], as well as by surface morphology or roughness on a microscopic level [107,108].

When surface roughness of implants, which have been clinically used and evaluated as successful implants, it was found that regardless of the type of implant materials used, if the surface roughness is manipulated to have a range from 1 to 20 μm, the implant's survival rate is excellent [109,110]. This finding leads toward a morphological compatibility, which will be discussed later in this book.

These characteristics undoubtedly affect how cells and tissues respond to various types of biomaterials. Of all the cellular responses, it has been suggested that cellular adhesion is considered the most important response necessary for developing a rigid structural and functional integrity at the bone/implant interface [111]. Cellular adhesion alters the entire tissue response to biomaterials [112].

On a macroscopic level (roughness > 10 μm) roughness influences the mechanical properties of the titanium/bone interface, the mechanical interlocking of the interface, and the biocompatibility of the material [113,114]. Surface roughness in the range from 10 nm to 10 μm may also influence the interfacial biology, since it is the same order as the size of the cells and large biomolecules [115]. Microroughness at this level includes material defects, such as grain boundaries, steps and kinks, and vacancies that are active sites for adsorption, and therefore influence the bonding of biomolecules to the implant surface [116]. Microrough surfaces promote significantly better bone apposition than smooth surfaces, resulting in a higher percentage of bone in contact with the implant. Microrough surfaces may influence the mechanical properties of the interface, stress distribution, and bone remodeling [117]. Increased contact area and mechanical interlocking of bone to a microrough surface can decrease stress concentrations resulting in decreased bone resorption. Bone resorption takes place shortly after loading smooth surfaced implants [118], resulting in a fibrous connective tissue layer, whereas remodeling occurs on rough surfaces [119].

Rich and Harris [107] reported that macrophages exhibited a rugophilia, or an affinity for rough surfaces, whereas fibroblasts failed to readily adhere to these same surfaces. This finding may complement the previous work indicating that rough surfaces promote inflammation via macrophage attraction, rather than wound healing by a connective tissue [107]. Studies by Brunette [120] and Chehroudi et al. [121,122] have demonstrated that cells of differing origins can orient themselves in the grooves of differing micromachined surfaces. It was determined that epithelial cells were more likely to attach to grooves of specific dimension than to adjacent smooth surfaces. Michaels et al. [123] determined that a higher percentage of osteoblast-like cells attached to rough CpTi surfaces produced by sand-blasting than to smoother surfaces polished with 1 μm diamond paste. Keller et al. [124] later confirmed this.

In order to achieve morphological compatibility [109,125], titanium implant surfaces need to be modified. They can be treated by additive methods, such as the titanium beads plasma spray procedure, to increase the effective surface area. They have also been modified by subtractive methods such as acid pickling, acid etching, sand-blasting, and other small particle-blasting to change the texture, as well as to increase the surface area. The development and use of these surface modifications have been based on that an improved osseointegration can be achieved by increasing the topography or roughness of the implant surface [126].

Three types of cylindrical implants (fiber-reinforced compost with porous surfaces, solid PMMA, and CpTi) were prepared and inserted in a transverse direction into the intercondular trabeculou bone area of distal femurs and proximal tibias of New Zealand White rabbits [127]. Histological observation revealed new bone growth into the porous surface of composite implant. Solid PMMA and CpTi implants were encapsulated mostly with the fibrous connective tissue. Implanted rough surfaces have long been associated with the accumulation of macrophages and other cells of the monocytic lineage such as foreign body giant cells and osteoclasts [127]. Chehroudi et al. [128] compared events at the interface of implant surface topographies with varied roughness in a rat subcutaneous model. Titanium-casted epoxy replicas are machined, etched, blasted, titanium-plasma-sprayed, sandblasted and etched, and micromachined, and polished surfaces were implanted for up to 11 weeks. Based on the results, it was concluded that there appears to be two routes to bone-like tissue formation on Ti implants in the rat subcutaneous model: macrophage-mediated and macrophage-independent dense collagenous-matrix-associated [128]. Bhola et al. [129] investigated the cellular response of osteocytes to commercially pure titanium (α) and its alloys (α + β and β) in a culture media and it was mentioned that results serve as a preliminary base-line to characterize the best alloy system for a comprehensive long-term investigation [129].

3.5.2. Cell Attachment, Adhesion, and Spreading

Ti implant systems have been exploited as bone anchored implants for many years. Although titanium is well tolerated by the body, the reason for the successful use of this material is not clear. Beneficial effects due to the oxide that spontaneously forms on Ti have been implicated [100,130]. The success is not due to Ti being passively incorporated into the body, since the body recognizes Ti as foreign and Ti elicits an inflammatory response. When a biological system encounters an implant, reactions are induced at the implant–tissue interface. Such interfacial reactions include that (i) the body wants to keep the implant isolated, (ii) a protective layer of macrophages, monocytes, and giant cells is formed, and (iii) a wall of collagen fibers (capsule) is established, and the type of material may influence the fibrous capsule thickness. Surface and interface properties of interest are chemical composition, contamination and cleanliness, microarchitecture and structure, and so forth. [131]. Fibroblasts lay down a dense fibrous tissue (collagen, elastin, and reticular) that is gradually replaced by a less dense, normal connective tissue, but the body cannot build a normal tissue all the way up to an implant.

The host hard/soft tissue response to biomaterials should be considered first as an inflammatory reaction, as mentioned before. Any biomaterial implanted into the body will be perceived as a threat. The host defenses will attempt to eliminate it. This will not happen if the biomaterial is inert and cannot be degraded. Eventually inert biomaterials will be integrated into the tissue or will become walled off. Biodegradable biomaterials are slowly resorbed over time and are eventually eliminated. Some biomaterials have chemical reactivity and will continue to stimulate over long periods of time. The aforementioned inflammatory processes should include four main stages: initial events (redness, swelling, and pain), cellular invasion (white cells invade tissues), tissue remodeling, repair (being orchestrated by macrophages; occurs differently in different tissues; bone may completely remodel; usually complete within 3–4 weeks), and resolution (extrusion, resorption, integration, and encapsulation). Furthermore, cellular invasion has a neutrophil action (main function is phagocytes; die at tissue site; release further inflammatory medicators; prostaglandins, leukotrinets) and macrophages (phagocytes; removal of dead cells; numbers and activity depend on the pressure of particulate material). Moreover, resolution is an attempt to return to the original condition: extrusion and resorption of implant material for re-establishment of homeostasis, and integration and encapsulation with a layer of fibrous tissue to establish a steady state [132,133].

The response, however, resembles normal wound healing regarding cell recruitment and persistence [134,135]. During the surgical procedure of implantation, the biomaterial most likely will encounter blood. Almost instantly following contact with blood the implant surface will be covered with plasma proteins that become adsorbed to the surface [136,137]. Ti in contact with serum or plasma is known to adsorb high-molecular-weight kininogen, Factor XII, fibrinogen, IgG, prekallikrein, and Clq [138,139]. It was reported that, after 5 s, platelets were found on Ti surfaces exposed to whole blood, while it took about 10 minutes before polymorphonuclear granulocytes adhered [140]. Protein–platelet [141], leukocyte–platelet [142], and protein–leukocyte [143] are possible interactions at the surface. Furthermore, release of inflammatory mediators at the surface may influence both recruitment and activation of cells [141]. The polymorphonuclear granulocytes are the first leukocytes to be recruited to a Ti surface exposed to blood [140]. Adhesion and activation are two processes polymorphonuclear granulocytes may go through upon material contact. Adhesion involves receptor occupation with appropriate surface ligands [143,144], and when polymorphonuclear granulocytes are challenged with different stimuli, they activate their nicotinamide adenine dinucleotide phosphate (NADPH) oxidase (which are a group of plasma membranes—associated enzymes formed in a variety of cells of mesodermal origin). By using oxygen, the NADPH oxidase produces reactive oxygen species that are used in the cell's defense against microorganisms [141,145].

Close contact between bone and implant has been observed with titanium implants [146–148] and coated Ti [149], but has also been reported with alumina oxide (Al_2O_3) [150] and zirconium implants [151]. Most authors report a noncellular layer of proteoglycans between bone and titanium [147]. There are indications that implant materials, including a thick proteoglycan layer formation, have a lower biocompatibility than implants producing a thin proteoglycan layer [152,153]. Most of the articles on implant/bone interactions are presented and discussed based on the interfacial reaction between the metal surface and the bone. However, this is not right, since the immediate contacting species of the implant surface is not metal, but its oxide. If the implant material is one of titanium materials, titanium oxide should be considered as an extreme surface, contacting the living hard/soft tissue. Titanium reacts immediately with oxygen when exposed to air, forming a very thin surface oxide film. This film, which increases during prolonged exposure to oxygen, consists primarily of TiO_2, but Ti_2O_3 and other oxides are also present [115,154]. Ti dioxide has physical/chemical characteristics that differ from metallic Ti, characteristics which are more closely related to ceramics than to metals. As TiO_2 particles have been used in chromatography, it is well established that titanium oxide surfaces bind cations, particularly polyvalent cations [154]. TiO_2 surfaces have a net negative charge at the pH values encountered in animal tissues (around pH 4.0). This binding of cations is based on electrostatic interactions between titanium-linked O^- on the implant surface and cations. The oxide is highly polarized and attracts water and water-soluble molecules in general [153].

Osteoblast cells adhesion to HA [155] and mesenchymal stem cells adhesion to HA [156] were investigated. Luo et al. [155] combined clodronate, one of bisphosphonates, to the surface of the HA scaffold by chelation and found that clodronate had no obvious effect on the cytocompatibility of HA, and clodronate-HA might be used as a bone scaffold with potential ability to improve osteogenesis. Wu et al. [156] combined a HA-coated substrate with a cellular vehicle for the delivery of bone morphogenetic protein-2 (BMP-2) synergistically enhancing the osteoconductivity of implant surfaces and concluded that the HA coated substrate could allow the attachment and growth of BMP-2 gene-modified BMSCs, and this combined application synergistically enhanced osteconductivity of the substrate surface, suggesting that the synergistic method may be of the osseointegration value in orthopedic and dental implant surgery.

During the first week after implantation of Ti in soft tissues, a fluid space, which contains proteins [157–159] and scattered inflammatory cells [160], separates the implant surface from the tissue. The majority of cells in the fluid space are not in direct contact with the surface during the first week of the healing [161]. However, during later time intervals, macrophages are adherent to the surface of Ti [160,162] and other biomaterials [163]. One factor which may influence the regenerating tissue around the implant is the activity of the macrophages and the release of mediators from macrophages adherent on the implant surface. It is possible that these cells act as "messenger cells," transmitting information about the implant surface structure and composition to the surrounding tissue [164,165].

Healy et al. [166] employed surface-sensitive spectroscopies, Auger electron, and X-ray photoelectron spectroscopy (XPS) techniques to characterize changes in Ti oxide composition, oxide stoichiometry, and adsorbed surface species as a function of exposure to human serum in a balanced electrolyte (serum/SIE), and 8.0 mM ethylenediamenetetraacetic acid in a balanced electrolyte (EDTA/SIE) at 37 V. It was reported that (i) before immersion, the oxide was near ideal TiO_2, covered by two types of hydroxyl groups: acidic OH(s) with oxygen doubly coordinated to Ti, and basic Ti-OH groups singly coordinated, and (ii) after extended exposure to both solutions, up to 5,000 hours (ca. 200 days), the surface concentration of OH groups increased and nonelemental P appeared. The adsorbed phosphate species were presumed to be either $Ti–H_2PO_4$ or $Ti-HPO^4$. Hence, it was suggested that Ti metal is not in direct contact with the biological milieu, but rather there is a gradual transition from the bulk metal, near-stoichiometric oxide, Ca- and P-substituted hydrated oxide, adsorbed lipoproteins and glycolipids, proteoglycans, collagen filaments, and bundles to cells [166]. This finding is very important to develop the gradual functioning implant surface structure, as will be described in later.

The protein adsorption behavior of thin films of calcium phosphate (CaP) bioceramic and Ti was investigated by Zeng et al. [167]. The thin films were produced with an ion beam sputter deposition technique using targets of HA, fluorapatite, and Ti. Fourier transform infrared spectroscopy (FTIR) with attenuated total internal reflectance was used to evaluate protein adsorption on these surfaces. It was shown that (i) surface composition and structure influenced the kinetics of protein adsorption and the structure of adsorbed protein, (ii) CaP adsorbed a greater amount of protein than the Ti surface and caused more alteration of the structure of adsorbed BSA than did the Ti surface, and (iii) the differences in protein adsorption behavior could result in very different initial cellular behavior on CaP bioceramic and Ti implant surfaces.

MacDonald et al. [168] surface-modified TiO_2 particles and investigated their effects on protein adsorption, using a model cell binding protein, human plasma fibronection (HPF), which is an important matrix glycoprotein that plays a major role in cell and protein attachment. TiO_2 surfaces were modified by heating Ti dioxide powder at

800 °C for 1 hour or treating with an oxidizing agent: peroxide ammonium hydroxide followed by peroxide in hydrochloric acid. Oxidized and control samples were further treated with butanol:water (by 9:1 fraction) for 30 min. It was found that (i) maximum HPF adsorption on modified or unmodified TiO_2 occurred within 30 min, with greater protein adsorption occurring on butanol-treated samples, (ii) desorption was minimal with all modifications, and (iii) by modifying the physico-chemical properties of TiO_2 surfaces, it may be possible to alter protein adsorption, and hence optimize cell attachment [168].

The effect of surface roughness (Ra: 0.320, 0.490, and 0.874 μm) of Ti–6Al–4V on the short- and long-term response of human bone marrow cells *in vitro* and on protein adsorption was investigated. Cell attachment, cell proliferation, and differentiation (alkaline phosphatase specific activity) were determined. The protein adsorption of BSA and fibronectin, from single protein solutions on rough and smooth Ti–6Al–4V surfaces, was examined with XPS and radiolabeling. It was reported that (i) cell attachment and proliferation were surface roughness sensitive and increased as the roughness of Ti–6Al–4V increased, (ii) human albumin was adsorbed preferentially onto the smooth substratum, and (iii) the rough substratum bound a higher amount of total protein (from culture medium supplied with 15% serum) and fibronectin (10-fold) than did the smooth one [169].

Eriksson et al. [100] treated CpTi surfaces (i) to have a rigid TiO_2 formation by boiling CpTi in H_2O–H_2O_2–NH_4OH (5:1:1) for 5 minutes, followed by heating at 700 °C, or (ii) to have a rough (facetted) Ti surface by etching in 10% HF (hydrofluoric acid) to grow a thick oxide film. CpTi surfaces were also treated in concentrated HNO_3 to grow a novel thin oxide, which resulted in a rough surface, too. It was observed that all surfaces consisted of TiO_2 covered by a carbonaceous layer. The surfaces were incubated with capillary blood for time periods of between 8 minutes and 32 hours. It was reported that (i) leukocyte adhesion to the surfaces increased during the first hours of blood-material contact and then decreased, (ii) polymorphonuclear granulocytes were the dominating leukocytes on all surfaces, followed by monocytes, (iii) cells adhering to rough surfaces were higher than cells on smooth surfaces, (iv) maximum respiratory burst response occurred earlier on the smooth than on the rough surfaces, and (v) topography had a greater impact than oxide thickness on most cellular reactions investigated, where the latter often had a dampening effect on the responses [100].

Events leading to integration of an implant into bone, and hence determining the long-time performance of the device, take place largely at the interface formed between the tissue and the implant [170]. The development of this interface is complex and is influenced by numerous factors, including surface chemistry and surface topography of the foreign material [171–173]. For example, Oshida et al. treated NiTi by acid-pickling in $HF:HNO_3:H_2O$ (1:1:5 by volume) at room temperature for 30 s to control the surface topology and selectively dissolve Ni, resulting in a Ti-enriched NiTi surface layer [174]. Zinger et al. [175] investigated the role of surface roughness on the interaction of cells with titanium model surfaces of well-defined topography using human bone-derived cells (MG63 cells) to understand the early phase of interactions through a kinetic morphological analysis of adhesion, spreading, and proliferation of the cells. SEM and double immunofluorescent labeling of vinculin and actin revealed that the cells responded to nanoscale roughness with a higher cell thickness and a delayed apparition of the focal contacts. A singular behavior was observed on nanoporous oxide surfaces, where the cells were more spread and displayed longer and more numerous filopods. On electrochemically microstructured surfaces, the MG63 cells were able to go inside, adhere, and proliferate in cavities of 30 or 100 μm in diameter, whereas they did not recognize the 10 μm diameter cavities. Cells adopted a 3D shape when attaching inside the 30 μm diameter cavities. It was therefore concluded that nanotopography on surfaces with 30 μm diameter cavities had little effect on cell morphology compared to flat surfaces with the same nanostructure, but cell proliferation exhibited a marked synergistic effect of microscale and nanoscale topography [175].

Rat bone marrow (RBM) stromal cells were cultured on either a smooth surface (roughness: 0.14 μm) or a rough surface (5.8 μm) of Ti–6Al–4V disks for 24 or 48 h. Cells on the smooth surface showed typical fibroblastic morphology, whereas cells on the rough surface were in clusters with a more epithelial appearance. RNA was extracted from the cells at both time points, and gene expression was analyzed by using a rat gene microarray. At 24 and 48 hours, a similar number of genes were both up- and down-regulated at least twofold on the rough surface compared to the smooth surface. It was noticed that (i) roughness did not appear to be a specific stimulator of osteogenesis because genes of both the bone and cartilage lineage were up-regulated on the tough surface, and (ii) surface roughness alters the expression of a large number of genes in marrow stromal cells, which are related to multiple pathways of mesenchymal cell differentiation [176]. A highly porous Ti–6Al–4V was fabricated by a polymeric sponge replication method [177]. A polymeric sponge, impregnated with Ti–6Al–4V slurry prepared from Ti–6Al–4V powders and binders, was subjected to drying and pyrolyzing to remove the polymeric sponge and binders. The porous Ti–6Al–4V made by this method had a three-dimensional trabecular porous structure with interconnected pores mainly ranging from 400 to 700 μm and a total porosity of about 90%. The compressive strength was 10.3 ± 3.3 MPa and the elastic constant 0.8 ± 0.3 GPa. It was also reported that MC3T3-E1 cells attached and spread well in the inner surface of pores [177].

Müller et al. [178] studied the adsorption of BSA on surfaces of dental enamel and of dental materials as a function of contact time between protein and surface, pH, wettability, and isoelectric point of the surface. It was found that (i) whereas the chosen ceramic and composite materials resemble very well the adhesion on natural enamel, a much stronger adhesion was found for the more hydrophobic surfaces, that is, gold, titanium, PMMA (polymethy methacrylate), and PTFE (polytetrafluoroethylene), (ii) on hydrophilic surfaces, adhesion is mainly influenced by the electrostatic forces between protein and surface, and (iii) on the very hydrophobic PTFE surface, the special interface structure between PTFE and water plays an important role which governs BSA adhesion [178]. Antithrombogenic biomaterials have been of great interest in the development of artificial organs and devices. Weng et al. [179] used titanium oxide coatings as the basis for covalent immobilization of a BSA layer by a photochemical method. It was reported that (i) platelet experiments of both qualitative and quantitative analysis showed that BSA immobilized surface was effective to inhibit platelet adhesion *in vitro* and (ii) the *in vivo* study also confirmed better hemocompatibility of the BSA immobilized surface after 90 days implantation [179].

The adsorption of BSA on to Ti powder has been studied as a function of protein concentration and pH, and in the presence of calcium and phosphate ions. It was reported that (i) the maximum adsorption at pH 6.8 is 1.13 ± 0.21 mg/m^2, (ii) for the pH dependence of adsorption, the amount adsorbed increases with decreasing pH (at pH 5.15 the maximum adsorption was 1.31 ± 0.2 mg/m^2), indicating that hydration effects are important, and (iii) adsorption increases and decreases in the presence of calcium (at pH 6.8 the maximum adsorption was 1.73 ± 0.23 mg/m^2) and phosphate (where at pH 6.8 the maximum adsorption was 0.64 ± 0.14 mg/m^2) ions, indicating that electrostatic effects are important [180].

The *in vitro* study was conducted to investigate the adsorption of albumin and fibronectin on titanium surfaces, and the effect of pre-adsorbed BSA and bovine fibronectin on osteoblast attachment. Maximum adsorption of BSA and fibronectin on Ti surfaces was observed after the incubation for 180 min. In the presence of pre-adsorbed proteins, osteoblast attachment on Ti surfaces was observed to be enhanced compared to control Ti surfaces. However, cell attachment was affected by the types of protein adsorbed. Pre-adsorbed albumin was observed to have no significant effect on the amount of osteoblast cells attached. In comparison to the control Ti surface and those pre-adsorbed with albumin, the Ti surfaces pre-adsorbed with fibronectin for 15 minutes were observed to significantly increase osteoblast cell attachment, whereas the Ti surfaces preadsorbed with fibronectin for 180 min did not affect cell attachment. In addition, cell morphology of the attached cells on protein preadsorbed Ti surfaces was not affected by the type of protein used. Based on these findings, it was concluded that (i) the concentration of fibronectin adsorbed on Ti surfaces was higher compared to albumin, and (ii) the concentration of fibronectin on Ti surfaces plays a role in governing cell attachment [170].

Webster et al. [181] claimed that $CaTiO_3$ is a strong candidate to form at the interface between hydroxylapatite (HA) and titanium implants during many coating procedures. The ability of bone-forming cells (osteoblasts) to adhere on titanium coated with HA, resulting in the formation of $CaTiO_3$, was investigated. For the formation of $CaTiO_3$, titanium was coated on HA disks and annealed either under air or a $N_2 + H_2$ environment. Results from cytocompatibility tests revealed increased osteoblast adhesion on materials that contained $CaTiO_3$ compared to both pure HA and uncoated titanium. The greatest osteoblast adhesion was observed on titanium-coated HA annealed under air conditions. Because adhesion is a crucial prerequisite to the subsequent functions of osteoblasts (such as the deposition of calcium-containing minerals), it was suggested that orthopedic coatings that form $CaTiO_3$ could increase osseointegration with juxtaposed bone needed to enhance implant efficacy and longevity [181].

Extensive studies on the microstructure, chemical composition, and wettability of thermally and chemically modified Ti–6Al–4V alloy disks were done and correlated with the degree of radiolabeled fibronectin-alloy surface adsorption and subsequent adhesion of osteoblast-like cells [182]. Heating, either in pure oxygen or atmosphere (atm), resulted in an enrichment of Al and V within the surface oxide formed on Ti–6Al–4V [183]. As for the surface contact angle (or wettability), it was reported that (i) pre-heating (oxygen/atm) or hydrogen peroxide treatment brought a thicker oxide layer with more hydrophilicity when compared with passivated controls, but (ii) post-treatment with butanol resulted in less hydrophilic surfaces than those by heating or hydrogen peroxide treatment. It was therefore indicated that (i) an increase in the absolute content of Al or V (heat), or both, or in the Al/V ratio (with little change in hydrophilicity; heat+butanol), or both, is correlated with an increase in the fibronectin-promoted adhesion of an osteoblast-like cell line, and (ii) the thermal treatment-induced enhancement of cell adhesion in the presence of the protein is due to its increased biological activity, rather than a mass effect alone, which appear to be associated with changes in chemical composition of the metallic surface [183].

Nanophase materials are unique materials that simulate dimensions of constituent components of bone since they possess particle or grain sizes of less than 100 nm [180], and their interactions with osteoblasts, compared to conventional metals, were *in vitro* studied to synthesize, characterize, and evaluate osteoblast adhesion on nanophase metals (specifically, Ti, Ti–6Al–4V, and Co–Cr–Mo alloys), which are widely used in orthopedic applications. It was found that (i) the osteoblast adhesion on nanophase was more than that on conventional metals, and (ii) nanometal surfaces possessed similar chemistry, and only altered in degree of nanometer surface roughness when compared to their respective conventional counterparts [184].

Improving the biological performance of engineered implants interfacing tissues is a critical issue in implantology and its related science and engineering. Micromotion at the soft tissue–implant interface has been shown to sustain an inflammatory response. To eliminate micromotion, it is desirable to promote cellular and extracellular matrix adhesion to the implant surface. Jain et al. [185] modified titanium surfaces topographically or chemically to affect cellular adhesion and to influence cellular interactions and function, and conducted an *in vitro* study to compare the independent effects of surface chemistry and topography on fibroblast-test specimen proximity. Titanium was sputter-coated in stepwise, increasing thicknesses (20–350 nm) onto a series of either smooth or microtextured polyethylene terephthalate (PET), resulting in a stepwise change from a PET surface to a Ti surface—as gradually functioning material. It was found that (i) fibroblast proximity to the coverslip surface increases as the Ti thickness increases on either smooth or textured test specimens, and (ii) fibroblasts were firmly attached to the ridge tops on the coated textured test specimens. Therefore, fibroblast apposition is strongly enhanced by microtextured surfaces and Ti rather than smooth surfaces and polyethylene terephthalate [185].

Osteoblast adhesion on the implant material surface is essential for the success of any implant in which osseointegration is required. Surface properties of implant material have a critical role in the cell adhesion progress. Zhang et al. [186] employed the microarc oxidizing and hydrothermally synthesizing methods to modify the TiO_2 layer on the titanium surface, on which the mouse osteoblastic cell line (MC3T3-E1) was seeded to evaluate their effect on cell behavior. The surface structure of microarc oxidized samples exhibited micropores with a diameter of 1–3 μm, whereas the micro-arc oxidation/hydrothermal synthesized samples showed additional multiple crystalline microparticles on the microporous surface. Both treated surfaces possessed higher energy than that of untreated titanium. It was concluded that the microarc oxidation and micro-arc oxidation/hydrothermal synthesization methods change the surface energy of the TiO_2 layer on the titanium surface, indicating that this may have an influence on the initial cell attachment [186].

Surface characteristics play a vital role in determining the biocompatibility of materials used as bone implants. It is well documented that calcium ion implantation of titanium enhances osteointegration and bone formation *in vivo*. In order to measure the precise effects of ion implantation of titanium on bone cells *in vitro*, alveolar bone cells were seeded on the surface of polished titanium disks implanted with calcium, potassium, and argon ions. Using radioisotopically tagged bone cells, it was found that (i) although the calcium ion implanted surface reduced cell adhesion, it nevertheless significantly enhanced cell spreading and subsequent cell growth, but (ii) in contrast, few differences in bone cell behavior were observed between the potassium- and argon-implanted titanium and the control nonimplanted titanium disks. Based on these findings, it was suggested that the calcium-implanted surface may significantly affect the biocompatibility of titanium implants by enhancing bone cell growth; it was therefore concluded that surface modification by ion implantation could thus prove to be a valuable tool for improving the clinical efficacy of titanium for bone repair and regeneration *in vivo* [187]. Bio-activation of the titanium surface by sodium plasma immersion ion implantation and deposition (PI^3&D) was compared to that of the untreated, Na beam-line implanted and NaOH-treated titanium samples [188]. It was found that (i) from a morphological point of view, cell adherence on the NaOH-treated titanium is the best, (ii) on the other hand, the cell activity and protein production were higher on the non-bioactive surfaces, and (iii) the active surfaces support an osteogenic differentiation of the bone marrow cells at the expense of lower proliferation, due to the high alkaline phosphatase activity per cell [188]. Muhonen et al. [189] investigated the responses of mature osteoclasts cultured on austenite and martensite phases of NiTi shape memory implant material, using the sensitivity of osteoclasts to the underlying substrate and actin ring formation as an indicator of the adequacy of the implant surface. It was reported that osteoclasts tolerated well the austenite phase of NiTi, but the chemically identical martensitic NiTi was not as well tolerated by osteoclasts (e.g., indicated by diminished actin ring formation), concluding that certain physical properties specific to the martensitic NiTi have an adverse effect onosteoclast survival in this NiTi phase [189].

Living bone cells are responsive to mechanical loading. Consequently, numerous *in vitro* models have been developed to examine the application of loading to cells. However, not all systems are suitable for the fibrous and porous three-dimensional materials, which are preferable for tissue repair purposes, or for the production of tissue engineering scaffolds. For three-dimensional applications, mechanical loading of cells with either fluid flow systems or hydrodynamic pressure systems has to be considered. The response of osteoblast-like cells to hydrodynamic compression, while growing in a three-dimensional titanium fiber mesh scaffolding material, was evaluated by Walboomers et al. [190]. Bone marrow cells were obtained from the femora of young (12-day-old) or old (1-year-old) rats, and precultured in the presence of dexamethasone and β-glycerophosphate to achieve an osteoblast-like phenotype. Subsequently, cells were seeded onto the titanium mesh scaffolds and subjected to hydrodynamic pressure, alternating from 0.3 to 5.0 MPa at 1 Hz, at 15-minute intervals for a total of 60 min per day for up to 3 days. After pressurization, cell viability was checked. Afterward, DNA levels, alkaline phosphatase (ALP) activity, and extracellular calcium content were measured. Finally, all specimens were observed with SEM. Cell viability studies indicated that (i) the applied pressure was not harmful to the cells, and (ii) the cells were able to detect the compression forces [190].

Improved methods to increase surface hardness of metallic biomedical implants are being developed in an effort to minimize the formation of wear debris particles that cause local pain and inflammation. However, for many implant surface treatments, there is a risk of film delamination due to the mismatch of mechanical properties between the hard surface and the softer underlying metal. Hence, Clem et al. [191] developed a new surface modification of titanium alloy (Ti–6Al–4V), using microwave plasma chemical vapor deposition to induce titanium nitride (TiN) formation by nitrogen diffusion. The result is a gradual transition from a TiN surface to the bulk titanium alloy, without a sharp interface that could otherwise lead to delamination. The vitronectin adsorption as well as the adhesion and spreading of human mesenchymal stem cells to plasma-nitrided titanium were evaluated, and they were equivalent to that of Ti–6Al–4V, while hardness is improved 3- to 4-fold. These *in vitro* results suggested that the plasma nitriding technique has the potential to reduce wear, and the resulting debris particle release, of biomedical implants without compromising osseointegration, thus minimizing the possibility of the implant loosening over time [191].

As we have seen above, the biological events occurring at the bone–implant interface are influenced by the topography, chemistry, and wettability of the implant surface. Advincula et al. [192] introduced other method to achieve the aforementioned specific aim. The surface properties of titanium alloy prepared by either surface sol–gel processing (SSP), or by passivation with nitric acid, were investigated. The bioreactivity of the substrates was assessed by evaluating MC3T3-E1 osteoblastic cell adhesion, as well as by *in vitro* formation of a mineralized matrix. It was found that (i) surface analysis of sol–gel-derived oxide on Ti–6Al–4V substrates showed a predominantly TiO_2 composition with abundant hydroxyl groups, (ii) the surface was highly wettable, rougher, and more porous compared to that of the passivated substrate, and (iii) significantly more cells adhered to the sol–gel-coated surface as compared with passivated surfaces after 1 and 24 hours following cell seeding, and a markedly greater number of mineralized nodules were observed on sol–gel coatings [192].

The effectiveness of ultraviolet (UV)/ozone irradiation in the cleaning procedure for titanium in dental implants was studied, on particularly the wettability and initial MTS (cell proliferation) assay cell adhesion of polished titanium. It was reported that (i) contact angles of the UV/ozone irradiation group were significantly smaller than those of the autoclave sterilization group, but were not influenced by the irradiation time and (ii) there was no significant difference in initial cell adhesion between the UV/ozone irradiation group and the autoclave sterilization group, suggesting that the UV/ozone irradiation might be useful in the cleaning of titanium surfaces, although further clarification concerning cellular physiology is required [193].

3.5.3. Cell Proliferation and Differentiation

Studies of blood plasma protein interactions with Ti oxides is one possible way to understand blood interactions and tissue integration better, since blood is the first medium encountered after the surgical procedure, and thus governs the subsequent cell attachment and wound healing. Adsorption of albumin and fibrinogen from human blood plasma onto CpTi surfaces with varying oxide properties was studied with an enzyme-liked immunosorbent assay. The intrinsic activation of blood coagulation (contact activation) was studied *in vitro* using a kallinkrein-sensitive substrate. It was reported that (i) low fibrinogen and high albumin adsorption was observed for all titanium samples, except for the radio frequency plasma-treated and water-incubated samples, which adsorbed significantly lower amounts of both, and (ii) smooth samples with a surface roughness with less than 1 nm showed some correlation between surface wettability and adsorption of fibrinogen and albumin, whereas rough surfaces (> 5 nm) did not [194]. The role of implant surface topography in cell attachment has been reviewed extensively [120,195]. Rough or textured porous surfaces promote cell attachment [196,197]. Surface roughness and composition have been considered the most important parameter for altering cell activity. There are observations that cell responses, such as adhesion, morphologym, and collagen synthesis differed on the two grades of CpTi. Between 4 and 24 h, the rate of cell attachment to CpTi (grade I) differed significantly, compared to cell attachment to CpTi (grade IV). At 24 hours, the percentage of collagen synthesized was significantly more on Grade 1 than on Grade 4. Alkaline phosphatase activity was similar on all substrates. The calcium content was significantly higher on Grade 1 than on 4 as well as on glass at 24 hours and at 4 weeks. Based on these observations, it was concluded that commonly used CpTi induced differential morphologic and phenotypic changes in human osteoblast-like cells depending on the material grade [198].

Khakbaznejad et al. [199] investigated on osteogenic cells from newborn rat calvariae which were cultured on titanium surfaces, on which cell orientation could be manipulated, to measure the orientation angles of cells. Substrata included smooth surfaces and smooth regions (gaps) flanked by grooves of 47-μm pitch and 3, 10, or 30 μm depth to create micromachined surfaces. There were several interesting findings reported. Grooves proved effective in orienting cells, but their orienting ability decreased above the ridge level. Cells on the smooth surface showed no preferred orientation. Cells in the gaps became oriented as a result of cell–cell interactions with the cells on the flanking grooves. Cells in the grooves produced oriented collagen fibers, but in the gaps, fibers could be parallel, perpendicular, or diagonal to the grooves. Collagen fibers on the smooth surfaces formed arrays of parallel fibers in a crisscross pattern. In long-term cultures, bone-like nodules were formed, but mostly above the ridge level. Based on these findings, it was reported that grooved surfaces can influence cell orientation both in cell populations above the cells in contact with the grooves and in cell populations adjacent to the grooves [199].

To investigate the roles of composition and characteristics of titanium surface oxides in cellular behavior of osteoblasts, the surface oxides of titanium were modified in composition and topography by anodic oxidation in two kinds of electrolytes: 0.2 M H_3PO_4, and 0.03 M calcium glycerophosphate + 0.15 M calcium acetate. It was found that (i) calcium and phosphorous ions are incorporated into the anodized surfaces in the form of phosphate and CaP, (ii) the geometry of the micropores in the anodized surfaces varied with diameters up to 0.5 μm in 0.2 M H_3PO_4 and to 2 μm in 0.03 M Ca-GP and 0.15 M CA, depending on voltages and electrolyte, and (iii) contact angles of all the anodic oxides were in the range of 60° to 90°, indicating a relatively hydrophobicity. As for cell culture studies, the absence of cytotoxicity and an increase of osteoblast adhesion and proliferation by the anodic oxides were found, and cells on the surfaces with micropores showed an irregular, polygonal growth, and more lamellipodia [200].

Saldaña et al. [201] evaluated the biocompatibility of the oxidized (700 °C × 1 hour and 500 °C × 1 hour) surfaces of Ti–6Al–4V by assessing cell adhesion, proliferation, and differentiation of primary cultures of human osteoblastic cells. Compared with the polished alloy, both thermal treatments increased osteoblast adhesion measured as cell attachment, β1 integrin, and FAK-Y397 expression, as well as cytoskeletal reorganization. It was found that (i) when compared with treatment at 500 °C, thermal oxidation at 700 °C enhanced cell adhesion, (ii) treatment at 700 °C transiently impaired cell proliferation and viability, which were not altered in alloys oxidized at 500 °C, (iii) several markers of osteoblastic differentiation such as procollagen I peptide, alkaline phosphatase, osteocalcin, and mineralized nodule formation were found either unaffected or differentially increased by alloys treated either at 500 °C or 700 °C, and (iv) thermal oxidation at 700 °C also increased osteoprotegerin secretion. It was therefore concluded that thermal oxidation treatments at 500 °C or 700 °C for 1 hour improve the *in vitro* biocompatibility of Ti–6Al–4V [201].

Osteoblast response to Ti implants depends not only on the chemistry of the implant but also on the physical properties of the implant surface, such as microtopography and roughness, as has been reviewed in the above. Early changes in cell morphology and gene expression during the early phase of osteoblast interaction with Ti–6Al–4V surfaces of two different roughnesses were examined. MG63 osteoblast-like cells were cultured for 2, 6, 24, and 72 hours on smooth (R_a = 0.18 μm) and rough (R_a = 2.95 μm) Ti–6Al–4V surfaces. Changes in gene expression for extracellular signal-regulated kinase 2 (Erk2), type I collagen, phospholipase C-γ2 (Plc-γ2), and β-actin were measured by Reverse Transcription Polymerase Chain Reaction (RT-PCR) after 6 and 24 hours in culture. It was found that the cell number was significantly higher on the smooth surface. Of the genes examined, only Erk2 and β-actin showed a change in expression with surface roughness. Both genes were upregulated on the rough surface at 6 hours. Hence, it was indicated that Ti–6Al–4V surface roughness affects osteoblast proliferation, morphology, and gene expression, and that these effects can be measured after periods as short as 2–6 hours [202].

Stainless steel, CpTi, and Ti–6Al–7Nb are frequently used metals in orthopedic internal fracture fixation. Particularly, clinilca uses of Ti–6Al–7Nb are becoming more popular due to its excellent wear resistance. The *in vitro* soft tissue compatibility of Ti–6Al–7Nb in comparison to stainless steel and CpTi, using a human fibroblast model, was conducted by Meredith et al. [203]. It was found that (i) cell morphology and growth rate were similar for stainless steel, electro-polished CpTi, and Ti–6Al–7Nb, with cells well spread-out and forming a confluent monolayer after 10 days, (ii) cell growth on standard CpTi was similar to the electropolished samples; however, they showed a less spread-out morphology, with more filopodia and surface ruffling present, and (iii) the endocytosis of β-phase particles originating from the standard Ti–6Al–7Nb surface was noted [203].

Polished Ti disks were implanted with high (1×10^{17} ions/cm^2), medium (1×10^{16} ions/cm^2), and low (1×10^{15} ions/cm^2) doses of Ca ions at 40 keV to promote an enhanced osseointegration. The effects of different levels of Ca implantation on morphology, attachment, and spreading of MG-63 cells seeded on the surface of the control (nonimplanted) Ti and Ca-Ti disks were examined. The effects of pre-immersion of the Ca (high)-Ti in tissue culture medium on cell attachment were measured and correlated with specific chemical changes at the Ti surface. It was reported that (i) although cell adhesion on high-dosed Ca–Ti was initially reduced, it nevertheless was not only restored, but substantially increased with progressing culture times, (ii) a significantly enhanced cell spreading, formation of focal adhesion plaques, and expression of integrins were measured on this particular surface, (iii) in contrast, no marked differences were observed in cell behavior on low- and medium-dosed Ca-Ti, (iv) pre-immersion studies indicated that the decrease in cell attachment to high-dosed Ca–Ti at early time periods may be linked to the presence of Ca- and P-rich particles on the surface, and (v) the absence of these particles at 24 hours was consistent with a significant increase in cell attachment [204].

A Ca-deficient carbonate apatite coating on titanium was prepared by pre-calcifying titanium in a saturated $Ca(OH)_2$ solution, and then immersing in a supersaturated CaP solution by Feng et al. [205]. The interaction of the protein with the apatite coating on Ti was investigated by SME with X-ray energy dispersion spectroscopy, XPS, X-ray diffraction, and FTIR. During immersion of the coating in the BSA solution, it was observed that calcium and phosphate ions dissolved and re-precipitated, resulting in the formation of the coating contamination BSA from the surface to subsurface layers. The adsorption modified the structure and morphology of the apatite and changed the protein configuration. It was also found that the protein chemically adsorbed onto surfaces containing calcium or phosphorous, showing that both Ca and P on the apatite coating were the protein binding sites [205].

Recently, Tetè et al. [206], using SEM and profilometric analysis, investigated the *in vivo* collagen fiber behavior around two different dental implant necks (machined titanium and ZrO_2 implants) in mandibular bone of adult pigs. It was concluded that (i) collagen fiber was similar, regardless of implant material, demonstrating a predominantly parallel or parallel-oblique pattern, and (ii) ZrO_2, which is used as a transgingival collar on some implants, showed connective tissue adhesion that was similar to that seen on the machined titanium surface, but demonstrated limited plaque formation and may provide better esthetics [206]. The same test combination of titanium and ZrO_2 was studied on the tendency to adhesion and colonization of two periodontal pathogens on both hard surfaces and soft tissues *in vivo* [207]. The study was designed as a prospective stratified randomized controlled clinical trial. Patients were scheduled to receive two implants with different types of abutments in the posterior mandible. Three months after implant placement, titanium and zirconium abutments were connected. Five weeks after abutment connections, the abutments were removed, probing depth measurements were recorded, and gingival biopsy samples were obtained. Abutments and biopsy specimens were analyzed. It was mentioned that zirconium abutments showed lower surface free energy than titanium abutments. It was further reported that zirconium oxide surfaces have comparable properties to titanium alloy surfaces in their tendency to adhesion and clononization of two periodontal pathogens on both had surfaces and in soft tissues [207].

Cell adhesion is a fundamental process that controls cell proliferation, migration, and differentiation and is crucial for biomaterial-tissue integration. Osteoblast attachment on the surfaces of implant materials is, therefore, essential for the proper function of any implant in which osteointegration is required. Faghihi et al. [208] investigated the effects of atomic order of specific crystallographic orientation of substrates on cell behavior. It was reported that (i) surface recognition by cell is influenced by the atomic structure of the surface leading to cell-type-specific adhesion, (ii) the degree of pre-osteoblast attachment is significantly higher on the Ti-(1 1 2 0), whereas the fibroblast adhesion is increased on the Ti-(1 0 1 0), suggesting that the role of the crystal structure in regulating and improving cell–substrate interactions relevant for the optimal function of bone implant materials [208]. Initial attachment of human oral keratinocytes cultured on mirror-surfaced CpTi and yttria-stabilzie tetragonal polycrystalline ZrO_2 was investigated [209] and concluded that ZrO_2 has a potential to form epithelial attachment like CpTi.

The cell attachment and gene expression of MC3T3-E1 cells on fibromectin-immobilized titanium was investigated and found that the immobilization of fibronectin on tresylated titanium promoted early matrix mineralization and bone formation [210]. The initial bone cell response to yttria-stabilized ZrO_2/alumina composite ceramics was studied and compared to CpTi, and found that the ZrO_2–alumina composite ceramics showed at least equivalent or slightly better biological responses of osteoblast-like cells than CpTi during a short-time cell culture period [211]. The influence of the porous Ti structure on the osteogenic cell behavior was investigated [212]. The porous Ti has the following characteristics: pore size between 50 and 400 μm, a porosity of 60%. Osteogenic cells obtained from the human alveolar bone were cultured until subconfluence and subcultured on solid Ti (control) and porous Ti for periods of up to 17 days. It was found that the amount of mineralized matrix was greater on porous Ti compared with the solid one, demonstrating that the porous Ti is an appropriate substrate for osteogenic cell adhesion, proliferation, and production of a mineralized matrix. Shapira et al. [213] studied the behavior of human osteoblast-like cells cultured on Ti–6Al–4V and Ti–6Al–7Nb disks with a rough or a machined surface. It was reported that (i) Ti–6Al–7Nb showed the highest alkaline phosphatase activity, the lowest activity was observed on the machined Ti–6Al–4V surface, and (ii) the highest level of osteocalcin was found in the cells cultured on rough Ti–6Al–7Nb, also higher levels of transforming growth factor were noted for cells cultured on the rough Ti–6Al–7Nb disks, suggesting that the Nb-containing alloy supports more rapid maturation of the osteoblast [213].

Titanium implant surfaces with rough microtopography exhibit increased pullout strength *in vivo*, suggesting that the bone-to-implant contact (BIC) was enhanced. This is supported by *in vitro* studies showing that on surfaces with rough microtopographies, osteoblasts secrete factors that enhance osteoblast differentiation, while decreasing osteoclast formation and activity [214]. A novel approach to electrochemical processing of a HA coating was explored by Hu et al. [215]. Vinyl acetate was added in the electrolytes of calcium and phosphorous in order to improve the adhesion between HA coating and titanium substrate. X-ray powder diffractometer (XRD) spectra indicated that the vinyl acetate did not interfere with the deposition of HA on the surface of titanium cathodes. Results obtained from XPS and SEM revealed that (i) both vinyl acetate and HA were deposited on the titanium cathodes, (ii) the vinyl acetate changed the HA crystalline morphology in the deposition layer, and (iii) the shape and growth direction of the HA crystals in the coating with vinyl acetate differed from those of HA deposition alone. It was moreover mentioned that a preliminary study of the bioactivity showed that osteoblastic cells exhibited higher cell proliferation potential on the HA/vinyl acetate coating than on that of pure HA [215].

Vehof et al. [216] prepared the osteogenic activity of CaP-coated and noncoated porous titanium (Ti) fiber mesh loaded with cultured syngeneic osteogenic cells after prolonged *in situ* culturing to compare in a syngeneic rat ectopic assay model. RBM cells were loaded onto the CaP-coated and noncoated Ti scaffolds using either a droplet or a suspension loading method. After loading, the RBM cells were cultured for 8 days *in vitro*. Thereafter, implants were subcutaneously placed in 39 syngeneic rats. The rats were euthanized and the implants retrieved at 2, 4, and 8 weeks postoperatively. Further, in the 8-week group, fluorochrome bone markers were injected at 2, 4, and 6 weeks. It was reported that (i) histological analysis demonstrated that only the CaP-coated meshes supported bone formation, (ii) the amount of newly formed bone varied, between single and multiple spheres, filling a significant part of the mesh porosity, (iii) in the newly formed bone, osteocytes embedded in a mineralized matrix could be clearly observed, but (iv) on the other hand, in the noncoated titanium implants, abundant deposition of calcium-containing material was seen. In CaP-coated implants, the accumulation sequence of the fluorochrome markers showed that bone formation started on the mesh fibers. It was concluded that the combination of a thin CaP coating, Ti-mesh, and RBM cells can generate ectopic bone formation after prolonged *in vitro* culturing [216].

Titanium (Ti) and its alloys continue to serve as successful implant materials for skeletal repair because of their physical properties and biocompatibility. The influence of organoapatite (which is an organic compound in which apatite crystals have been nucleated and grown on a polymer), grown directly onto an L-shaped Ti mesh, on preosteoblastic cellular colonization was investigated. Unseeded mesh samples were placed on subconfluent layers of MC3T3-E1 murine calvaria cells and cultured for up to 2 weeks. It was found that (i) cells demonstrated accelerated colonization of the three-dimensional organoapatite-Ti mesh substrates over bare Ti controls, (ii) cells also showed significantly increased proliferation on the organoapatite-Ti mesh over bare Ti controls, and (iii) cellular differentiation, measured by alkaline phosphatase and osteocalcin expression, was observed at late stages of the experiment with no notable differences between the organoapatite-Ti mesh and bare Ti controls, suggesting that organoapatite grown onto porous Ti substrates is capable of inducing accelerated colonization of unseeded implant structures by osteogenic cells [217].

Rodriguez et al. [218] modified titanium surfaces by anodization in a mixed electrolyte of calcium glycerophosphate and calcium acetate. Hydrothermal treatments were performed on two of the anodized groups for either 2 or 4 hours. *In vitro* osteoblast response to anodized oxide and the hydrothermal treated oxide after anodization was evaluated. It was found that (i) calcium and phosphorus ions were deposited on the Ti oxide during anodization, (ii) anodized surfaces following a 4-hour hydrothermal treatment were observed to promote the growth of apatite-like crystals, as compared with anodized surfaces after a 2-hour hydrothermal treatment, (iii) cellular function and onset of mineralization, as indicated by protein production and osteocalcin production, respectively, were also observed as enhanced on hydrothermal-treated surfaces. It was thus concluded that CaP and apatite-like crystals could be deposited on Ti surfaces using anodization and a combination of anodization and hydrothermal treatment, and the phenotypic expression of an osteoblast was enhanced by the presence of CaP or apatite-like crystals on anodized or hydrothermally treated Ti surfaces [218].

The topographic effects of HA and titanium (Ti) surfaces having identical micropatterns were determined as to whether there was a synergistic interaction between surface chemistry and surface topography. Surface microgrooves with six different groove widths (4, 8, 16, 24, 30, and 38 μm) and three different groove depths (2, 4, and 10 μm) were made on single crystalline silicon wafers using microfabrication techniques. Ti and HA thin films were coated on the microgrooves by radio-frequency magnetron sputtering, followed by seeding human osteoblast-like cells and culturing on the microgrooved surfaces for up to 7 days. It was reported that (i) contact guidance and cell shape changes were observed on the HA and Ti microgrooves, and (ii) no difference in the orientation angle between HA and Ti microgrooves was found, suggesting that surface chemistry was not a significant influence on cell guidance [219].

The homogeneous deposition of Ca–P can be coated on porous implants by immersion in the simulated physiologic solution. In addition, various Ca–P phases, such as octacalcium phosphate or bone-like carbonated apatite, can be applied. Barrère et al. [220] conducted experiments (i) to investigate the osteoinduction of octacalcium phosphate-coated and noncoated porous tantalum cylinders, and of dense titanium alloy cylinders (5 mm in diameter and 10 mm in length) in the back muscle of goats at 12 and 24 weeks, and (ii) to compare the osteogenic potentials of bone-like carbonated apatite-coated, octacalcium phosphate coated, and bare porous tantalum cylinders in a gap of 1 mm created in the femoral condyle of a goat at 12 weeks. It was found that (i) in the goat muscle, after 12 weeks, the octacalium phosphate-coated porous cylinder had induced ectopic bone, as well as bone within the cavity of the octacalcium phosphate-coated dense titanium cylinder, (ii) in the femoral condyle, bone did not fill the gap in any of the porous implants, but (iii) in contrast with the two other groups, octacalcium phosphate-coated porous cylinders exhibited bone formation in the center of the implant [220].

Studies examining osteoblast response to controlled surface chemistries indicate that hydrophilic surfaces are osteogenic. The TiO_2 surfaces, however, produced until now exhibit low surface energy because of adsorbed hydrocarbons and carbonates from the ambient atmosphere, or roughness induced hydrophobicity. Zhao et al. [221] used hydroxylated/hydrated Ti surfaces in order to retain high surface energy of TiO_2. It was reported that (i) osteoblasts grown on this modified surface exhibited a more differentiated phenotype, characterized by increased alkaline phosphatase activity and osteocalcin, and generated an osteogenic microenvironment through higher production of PGE2 and TGF-β1, and (ii) 1α,25(OH)2D3 increased these effects in a manner that was synergistic with high surface energy, suggesting that increased bone formation observed on modified Ti surfaces *in vivo* was due in part to stimulatory effects of high surface energy on osteoblasts [221].

To further understanding the biological mechanisms underlying bone-titanium integration and biomechanical properties of the integrated bone, Takeuchi et al. [222] cultured RBM-derived osteoblastic cells on either the machined titanium disk or acid-etched titanium disk. It was found that (i) the modulus of elasticity (MOE) of the mineralized tissue was also three times greater on the acid-etched surface than on the machined surface, and (ii) after 28 days of culture, the mineralized nodule area was significantly lower on the acid-etched surface than on the machined surface, while total calcium deposition did not differ between the two surfaces, indicating denser mineral deposition on the acid-etched surface. Scanning electron microscopic images revealed that tissue cultured on the acid-etched titanium exhibited plate-like, compact surface morphology, while the tissue on the machined titanium appeared porous and was covered by fibrous and punctate structures. It was therefore concluded that culturing osteoblasts on rougher titanium surfaces enhances the hardness and elastic modulus of the mineralized tissue associated with the condensed mineralization, accelerated collagen synthesis, and upregulated expression of selected bone-related genes [222]. An electrochemical anodization treatment was used to produce a network oxide layer on the Ti surface. Human bone marrow mesenchymal stem cells were made to express green fluorescent protein. The green fluorescent protein signal was measured *in situ* to assess cell growth on Ti surfaces. It was found that the formation of the TiO_2 nano-network on the Ti surfaces can increase the human bone marrow mesenchynal stem cell growth *in vitro* and *in vivo* [223].

3.5.4. Bone Ingrowth

The oral epithelium and connective tissue were able to form a peri-implant epithelium similar in appearance to that around natural teeth [224]. In studies of peri-implant mucosa conducted in nine-month old beagle dogs, placement of one-stage and two-stage implants demonstrated that the mucosal barrier that formed had a definite epithelial, and the connective tissue component was similar in dimension in both the one-stage and two-stage implants [225]. It was proposed that a certain minimum width of the peri-implant mucosa was required, and that bone resorption would occur if the soft tissue dimension was not satisfied, being similar to the phenomenon of the biologic width that occurs in natural human dentition [226]. The connective tissue lateral to the junctional epithelium comprises the dense collagenous tissue with few vascular structures and scattered inflammatory cells. The "zone of connective tissue integration" between the bone crest and the junctional epithelium is characterized as a collagen rich and cell poor scar-like connective tissue. There was a narrow zone close to the implant that had mainly collagen fibers running parallel to the surface of the implant and attaching to the periosteum of the bone [225]. Using light microscopy, it was noted that the inner peri-implant epithelium ended 1–2 mm from the bone [227]. Using transmission electron microscopic studies, it was noted that the outermost epithelial cells close to the implant exhibited condensed structures resembling hemidesmosomes [228]. Good adhesion between the implant surface and the soft tissue is extremely important to assure the survival of dental implants [229]. Percuaneous and permucosla implants require a strong support from the underlying connective tissue if an epithelial downgrowth and subsequent failure are to be avoided [230]. Systematic and continuous monitoring of peri-implant tissues during maintenance care is recommended for the early diagnosis of peri-implant disease [231]. The tissue reaction has been shown to vary with micrometer range changes in the substratum [232]. Studies have shown that changes in the range of 130 nm are adequate to produce changes in contact guidance of the cells [223]. Surface roughness may have had a significant effect on the cell density and proliferation. Some studies concluded that surface microtexture influences the attachment and growth of human gingival fibroblasts [234,235], while others suggested that the surface roughness does not influence soft tissue attachment [236]. Significantly greater numbers of cells were attached to rougher milled and sintered surfaces than to polished surfaces, possibly indicating higher proliferation capacity [237].

The distribution of released metal in the surrounding tissue is important information to estimate the relation between the dissolution content and tissue response. However, the distributions of released metal have not been studied well because of the difficulty in detecting the very low concentration of rarely contained metal elements in the surrounding tissue. Soft tissues implanted with Cu, Ni, Fe, Ag, Ti, NiTi, 304 (18Cr–8Ni) and 316 (18Cr–8Ni–2Mo) stainless steel wires were investigated with XSAM (X-ray scanning analytical microscope) and compared with histological observation. The relationship between the distribution metal elements and the tissue response was evaluated. Severe damage was observed around Ni and Cu implants, while fibrous connective tissue was formed around the Fe implant. The dissolved concentration was approximately 10–20 mM for Ni and Cu and was considered to be on the order of ten times higher in Fe. It was concluded that (i) the toxicity at the same concentration followed the sequence (from greater toxicity to least): Ni > Cu > Fe, and (ii) for Ag, Ti, NiTi, 304 and 316 stainless steel implants, significant dissolution and severe tissue damage were not observed [238].

Sundgren et al. [239] used Auger electron spectroscopy to study the interface between human tissue and implants of Ti and stainless steel. Both the thickness and the nature of the oxide layers on the implant have been found to change during the time of implantation. The stainless steel implants have a surface oxide about 50 Å thick prior to implantation. The metal atoms in the oxide are mainly Cr, with which Cr_2O_3 may be formed. For implants located in cortical bone, the thickness of the interfacial oxide layer remains unaffected, while it increases by a factor of 3–4 on samples located in bone marrow. In both these cases, Ca and P are incorporated in the oxides. Implants located in soft tissue have an interfacial oxide with a thickness of about one and a half times that of an unimplanted sample. On these samples, C and P are not incorporated in the oxide layer. Also, for Ti an increase in oxide thickness and an incorporation of Ca and P are found. In the cases with Ti implants, it is also demonstrated that the oxidation process occurs over a long period of time, up to several years. For the elements incorporated in these interfacial oxide layers on both stainless steel and Ti implants, it is found that P is strongly bound to oxygen, suggesting the presence of phosphate groups in the oxide. Other species that can oxidize the implants are H_2O_2 and free radicals, such as O_2^- or OH^-. Such species are normally produced during the inflammatory reactions [239].

The immuno-inflammatory responses to stainless steel (21 implants in 20 patients) and Ti plates (22 implants in 20 patients) used in the treatment of long bone fractures were studied. All fractures healed without complications. It was reported that (i) in the soft tissue adjacent to the surface of the implants, a dark discoloration of the tissue was visible in 18 out of 21 stainless steel implants and 20 out of 22 Ti plates, and (ii) tissue specimens of all patients contained positive staining for macrophages (CD68-positive cells), demonstrating clearly the presence of a marked inflammation and tissue reaction in the soft tissue covering stainless steel and Ti plates which were used for internal fixation of bones, independently from the material [240].

Successful clinical performance of machine/turned CpTi implants has resulted in a widespread usage of them. However, in bone of poor quality and quantity, the results have not always been so good, motivating the development of "novel types of osseointegrated implants." The development of Ti implants has depended on new surface processing technologies. Recently developed clinical oral implants have been focused on topographical changes of implant surfaces, rather than alterations of chemical properties [241–245]. These attempts may have been based on the concept that mechanical interlocking between tissue and implant materials relies on surface irregularities in the nanometer to micrometer level. Recently, published *in vivo* investigations have shown significantly improved bone tissue reactions by modification of the surface oxide properties of Ti implants [246–252]. It was found that in animal studies, bone tissue reactions were strongly reinforced with oxidized titanium implants, characterized by a titanium oxide layer thicker than 600 nm, a porous surface structure and an anatase type of Ti oxide with large surface roughness compared with turned implants [251,252]. This was later supported by work done by Lim et al. [98], who found that the alkali-treated CpTi surface was covered mainly with anatase type TiO_2, and exhibited hydrophilicity, whereas the acid-treated CpTi was covered with rutile type TiO_2 with hydrophobicity. Besides this characteristic crystalline structure of TiO_2, it was mentioned that good osseointegration, bony apposition, and cell attachment of Ti implant systems are partially due to the fact that the oxide layer [253–256].

Turned (as-machined implants) with amorphous TiO_2, anatase TiO_2 with S, amorphous TiO_2 with P, and anatase TiO_2 with Ca were prepared by the microarc oxidation method. Eighty implants were inserted in the femora and tibiae of 10 mature New Zealand white rabbits for 6 weeks. It was reported that (i) the removal torque values showed significant differences between S implants and controls, Ca implants and controls, Ca implants and P implants but did not show significant differences between the others, and (ii) the bone to metal contact around the entire implants demonstrated a 186% increase in S implants, 232% increase in P implants, and 272% increase Ca implants when compared to the paired control groups. It was therefore concluded that surface chemistry and topography separately or together play important roles in bone response to the oxidized implants [245].

The effects of pure commercial titanium implants on the process of primary mineralization were studied by Kohavi et al. [257] by insertion of titanium implants into rat tibial bone after ablation. The effects of the titanium were studied through the behavior of extracellular matrix vesicles. It was found that the insertion of titanium implants was followed by an increase in the number of extracellular matrix vesicles, as well as vesicular diameter, and by a decrease in vesicular distance from the calcified front when compared to normal healing. It was therefore suggested that (i) the process of extracellular matrix vesicles maturation around titanium implants was delayed when compared to normal primary bone formation during bone healing, and (ii) the delay in mineralization was compensated by an increase in vesicle production, resulting in an enhancement of primary mineralization by the titanium [257].

Jasty et al. [258] investigated bone ingrowth into uncemented hemispherical canine acetabular components, porous coated with Co–Cr spheres, and compared them to those porous coated with titanium fiber mesh. Good bone ingrowth was noted in both types of porous coatings at 6 weeks after surgery, with no difference in the histologic quality of the ingrowth bone. Quantification of bone ingrowth showed that significantly more bone grew into the titanium fiber mesh porous-coated components. It was demonstrated that the mean values of the amount of bone ingrowth, the area density of the ingrowth bone inside the pores, the ingrowth bone penetration depth, and the degree of the periphery of the porous layer with bone ingrowth of titanium mesh exceeded those values with Co–Cr spheres [258].

Bony ingrowth to control (nontreated) and heat-treated 316L stainless steel and Ti–6Al–4V implants, which were placed into the medullary canal of the femur in rats, was studied by mechanical, chemical and Auger electron spectroscopic microanalysis. Control samples of both materials are autoclaved at 280 °C. Heat treatment was done at 550 °C for 1.5 hours. It was found that, at all-time intervals up to 35 days postimplantation, the shear strengths of the heat-treated Ti–6Al–4V and stainless steel implants were significantly higher (1.6-fold–3.4-fold) than in control implants. Using Auger electron spectroscopy depth profiling methods, it was also found that the heat treatment modified the implant surface composition significantly, resulting in a thicker oxide layer and other chemical changes. It is therefore concluded that preoxidation of metallic implants prior to their insertion alters their chemical surface property and augments bony ingrowth to them [259].

Interstitial bone ingrowth is extremely important for optimum fixation of implanted materials under load-bearing conditions. Three types of biomaterial tests pieces were manufactured in solid and open-pore structures, and implanted into dog femoral condyles. Bone formation and remodeling were observed histologically and roentgenologically for 24 weeks thereafter. It was reported that (i) at 24-week postimplantation, the thick fibrous tissue surrounded by corticalized bone was formed around both solid smooth-surfaced alumina and titanium implants, but (ii) on the other hand, with an implant made of an artificial osteochondral composite material, thickening of ingrowth trabeculae could be observed as early as 4 weeks, (iii) bone ingrowth into the titanium fiber mesh was abundant and increased with time after implantation. This interstitial bone ingrowth resulted in the complete integration of the implant and the viable host bone. It was thus suggested that interstitial bone ingrowth has great significance; even new bone formation and remodeling follows Wolff's law [260] after the completion of the bonding between the bone and implanted material under load-bearing conditions. The artificial osteochondral composite material could lead to complete integration of the implant and viable bone, suggesting that it is a promising material for joint replacements. Moreover, the tibial joint surface which bore against the polyvinyl alcohol hydrogel surface of this implant, remained intact, suggesting that this composite is a very promising biomaterial for use in joint prostheses [261].

The histological study was conducted on the surrounding tissues of two screw-shaped titanium plasma-sprayed implants, retrieved due to the fractured abutment after 18 and 42 months. The microscopical examination showed that a large part of the implant surface on both implants was covered by compact, mature lamellar bone, with the presence of many Haversian systems and osteons. With von Kossa staining, at the interface with the implant, the bone was highly mineralized, and any connective tissue or inflammatory cells were not present at the interface [262].

The micromotion chamber for implantation in the rabbit tibia consists of two titanium components that have a 1 mm continuous (not independent) pore for bone ingrowth. The fixed, outer cylinder of the chamber contains a movable inner core that can be manually rotated. A comparison was made between the histological and scintigraphic results of bone ingrowth into chambers having a congruently shaped interface that was moved at 20 cycles/d, with amplitude of either 0.5 or 0.75 mm. It was found that (i) histological sections from both amplitude groups contained extensive new woven and trabecular bone, embedded in a fibrovascular network; however, (ii) the chambers with a larger amplitude of motion yielded less bone ingrowth than those with a smaller amplitude. It was therefore suggested that short, discrete periods of motion can stimulate the formation of fibrous tissue rather than bone, using the parameters chosen in this model [263].

Li et al. [264] investigated the effect of the surface macrostructure of a dimpled CpTi implant on bone ingrowth *in vivo* by means of histological examination and a push-out test. Cylindrical implants were inserted in one femur of each experimental rabbit and the animals were killed at 1.5, 3, and 13 months after implantation. The femur with the implant of each animal was then examined in a push-out test. The fracture surfaces of the bone–implant interface were examined after the push-out test under light and electron microscopy. It was reported that the dimpled CpTi surface enhanced mechanical retention of the CpTi implant in bone due to interlocking between vital bone and the dimples [264].

A nonsubmerged ITI-Bonefit implant, after a loading period of 4 years, was examined. It was reported that the behavior of peri-implant bone was tightly related to the magnitude and concentration of stresses which were transmitted to the implant [265]. These peri-implant stresses are subject to several variables: opposing occlusion, bite force, number of implants available to carry the load, position of the implant within the prostheses, rigidity of the prosthesis, and implant geometry [265]. Moreover, torque or bending moments can be applied to implants, for example, by excessively cantilevered bridges and can produce a breakdown at the interface, a resorption of bone, a loosening of the screw, or a fracture of the bar/bridge, or both [266]. It is also significant that the fracture was associated with a severe and rapid marginal bone height loss, and with an almost 100% bone–implant contact [267].

The *in vivo* effect of biomimetic CaP coating of titanium implants on peri-implant bone formation and bone/implant contact was investigated by Schliephake et al. [268]. Five types of implants were used: Ti–6Al–4V implants with a polished surface; Ti–6Al–4V implants with collagen coating; Ti–6Al–4V implants with a mineralized collagen layer; Ti–6Al–4V implants with a sequential coating of HA and collagen; and Ti–6Al–4V implants with HA coating only. All implants were press fit inserted into 4.6 mm trephine burr holes in the mandibles of 10 beagle dogs. The implants of five animals each were evaluated after a healing period of 1 month and 3 months, respectively, during which time sequential fluorochrome labeling of bone formation had been performed. Bone formation was evaluated by morphometric measurement of the newly formed bone around the implants and the percentage of implant bone contact. It was reported that (i) after 1 month, there was a significantly higher percentage of mean bone/implant contact in the HA-coated implants compared to those with polished surfaces and those with the collagen-coated surface, but (ii) after 3 months, these differences were not present anymore, and (iii) bone apposition was significantly higher next to implants with sequential HA/collagen coating compared to the polished surfaces and mineralized collagen layer. It is concluded that the HA coating to titanium implants has increased bone–implant contact in the early ingrowth period, and the addition of collagen to an HA coating layer may hold some promise when used as a sequential HA/collagen coating with mineralized collagen as the surface layer [268].

A major consideration in designing dental implants is the creation of a surface that provides strong attachment between the implant and bone, connective tissue, or epithelium. In addition, to maintain plaque-free implants, it is important to inhibit the adherence of oral bacteria on titanium surfaces exposed to the oral cavity. Therefore, Groessner-Schreiber et al. [269] examined antimicrobial characteristic TiN. Mouse fibroblasts were cultured on smooth titanium disks that were either magnetron-sputtered with a thin layer of TiN or thermal oxidized, or modified with laser radiation (using an Nd:YAG laser). It was reported that (i) fibroblasts on oxidized titanium surfaces showed a more spherical shape, whereas cells on laser-treated titanium and on TiN appeared intimately adherent to the surface, and (ii) when compared to all other surface modifications, fibroblast metabolism activity and total protein were significantly increased in the fibroblasts cultured on titanium surfaces coated with TiN, suggesting that a TiN coating might be suitable to support tissue growth on implant surfaces [269].

Osteoconductive apatite coatings represent an established technology for enhancing the integration of orthopedic Ti implants with living bone. The *in vivo* evaluation of a biomimetic apatite coating was performed. A dense and substantially pure ceramic coating with a crystal size of less than 1 μm was fabricated by using a mixed solution including all major inorganic ions (Na^+, K^+, Mg^{2+}, Ca^{2+}, Cl^-, HPO_4^{2-}, HCO_3^-, and SO_4^{2-}). The biomimetic apatite coating was grown on Ti 6Al 4V at 45°C for 4 days. Three types of measurements were taken on linear ingrowth %, area ingrowth percentage, and continuous bone apposition percentage. It was demonstrated that (i) under controlled conditions, the apatite coating appears to resorb in eight weeks, and stimulated early osseointegration with the metal surface with a reduction in fibrous tissue encapsulation, and (ii) this coating may, therefore, be useful in facilitating early bone ingrowth into porous surfaces without the potential for coating debris, macrophage infiltration, fibrous tissue encapsulation, and eventual coating failure, as may occur with current plasma-sprayed HA coating techniques [270].

Roughened titanium surfaces have been favorably fabricated and widely used for dental implants, as has been seen above. In recent years, there has been the tendency to replace Ti plasma-sprayed surfaces by sandblasted and acid-etched surfaces in order to enhance osseous apposition. Another approach has been the utilization of HA-coated implants. Knabe et al. [271] examined the effect of two roughened Ti dental implant surfaces on the osteoblastic phenotype of human bone-derived cells and compared this behavior to that for cells on an HA-coated surface. Test materials were an acid-etched and sandblasted Ti surface, a porous Ti plasma-sprayed coating, and a plasma-sprayed porous HA coating (HA). Smooth Ti machined surfaces served as the control. Human bone-derived cells were grown on the substrata for 3, 7, 14, and 21 days, counted, and probed for various bone-related mRNAs and proteins (type I collagen, osteocalcin, osteopontin, osteonectin, alkaline phosphatase, and bone sialoprotein). It was reported that (i) dental implant surfaces significantly affected cellular growth and the temporal expression of an array of bone-related genes and proteins, (ii) HA-coated Ti had the most effect on osteoblastic differentiation, inducing a greater expression of an array of osteogenic markers than recorded for cells grown on acid-etched and sandblasted Ti and porous Ti plasma-sprayed Ti, thus suggesting that the HA-coated surface may possess a higher potency to enhance osteogenesis, and (iii) acid-etched and sandblasted Ti surfaces induced greater osteoblast proliferation and differentiation than porous Ti plasma-sprayed Ti [271].

Lu et al. [272] evaluated the osteoconduction of Ti–6Al–4V surfaces under various conditions, including micropatterned, alkali-treated, micropatterned, plus alkali-treated, and surfaces without any treatment as the control. The *in vitro* CaP formation on titanium surfaces was in static and dynamic SBF. An *in vivo* comparison was conducted in the medullary cavity of a dog femur, which could provide the same physiological environment for specimens with different surface conditions. It was reported that (i) there was good conduction of CaP on the alkali-treated surfaces, and also better CaP deposition on the microhole surface than that found on the flat surfaces in the dynamic SBF, and (ii) the beneficial effect of alkaline treatment on osteoconduction was confirmed. The *in vivo* experiments also indicate a synergistic effect of the alkaline treatment and the topographic pattern on osteoconduction [272], as suggested by basic studies done by Lim et al. [98].

Early bone ongrowth is known to increase primary implant fixation and reduce the risk of early implant failure. Arg-Gly-Asp (arginine-glycine-aspartate, RGD) peptide has been identified as playing a key role in osteoblast adhesion and proliferation on various surfaces. Elmengaard et al. [273,274] evaluated the effect of RGD peptide coating on the bony fixation of orthopedic implants. Sixteen unloaded cylindrical plasma sprayed Ti–6Al–4V implants, coated with cyclic RGD peptide, were press-fit inserted in the proximal tibia of eight mongrel dogs for 4 weeks. Uncoated control implants were inserted in the contralateral tibia. Results were evaluated by histomorphometry and mechanical push-out tests. It was shown that (i) a significant two-fold increase was observed in bone ongrowth for the RGD-coated implants, (ii) fibrous tissue ongrowth was significantly reduced for the RGD-coated implants, (iii) bone volume was significantly increased in a 0–100 μm zone around the implant; the increased bony anchorage resulted in moderate increases in mechanical fixation, as the apparent shear stiffness was significantly higher for RGD-coated implants, and (iv) increases in median ultimate shear strength and energy to failure were also observed. It was hence suggested that cyclic RGD coating increases early bony fixation of unloaded press-fit titanium implants [273,274].

It has been extensively discussed about the interfacial reaction of placed implant with hard tissue, but its reaction with soft tissue should be equally important. Tissues containing Ti dental implants were examined on the chemical state of Ti transferred from the placed implant into surrounding soft tissue [275]. No tissues that contacted CpTi cover screws for several months were excised in a second surgery whereby healing abutments were set. Six tissues that surrounded implants retrieved due to their failure were also exercised. It was concluded that (i) the existence of Ti in the tissue did not cause implant failure. Intraosseous transcutaneous amputation prostheses reply on the integrity of soft tissue–implant interface as a barrier to exogenous agents, and the prevention of avulsion and marsupialization [275]. Chen et al. [276] had conducted *in vivo* evaluation of soft tissue attachment to Ti–6Al–4V transcutaneous custom-made screws treated by a microarc oxidation method. The experimental model comprised implantation of 16 transcutaneous screws in the medial aspect of the left tibia of eight female goats. It was reported that (i) significant higher soft tissue attachment was observed in the microarc oxidized Ti–6Al–4V alloy group compared to the control, and (ii) the *in vivo* data indicated that modified Ti–6Al–4V alloy could be a useful biomaterial for tissue engineering and benefit applications where bone-anchored transcutaneous implants are used [276].

3.5.5. Bone Healing and Grafting

For both dental and orthopedic implant surgeries, bone healing is the most common and major step immediately after implant placements. There is union bone fracture and nonunion bone fracture. For these implant surgeries, it is important to understand the nonunion bone healing mechanism. There are principle steps of peri-implant bone healing. The first and most important healing phase, osteoconduction, relies on the recruitment and migration of osteogenic cells to the implant surface, through the residue of the peri-implant blood clot. This formation of hematoma is similar to that seen elsewhere in the body. This is a clot of blood originating from the lacerated blood vessels in the bone and the periosteum. Among the most important aspects of osteoconduction are the knock-on effects generated at the implant surface, by the initiation of platelet activation, which result in directed osteogenic cell migration. Necrotic bone is then resorbed by osteoclasts, and the hematoma by macrophages. As the hematoma is resorbed, the granulation tissue develops from the periosteum and endosteum. When this has completed, pluripotent cells migrate into the granulation tissue. These cells become chondrocytes, and later osteocytes, producing cartilage and bone, respectively. The second healing phase (bone formation) results in a mineralized interfacial matrix equivalent to that seen in the cement line in natural bone tissue. These two healing phases, osteoconduction and *de novo* bone formation, result in contact osteogenesis and, given an appropriate implant surface, bone bonding. The structure surrounding the fracture site is now slightly harder; this is a provisional callus. The area can be called a proper callus as time goes on, and more and more woven bone is made by the osteoblasts. This woven bone is initially remodeled into lamellar bone. With time, the bone is remodeled over the next few months, and the callus becomes smaller, as the trabeculae are formed along lines of stress [277].

A material implanted in bone is always inserted into coagulating blood. Protein and cell interactions during this initial implantation time will govern later healing. Many studies have focused on the tissue surrounding implants. Eriksson et al. [278] developed a method for evaluation of healing around implants in bone by studying cells adhering to the implant surface. Hydrophilic (in other words, active) titanium disks were inserted into rat tibiae. Samples were retrieved after 1, 2, 4, and 8 days of implantation and were analyzed by fluorescence microscopy techniques and SEM. Both proliferating and apoptotic cells were found on the surface. Generally, cells closest to the implant surface were nonviable, whereas cells in the fibrin network a distance from the surface were viable. Bone morphogenetic protein-2 (BMP-2) is an osteogenic substance. An increase in BMP-2-positive cells was seen during the implantation period, and a population of large BMP-2-positive cells appeared on the surface after 4 days of implantation. Hence, it was evaluated that this unique method was a suitable tool for rapid evaluation of the initial healing around implant material [278].

Osborn et al. [279] classified bio-response to endosseous implants into the following three groups: (i) bio-tolerant type, characterized by distance-osteogenesis, (ii) bio-inert type, characterized by contact-osteogenesis, and (iii) bio-reactive type, characterized by physico-chemical linkage between the implant and the surrounding bone. Rutile type oxide, which is formed on titanium as one of TiO_2s, is described as a stable crystalline form similar to ceramics in its bio-reactive behavior [280]. However, it is well recognized that Ti is known as a biotolerant biomaterial (which exhibits "distance osteogenesis," so that although such biomaterials are not rejected from the living tissue, they do not connect to the bone directly because they are covered with connective tissue), and when inserted to the living hard tissue, bone regeneration can be achieved either by the bone conductive mechanism (using HA, tricalcium phosphate, decalcified frozen dried bone, or autologous-bone) or bone inductive mechanisms (using BMP on the scaffold or platelet-rich plasma on the scaffold) [281].

TiN has been used in many fields as a coating for surgical instruments, with the purpose of creating materials more resistant to wear and corrosion, and also reducing adhesion. Titanium implants (180 implants with 2 mm × 2 mm) were divided into the following three groups: Group 1 ($n = 60$): 30 machined and 30 machined TiN-coated, Group 2 ($n = 60$): 30 sandblasted and 30 sandblasted TiN-coated, and Group 3 ($n = 60$): 30 titanium plasma sprayed, 30 titanium plasma sprayed and coated with TiN. The animals were killed after 5, 10, 20, 30, or 60 days. It was reported that (i) the healing around the TiN-coated implants was similar to that observed around the uncoated surfaces, and (ii) the TiN coating demonstrated a good biocompatibility [282].

The differences in the healing of cortical and cancellous bone around CpTi screw-type implants with two different surfaces (machined and anodized) were investigated in rabbit tibiae [283]. In the tibiae of rats, a total of 24 implants was surgically placed in randomized arrangement; the upper transverse canal was positioned in the cortical bone region, and the lower transverse canal was positioned in the cancellous bone region. After a 1-month healing period, un-decalcified ground sections were subjected to histologic and histomorphometric analyses. It was reported that (i) the percentage of BIC inside the upper canals was 16.45% for controls (machined surface) and 24.85% for anodized implants, (ii) BIC inside the lower canals was 7.01% for controls and 11.35% for anodized implants, (iii) the percentage of bone area inside the upper canals was 10.94% for controls and 27.95% for anodized implants, and (iv) the percentage of bone area inside the lower canals was 3.16% for controls and 4.66% for anodized implants. Hence, it was concluded that anodized surface modification of titanium implants is beneficial to both cortical and cancellous bone healing [283].

Franco et al. [284] found similarly the beneficial effect of anodizing the titanium implant surface for the bone healing process. The surface of CpTi was treated by multi-phase anodic spark deposition coating to make the surface layer to be enriched with Ca and P ions. Two mongrel dogs received bilateral implantation of three CpTi cylinders in humerus, with anodized and untreated (machined-control). After 8 weeks postimplantation, bone fragments containing implants were subject to histologic and histomorphometric analyses. It was reported that (i) in most cases, collagen fiber bundles were detected adjacent and oriented parallel to Ti surfaces, (ii) such connective tissue formation exhibited focal areas of mineralized matrix lined by active osteoblasts, (iii) the mean percentage of BIC were 2.3% for anodized and 0.4% for control implants. It was further concluded that the trend of anodizing treated surfaces to support contact osteogenesis in an experimental model that produces low BIC values [284]. Colnot et al. [285], using the mouse model, investigated effects of the implant surface on the early stages of bone healing. The healing around Ti–6Al–4V and other materials were assessed with qualitative cellular and molecular evaluations to show osteoblast differentiation and new bone deposition. Based on the results, it was concluded that the implant surface and microenvironment around implants favored osteogenesis.

Bone healing is also affected by mechanical environment [286,287]. Ti-7.5Mo (having a high-strength/modulus ratio) can be considered as a candidate for orthopedic applications. Ti-7.5Mo and Ti–6Al–4V implants were placed into the left and right rabbit femurs for 6, 12, and 26 weeks. It was reported that (i) the amount of new bone encircling the Ti-7.5Mo implant was approximately two-folds of that at Ti–6Al–4V by 26 weeks postimplantation, and (ii) this facilitation of bone formation could be associated with the unique properties such as a low modulus (less rigidity) and the composition of Mo [286]. During the implant healing, mechanical force is transmitted to osteogenic cells via implant surfaces with various topographies [287]. Rat bone-marrow-derived osteoblastic cells were cultured on titanium disks with machined and acid-etched surfaces. A loading session consisted of a 3 minute application of a 10- or 20-μm-amplitude vibration. It was found that (i) alkaline phosphatase activity and gene expression increased only when the cells were loaded in three sessions/day on machined surfaces, regardless of the vibration amplitude, whereas they were increased with one loading session/day on the acid-etched surface, and (ii) the loading did not affect the osteoblast proliferation on the surface, but selectively enhanced the cell spreading on the machined surface. Based on these findings, it was concluded that (i) osteoblastic differentiation is promoted by mechanical stimulation on titanium, and that promotion is disproportionate, depending on the titanium surface topography, and (ii) the frequency of mechanical stimulation, rather than its amplitude, appears to have a crucial role [287].

Bone grafting is performed to unite fractures, to fuse joints, and to repair skeletal defects. These are typically classified into two groups: biograft materials and artificial materials. Biograft materials are further grouped into (i) *autologous grafts*, which are obtained directly from the patient; autologous bone graft possesses maximum biocompatibility thus is generally considered to be the best material available for bone grafting, (ii) *allogenous grafts*, which are obtained from a donor of the same species and are commonly employed as the "second alternative" when an autograft is not possible; allogenous bone is also favored when the bone defect is extensive and the quality and quantity of autologous bone is insufficient; the primary problem with allogenous grafts is immunological, and (iii) *xenogenous graft*, which are bone materials obtained from another species; xenogenous bone is primarily harvested from cows; these grafts must be specially treated before use because of genetic incompatibility.

The artificial graft materials are also further classified into: (i) *natural products* such as Paris plaster, coral, and so forth, and (ii) *chemical products* which can includes sintered HA , β-TCP (tricalcium phosphate), self-hardening CaP, or others. It is widely recognized that requirements for successful bone re-generating materials should include, safety, preservability, handling property, washout resistance, shape-plasticity, shape-integrity, biocompatibility, and osteoformability (osteoconductivity or osteoinductivity).

3.5.6. Osseointegration

Broadly speaking, two types of anchorage mechanisms have been described: biomechanical and biochemical. Biomechanical binding is when bone ingrowth occurs into micrometer-sized surface irregularities. The term osteointegration is probably, realistically, the biomechanical phenomenon. Biochemical bonding may occur with certain bioactive materials where there is primarily a chemical bonding, with possible supplemental biomechanical interlocking. The distinct advantage with the biochemical bonding is that the anchorage is accomplished within a relatively short period of time, while biomechanical anchorage takes weeks to develop. This would clinically translate into the possibility of earlier restorative loading of implants. Most commercially available implants depend on biomechanical interlocking for anchorage. All implants must exhibit biomechanical as well as morphological compatibility. As we have seen previously, Ti implants coated with CaP, or inorganic or organic bone-like apatite, possess both anchorage mechanisms, because (i) coated surfaces are normally rough which can facilitate the biomechanical anchorage (morphological compatibility), and (ii) coated materials *per se* accommodate biochemical bonding (biological compatibility). In orthodontic mechano-therapy, the anchorage mechanism is slightly different from ordinary implants. Saito et al. [288] investigated the anchorage potential of titanium implants with the use of a sectional arch wire technique for orthodontic mesiodistal tooth movement, as assessed by the osseointegration of implants and tooth movement. Two implants were surgically placed in healed mandibular extraction sites of the second and third premolars on each side in four adult male beagle dogs. It was reported that (i) there was no statistical difference in the percentage of peri-implant bone volume between the loaded and unloaded sides, and (ii) there was also no statistical difference between the compression and tension sides in both loaded and unloaded implants, suggesting that the implants maintained rigid osseointegration. It was, hence, concluded that endosseous titanium implants can function as anchors for long-term orthodontic mesiodistal movement [288].

Bone fusing to titanium was first reported in 1940 by Bothe et al. [289]. Brånemark began extensive experimental studies in 1952 on the microscopic circulation of bone marrow healing. These studies led to dental implant application in early 1960, 10-year implant integration was established in dogs without significant adverse reactions to hard or soft tissues. Studies in humans began in 1965, were followed for 10 years, and reported in 1977 [290]. Osteointegration, as first defined by Brånemark, denotes at least some direct contact between vital bone with the surface of an implant at the light microscopic level of magnification [291]. The percentage of direct bone-implant contact is variable. To determine osseointegration, the implant must be removed and evaluated under a microscope. Rigid fixation defines the clinical aspect of this microscopic bone contact with an implant and is the absence of mobility with 1 to 500 g force applied in a vertical or horizontal direction. Rigid fixation is the clinical result of a direct bone interface, but has also been reported with fibrous tissue interfaces [291]. Osteointegration was originally defined as a direct structural and functional connection between ordered living bone and the surface of a load-carrying artificial implant (which is typically made of titanium materials). It is now said that an implant is regarded as osteointegrated when there is no progressive relative movement between the implant and the bone with which it has direct contact. In practice, this means that in osteointegration there is an anchorage mechanism, whereby nonvital components can be reliably and predictably incorporated into living bone and that this anchorage can persist under all normal conditions of loading. Bioactive (or biochemical) retention can be achieved in cases where the implant is coated with bioactive materials, like HA. These bioactive materials stimulate bone formation leading, to a physio-chemical bond. If it is recognized that the implant is ankylosed with the bone, it is sometimes called a biointegration instead of osteointegration [292].

For profound understanding of the osteointegration mechanism, there are several works reported. Fourteen titanium dental implants (TioblastTM) were implanted singly in the proximal tibia of New Zealand rabbits for 120 days. A bone defect was surgically produced and filled with Bio-Oss® (which is a natural, osteoconductive bone substitute that promotes bone growth in periodontal and maxillofacial osseous defects) around six of these implants. After the animals were sacrificed and their organs harvested, bone segments were fixed, and methacrylate embedded after the push-in test had been performed. The results showed that (i) the implants were apically and coronally surrounded by bone, whether Bio-Oss® was used or not, (ii) fractures were evident through the newly formed bone and between the pre-existing and newly formed bone, and (iii) detachment between the implant and the bone occurred at the coronal extremity of the implants and along its cervical region. Based on these findings, it was concluded that the bone–titanium interface has a high resistance to loading, exhibiting a greater resistance than the newly formed bone [293].

The effect of a dual treatment of titanium implants and the subsequent bone response after implantation were investigated by Rønold et al. [294]. Coin-shaped CpTi implants were placed into the tibias of 12 rabbits. The implant was dually blasted with TiO_2 particles of two different sizes (i.e., finer particles of 22–28 μm in size, and coarser particles of 180–220 μm in size). It was found that (i) the Ti surface blasted with coarse particles showed a significantly better functional attachment than the fine surface, and (ii) the Ti surface blasted with fine particles showed lower retention in bone, indicating that there is a positive correlation between the topographical and mechanical evaluation of the surfaces [294].

In cementless fixation systems, surface character is an important factor. Alkali and heat treatments of titanium have been shown to produce strong bonding to bone and a higher ongrowth rate. With regard to the cementless hip stem, Nishiguchi et al. [295] examined the effect of alkali and heat treatments on titanium rods in an intramedullary rabbit femur model. Half of the implants were immersed in the 5 mol/L sodium hydroxide solution and heated at 600 °C for 1 h, and the other half were untreated. The bone–implant interfaces were evaluated at 3, 6, and 12 weeks after implantation. Pull-out tests showed that the treated implants had a significantly higher bonding strength to bone than the untreated implants at each time point. As postoperative time elapsed, histological examination revealed that new bone formed on the surface of both types of implants, but significantly more bone made direct contact with the surface of the treated implants. At 12 weeks, ~56% of the whole surface of the treated implants was covered with the bone. Based on aforementioned results, it was concluded that (i) alkali-treated and heat-treated titanium create strong bone bonding and a high affinity to bone, as opposed to a conventional mechanical interlocking mechanism, and (ii) alkali and heat treatments of titanium may be suitable surface treatments for cementless joint replacement implants [295].

Several factors influence the healing process and the long-term mechanical stability of cementless fixed implants, such as bone remodeling and mineralization processes [296]. Histomorphometric and bone hardness measurements were taken in implants inserted in sheep femoral cortical bone at different times to compare the *in vivo* osseointegration of titanium screws with the following surface treatments: machined (Ti-MA); acid-etched with 25 vol% of HNO_3 solution for 1 hour (Ti-HF); hydroxyapatite vacuum plasma spray (Ti-HA); and Ca–P anodization (with 0.06 ml/L β-glycerophosphate plus 0.3 ml/L calcium acetate at 275V and 50 mA/cm^2), followed by a 300 °C autoclave-hydrothermal treatment for 2 hours (Ti-AM/HA). It was reported that (i) the BIC of Ti-HF was lower than that of the other surface treatments at both experimental times, (ii) significant differences in MAR (mineral apposition rate) were also found between the different experimental times for Ti-MA and Ti-HF, demonstrating that bone growth had slowed inside the screw threads of Ti-HA and Ti-AM/HA after 12 weeks, (iii) no bone microhardness changes in preexisting host bone were found, while Ti–MA showed the lowest value for the inner thread area at 8 weeks. Based on these findings, it was confirmed that osteointegration may be accelerated by adequate surface roughness and a bioactive ceramic coating, such as Ca–P anodization followed by a hydrothermal treatment, which enhances bone interlocking and mineralization [296].

Fujibayashi et al. [297] demonstrated that bone formation took place after 12-month implantation in the muscles of beagle dogs and reported that chemically and thermally treated plasma-sprayed porous titanium surfaces exhibited an intrinsic osteoinductivity. Takemoto et al. [298] tested on porous plasma-sprayed Ti blocks with the following characteristics: porosity of 41%, pore size of a ranging between 300 and 500 μm, and yield compressive strength of 85.2 MPa. Three types of surface treatments were applied (i) alkali (in the NaOH solution at 60 °C for 24 hours) and heat treatment (600 °C for 1 hour, followed by a furnace cooling), (ii) alkali, hot water, and heat treatment, and (iii) alkali, dilute 40 °C HCl for 24 hours, hot water, and heat treatment. The osteoinductivity of the materials implanted in the back muscles of adult beagle dogs was examined at 3, 6, and 12 months. It was found that (i) the alkali-acid/heat-treated porous bioactive titanium implant had the highest osteoinductivity, with induction of a large amount of bone formation within 3 months, (ii) the dilute HCl treatment was considered to give both chemical (titania formation and sodium removal) and topographic (etching) effects on the titanium surface, and (iii) adding the dilute HCl treatment to the conventional chemical and thermal treatments is a promising candidate for advanced surface treatment of porous titanium implants [298,299].

A number of experimental and clinical data on so-called oxidized implants have reported promising outcomes, as we have previously reviewed. However, little has been investigated on the role of the surface oxide properties and osseointegration mechanism of the oxidized implant. Sul et al. [300] recently proposed two action mechanisms for osseointegration of oxidized implants, that is, (i) mechanical interlocking through bone growth in pores/other surface irregularities, and (ii) biochemical bonding. Two groups of oxidized implants were prepared using a microarc oxidation process and were then inserted into rabbit bone. One group consisted of magnesium ion incorporated implants, and the other consisted of TiO_2 stoichiometry implants. It was reported that (i) after 6 weeks of follow up, the mean peak values for removal torque of the Mg-incorporated Ti implants dominated significantly over the TiO_2/Ti implants, (ii) bonding failure generally occurred in the bone away from the bone to implant interface for the Mg-incorporated Ti implant and mainly occurred at the bone to implant interface for the TiO_2/Ti implant which consisted mainly of TiO_2 chemistry and significantly rougher surfaces, as compared to the Mg-incorporated Ti implant, and (iii) between bone and the Mg-incorporated-Ti implant surface, ionic movements and ion concentrations gradient were detected. It was therefore concluded that the surface chemistry-mediated biochemical bonding can be theorized for explaining the oxidized bioactive implants [300]. Lim and Oshida [98] investigated the surface characteristics of acid-treated and alkali-treated CpTi. It was reported that (i) acid-treated CpTi was covered with rutile-type TiO_2 with high hydrophobicity (in other words, less surface activity), whereas (ii) oxide film formed on the alkali-treated CPTi surface was identified to be an anatase-type dominantly with a trace amount of rutile, which exhibited high hydrophilicity (i.e., high surface energy).

For the last 15 years, orthopedic implants have been coated with HA to improve implant fixation. The osteoconductive effect of HA coatings has been demonstrated in experimental and clinical studies. However, there are ongoing developments to improve the quality of HA coatings. Aebli et al. [301] investigated whether a rough and highly crystalline HA coating applied by vacuum plasma spraying had a positive effect on the osteointegration of special, high-grade titanium (Ti) implants with the same surface roughness. Ti alloy implants were vacuum plasma spray-coated with high grade Ti or HA. The osseointegration of the implants was evaluated by light microscopy or pullout tests after 1, 2, and 4 weeks of unloaded implantation in the cancellous bone of 18 sheep. It was found that (i) the interface shear strength increased significantly over all time intervals, (ii) by 4 weeks, values had reached ~10 N/mm^2, but (iii) the difference between the coatings was not significant at any time interval, and (iv) direct bone–implant contact was significantly different between the coatings after 2 and 4 weeks, and reached 46% for Ti and 68% for HA implants by 4 weeks. Therefore, it was indicated that the use of a rough and highly crystalline HA coating, applied by the vacuum plasma spray method, enhances early osteointegration [301].

Stewart et al. [302] investigated the effects of a plasma-sprayed hydroxyapatite/tricalcium phosphate (HA/TCP) coating on osteointegration of plasma-sprayed titanium alloy implants in a lapine, distal femoral intramedullary model. The effects of the HA/TCP coating were assessed at 1, 3, and 6 months after implant placement. The HA/TCP coating significantly increased new bone apposition onto the implant surfaces at all-time points. The ceramic coating also stimulated intramedullary bone formation at the middle and distal levels of the implants. There was no associated increase in pull-out strength at either 3 or 6 months; however, postpullout evaluation of the implants indicated that the HA/TCP coating itself was not the primary site of construct failure. Rather, failure was most commonly observed through the peri-prosthetic osseous struts that bridged the medullary cavity. It was therefore concluded that the osteoconductive activity of HA/TCP coating on plasma-sprayed titanium alloy implant surfaces may have considerable clinical relevance to early host–implant interactions, by accelerating the establishment of a stable prosthesis–bone interface [302].

The *in vivo* behavior of a porous Ti–6Al–4V material that was produced by a positive replica technique, with and without an octacalcium phosphate coating, has been studied both in the back muscle and femur of goats by Habibovic et al. [303]. Macro- and microporous biphasic CaP ceramic, known to be both osteoconductive and able to induce ectopic bone formation, was used for comparison. The three groups of materials (Ti–6Al–4V, octacalcium-phosphate-coated Ti–6Al–4V and biphasic CaP ceramic) were implanted transcortically and intramuscularly for 6 and 12 weeks in 10 adult. Dutch milk goats in order to study their osteointegration and osteoinductive potential. It was found that (i), in femoral defects, both octacalcium-phosphate-coated Ti–6Al–4V and biphasic CaP ceramic performed better than the uncoated Ti–6Al–4V at both time points, (ii) biphasic CaP ceramic showed a higher bone amount than octacalcium-phosphate-coated Ti–6Al–4V after 6 weeks of implantation, while after 12 weeks, this difference was no longer significant, (iii) ectopic bone formation was found in both octacalcium-phosphate-coated Ti–6Al–4V and biphasic CaP ceramic implants after 6 and 12 weeks, and (iv) the ectopic bone formation was not found in uncoated titanium alloy implants, suggesting that the presence of CaP is important for bone induction [303].

The osteointegration of the copper vapor laser-superfinished titanium alloy (Ti–6Al–4V) implants with pore sizes of 25, 50, and 200 μm was evaluated in a rabbit intramedullary model by Stangl et al. [304]. Control implants were prepared by corundum blasting. Each animal received all four different implants in both femora and humeri. Using static and dynamic histomorphometry, the bone–implant interface and the peri-implant bone tissue were examined 3, 6, and 12 weeks postimplantation. Among the laser-superfinished implants, it was reported that total bone–implant contact was the smallest for the 25-μm pores and was similar for 50 and 200-μm pore sizes at all-time points, and however, all laser-superfinished surfaces were inferior to corundum-blasted control implants in terms of bone–implant contact. Implants with 25-μm pores showed the highest amount of peri-implant bone volume at all-time points, indicating that the amount of peri-implant bone was not correlated with the quality of the bone–implant interface. Accordingly, it was concluded that although laser-superfinished implants were not superior to the corundum-blasted control implants in terms of osteointegration, understanding of the mechanisms of bone remodeling within pores of various sizes was advanced, and optimal implant surfaces can be further developed with the help of modern laser technology [304].

There is another work using the laser technology for surface modification. Götz et al. [305] examined the osteointegration of laser-textured Ti–6Al–4V implants with pore sizes of 100, 200, and 300 μm, specifically comparing 200-μm implants with polished and corundum-blasted surfaces in a rabbit transcortical model. Using a distal and proximal implantation site in the distal femoral cortex, each animal received all four different implants in both femora. The bone/implant interface and the newly formed bone tissue within the pores and in peri-implant bone tissue were examined 3, 6, and 12 weeks postimplantation by static and dynamic histomorphometry. It was shown that (i) additional surface blasting of laser-textured Ti–6Al–4V implants with 200-μm pores resulted in a profound improvement in osteointegration at 12-week postimplantation, (ii) although lamellar bone formation was found in pores of all sizes, the amount of lamellar bone within the pores was linearly related to the pore size, (iii) in 100-μm pores, bone remodeling occurred with a pronounced time lag relative to larger pores, and (iv) implants with 300-μm pores showed a delayed osteointegration compared with 200-μm pores. Therefore, it was concluded that 200 μm may be the optimal pore size for laser-textured Ti–6Al–4V implants, and that laser treating in combination with surface blasting may be a very interesting technology for the structuring of implant surfaces [305].

There are some researches done on method or technique to evaluate/examine the osteointegration [306–309]. Since bone should be observed to grow into the porous structure of the coating, yielding direct evidence of a mechanism of the bone/implant interface, it was proposed to employ the advanced various analytical devices including dual-beam focused ion beam microscopy, SEM, transmission electron microcopy, and X-ray energy dispersive spectrometer [306]. Stenport et al. [307] conducted comparison tests of tissue integration to CpTi and Ti–6Al–4V implants using various three-dimensional biomechanical and two-dimensional histomorphometrical techniques, and mentioned the loosening torque during *in vivo* removal torque in rabbits. It was found that significantly higher mean value of removal torque and shear strength test were observed for the CpTi implants compared to Ti–6Al–4V implants. In order to chronologically examine the titanium–bone interfaces and to clarify the process of osteointegration, Morinaga et al. [308] utilized light microcopy, transmission electron microscopy (TEM), quantitative tomography (QCT), and microcomputed tomography (micro-QCT). Experimental implants (Ti-coating plastic implants) were placed into tibiae of 8-week old rats. It was reported that (i) bone formation in osteointegration of Ti implants did not occur from the surfaces of the implant or preexisting bone, but it was likely that bone formation progressed at a site a small distance away from the surface, (ii) small bone fragments adhered to each other and transformed into reticular-shaped bone, and finally these bones became lamellar bone [308]. Kerner et al. [309] assessed *in vivo* new bone formation around Ti–6Al–4V alloy implants chemically grafted with macromolecules bearing ionic sulfonate or carboxylate groups, or both. Unmodified and grafted Ti–6Al–4V implants were placed bilaterally into rabbit femoral condyle. It was found that (i) the BIC was the lowest (13.4%) for the implants modified with grafted carboxylate only, (ii) the value of BIC on the implants with 20% sulfonate was significantly lower than that observed on 100% sulfonate surfaces, (iii) after both 4 and 12 weeks postimplantation, the BIC value for implants with more than 50% sulfonate was similar to that obtained with the unmodified Ti–6Al–4V, and (iv) the grafted Ti–6Al–4V alloy exhibiting either 100% sulfonate or carbonxylate and sulfonate (50% each) groups promoted bone formation. Such materials are of clinical interest because, they do not promote bacteria adhesion but, they support new bone formation, a condition which can lead to osseointegration of bone implants while preventing peri-implant infections [309].

The design, surface characteristics, and strength of metallic implants are dependent on their intended use and clinical application. Surface modifications of materials may enable reduction of the time taken for osseointegration and improve the biological response of bio-mechanically favorable metals and alloys. Titanium aluminum nitride

(TAN) coated and plain rods of stainless steel and CpTi were implanted into the mid-shaft of the femur of Wistar rats. The femurs were harvested at four weeks and processed for scanning electron and light microscopy. It was reported that (i) all implants exhibited a favorable response in bone with no evidence of fibrous encapsulation and (ii) although there was no significant difference in the amount of new bone formed around the different rods (osseoconduction), there was a greater degree of shrinkage separation of bone from the coated rods than from the plain rods ($p = 0.017$ stainless steel and $p = 0.0085$ titanium), indicating that the TAN coating may result in reduced osseointegration between bone and implant [310].

3.6. Loosening Implants and Infection

The risk of bacterial infections associated with open surgery or the implantation, or both, remains to be a major drawback in implantology and these implant-associated infections cause to loosen placed implants [311–314].

Besides the risk of infection, dental/medical implants can fail due to wear, fatigue, chemical degradation, and others which might lead to osteolysis and loosening implants [315].

Early implant instability has been proposed as a critical factor in the onset and progression of aseptic loosening and periprosthetic osteolysis in total joint arthroplasties. As was seen in Chapter 6, macrophages stimulated with cyclic mechanical strain release inflammatory mediators. But, little is known about the response of these cells to mechanical strain with particles, which is often a component of the physical environment of the cell. Fujishiro et al. [316] studied the production of prostaglandin E2 (PGE2), an important mediator in aseptic loosening and periprosthetic osteolysis in total joint arthroplasties, for human macrophages treated with mechanical stretch alone, titanium particles alone, and mechanical stretch and particles combined. A combination of mechanical stretch and titanium particles resulted in a statistically synergistic elevation of levels of PGE2 compared with the levels found with either stretch or particles alone. It was hence suggested that, while mechanical strain may be one of the primary factors responsible for macrophage activation and periprosthetic osteolysis, mechanical strain with particles load may contribute significantly to the osteolytic potential of macrophages *in vitro* [316].

Corrosion of implant alloys releasing metal ions has the potential to cause adverse tissue reactions and implant failure. Lin et al. [317] hypothesized that macrophage cells and their released reactive chemical species affect the corrosion property of Ti–6Al–4V. It was reported that (i) there was no difference in the charge transfer in the presence and absence of cells, and (ii) the alloy had the lowest charge transfer and metal ion release with activated cells was as follows: Ti $<$ 10 ppb, V $<$ 2 ppb, attributing to an enhancement of the surface oxides by the reactive chemical species. It was concluded that macrophage cells and reactive chemical species reduced the corrosion of Ti–6Al–4V alloys [317].

Prosthetic and osteosynthetic implants from metal alloys will be indispensable in orthopedic surgery, as long as tissue engineering and biodegradable bone substitutes do not lead to products that will be applied in clinical routine for the repair of bone, cartilage, and joint defects. Therefore, the elucidation of the interactions between the peri-prosthetic tissues and the implant remains of clinical relevance, and several factors are known to affect the longevity of implants. Sommer et al. [318] studied the effects of metal particles and surface topography on the recruitment of osteoclasts *in vitro* in a co-culture of osteoblasts and bone marrow cells. It was reported that (i) the cells were grown in the presence of particles of different sizes and chemical compositions, or on metal disks with polished or sandblasted surfaces, respectively, (ii) at the end of the culture, newly formed osteoclasts were counted, (iii) osteoclastogenesis was reduced when particles were added directly to the co-culture, and (iv) in co-cultures grown on sand-blasted surfaces, osteoclasts developed at higher rates than they did in cultures on polished surfaces. It was therefore summarized that the wear particles and implant surfaces affect osteoclastogenesis, and thus may be involved in the induction of local bone resorption and the formation of osteolytic lesions, leading eventually to the loosening of orthopedic implants [318]. Nanomaterial safety and toxicity are of great importance for nanomaterial-based medical implants and a better understanding of the fate of nanomaterials after production and after implantation is clearly necessary. Yang et al. [319] pointed out that, in terms of implant degradation, nanoscale materials can be generated and released into peripheral host tissues regardless of their constituent grain sizes (or other characteristic features, such as particle size) and unfortunately, the biological responses to and toxicity of nanoscale implant materials have not been sufficiently investigated.

The load of the implant should preferably be in the longitudinal direction. Thus it is important to avoid rotational or cantilever forces, once the implant has integrated. If forces are distributed in the longitudinal direction, even very high loads can be withstood by the implant during many years of function [320]. The loss of integration can be obtained by overload, torsional forces, or direct trauma to the implant. Overload might be the result of the long extensions of the bar construction or by misplaced implants. Minor torsion forces might induce microfractures in the bone that with time can rupture the delicate integration. The lack of adequate counterforces during tightening of the abutment might result in immediate implant loss. Tightening of individual magnets used as retentions without counterhold might as well cause implant failures [320]. The quantity of bone, and also the quality of bone might determine the force necessary to lose and implant. The most well-known cause for implant failure is the bone that has been irradiated as part of cancer treatment. Chemotherapy also affects implant survival to a similar degree as radiotherapy. Other factors that might affect implant survival are osteoporosis, steroid medication, and diabetes mellitus [321].

References

1. Misch, C.E., 1999, *Implant Dentistry*, 2nd ed. An Affiliate of Elsevier, St. Louis, MO.
2. Burden, D.J. and Eedy, D.J., 1991, Orthodontic headgear related to allergic contact dermatitis; a case report. *Br Dent J* 170:447–448. doi: http://dx.doi.org/10.1038/sj.bdj.4807585
3. Veien, N.K., Borchorst, E., Mattel, T. and Laurberg, G., 1994, Stomatitis or systemically induced contact dermatitis from metal wire in orthodontic materials, *Contact Derm* 30:210–213. doi: http://dx.doi.org/10.1111/j.1600-0536.1994.tb00645.x

4. www.medibix.com
5. BS ISO 7206 Implants for surgery. Partial and total hip joint prostheses. Determination of resistance to static load of modular femoral heads. www.bsi-global.com
6. Kasemo, B. and Lausmaa, J., 1988, Biomaterial and implant surfaces: A surface science approach, *Int J Oral Maxillofac Implants* 3:247–259.
7. Albrektsson, T., Brånemark, P.I., Hansson, H.A. and Lindstrom, J., 1981, Osseointegrated titanium implants. Requirements for ensuring a long-lasting, direct bone-to-implant anchorage in man, *Acta Orthop Scand* 52:155–170. doi: http://dx.doi.org/10.3109/17453678108991776
8. Albrektsson, T., 1983, Direct bone anchorage of dental implants, *J Prosthet Dent* 50:255–261. doi: http://dx.doi.org/10.1016/0022-3913(83)90027-6
9. Venugopal, B. and Luckey, T.D., 1978, *Metal Toxicity in Mammals,* Plenum Press, New York, NY.
10. Plenk, H. and Zitter, H., 1996, Material considerations, In: G.Watzek ed., *Endosseous Implants: Scientific and Clinical Aspects*, Quintessence, Hanover Park, IL.
11. Lemons, J.E., 1988, Dental implant retrieval analyses, *J Dent Educ* 52:748–756.
12. Lemons, J.E., Lucas, L.C. and Johansson, B., 1992, Intraoral corrosion resulting from coupling dental implants and restorative metallic systems, *Implant Dent* 1:107–112. doi: http://dx.doi.org/10.1097/00008505-199205000-00002
13. Zitter, H. and Plenk, H., 1987, The electrochemical behavior of metallic implant materials as an indicator of their biocompatibility, *J Biomed Mater Res* 21:881–896. doi: http://dx.doi.org/10.1002/jbm.820210705
14. Schroeder, A., Sutter, F. and Krekeler, G., 1991, *Oral Implantology*. Geor Thieme Verlag Stuttgart, New York, NY, pp. 45–48.
15. www.soils.wisc/edu
16. Sakurai, H., 2000, *Why are Metals Important to Human Body?* Kodansha, Tokyo, pp. 59–65.
17. Fuwa, K., 1980, *Living Organisms and Heavy Metals*. Kodansah-Scientific, Tokyo, pp. 33–56.
18. Hallab, N.J., Anderson, S., Caicedo, M., Brasher, A., Mikecz, K. and Jacobs, J.J., 2005, Effects of soluble metals on human peri-implant cells, *J Biomed Mater Res A* 74:124–140. doi: http://dx.doi.org/10.1002/jbm.a.30345
19. Maurer, A.M., Merritt, K. and Brown, S.A., 1994, Cellular uptake of titanium and vanadium from addition of salts or fretting corrosion in vitro, *J Biomed Mater Res* 28:241–246. doi: http://dx.doi.org/10.1002/jbm.820280215
20. Evans, E.J. and Benjamin, M., 1987, The effect of grinding conditions on the toxicity of cobalt-chrome-molybdenum particles in vitro, *Biomaterials* 8:377–384. doi: http://dx.doi.org/10.1016/0142-9612(87)90009-3
21. Yang, R.S., Tsai, K.S. and Liu, S.H., 2004, Titanium implants enhance pulmonary nitric oxide production and lung injury in rats exposed to endotoxin, *J Biomed Mater Res A* 69:561–566. doi: http://dx.doi.org/10.1002/jbm.a.30041
22. http://en.wikipedia.org/wiki/Toxicity
23. Shanbhag, A., Jacobs, J.J., Black, J., Galante, J.O. and Glant, T.T., 1994, Macrophage/particle interactions: Effects of size, composition and surface area, *J Biomed Mater Res* 28:81–90. doi: http://dx.doi.org/10.1002/jbm.820280111
24. Takeda, K., Shinkai, Y., Suzumi, K., Yanagita, S., Umezawa, M., Yokota, S., Tainaka, H., Oshio, S., Ihara, T. and Sugamata, M., 2011, Health effects of nanomaterials on next generation, Yakugaku Zasshi: *The Pharm Soc Japan* 131:229–236. doi: http://dx.doi.org/10.1248/yakushi.131.229

25. Morais, L.S., Serra, G.G., Muller, C.A., Andrade, L.R., Palermo, E.F.A., Elias, C.N. and Meyers, M., 2007, Titanium alloy mini-implants for orthodontic anchorage: Immediate loading and metal ion release, *Acta Biomaterialia* 3:331–339. doi: http://dx.doi.org/10.1016/j.actbio.2006.10.010
26. Wood, J.F.L., 1974, Patient sensitivity to alloy used in partial denture, *Br Dent J* 136:423–424. doi: http://dx.doi.org/10.1038/sj.bdj.4803203
27. Menne, T., Christophersen, J. and Green, A., 1989, Epidemiology of nickel dermatitis. In: H.I. Maibach, T.Menne ed., *Nickel and the Skin: Immunology and Toxicology*. CRC Press, Boca Raton, FL. pp. 109–116.
28. Romaguera, C., Grimalt, F. and Vilaplana, J., 1988, Contact dermatitis from nickel: An investigation of its source, *Contact Dermatitis* 19:52–57. doi: http://dx.doi.org/10.1111/j.1600-0536.1988.tb02868.x
29. Meijer, C., Bredberg, M., Fischer, T. and Widstrom, L., 1995, Ear piercing and nickel and cobalt sensitization, in 520 young Swedish men doing compulsory military service, *Contact Dermatitis* 32:147–179. doi: http://dx.doi.org/10.1111/j.1600-0536.1995.tb00804.x
30. Gammelgaard, B., Fullerton, A., Avnstorp, C. and Menne, T., 1992, Permeation of chromium salts through human skin in vitro, *Contact Dermatitis* 27:302–310. doi: http://dx.doi.org/10.1111/j.1600-0536.1992.tb03284.x
31. Frigerio, E., Pigatto, P.D., Guzzi, G. and Altomare, G., 2011, Metal sensitivity in patients with orthopaedic implants: A prospective study, *Contact Dermatitis* 64:273–279. doi: http://dx.doi.org/10.1111/j.1600-0536.2011.01886.x
32. Peters, M.A., Schroeter, A.L., van Hale, H.M. and Broadbent, J.C., 1984, Pacemaker contact sensitivity, *Contact Dermatitis* 11:214–222. doi: http://dx.doi.org/10.1111/j.1600-0536.1984.tb00986.x
33. Layor, P.A., Revell, P.A., Gray, A.B., Wright, S., Railton, G.T. and Freeman, M.A., 1991, Sensitivity to titanium. A case of implant failure? *J Bone Joint Surg* 73:25–28.
34. http://www.melisa.org
35. Magnusson, B. and Kligman, A.M., 1969, The identification of contact allergens by animal assay; the Guinea pig maximization test, *J Invest Dermatol* 52:268–276.
36. Goodwin, B.J.G., Crecel, R.W.R. and Johnson, A.W., 1981, A comparison of three guinea-pig sensitization procedures for the detection of 19 reported human contact sensitizers, *Contact Dermatitis* 7:248–258. doi: http://dx.doi.org/10.1111/j.1600-0536.1981.tb04060.x
37. Mor, S., Ben-Efraim, S., Leibovici, J. and Ben-David, A., 1988, Successful contact sensitization to chromate in mice, *Int Arch Allergy Appl Immunol* 85:452–457. doi: http://dx.doi.org/10.1159/000234550
38. Vreeburg, K.J.J., de Groot, K., van Hoogstraten, I.M.W., von Blomberg, B.M.E. and Scheper, R.J., 1991, Successful induction of allergic contact dermatitis to mercury and chromium in mice, *Int Arch Allergy Appl Immunol* 96:179–183. doi: http://dx.doi.org/10.1159/000235491
39. Basketter, D.A. and Sholes, E.W., 1992, Comparison of the local lymph node assay with the guinea-pig maximization test for the detection of a range of contact allergens, *Food Chem Toxicol* 30:65–69. doi: http://dx.doi.org/10.1016/0278-6915(92)90138-B
40. Samits, M.H., Katz, S.A., Sheiner, D.M. and Lewis, J.E., 1975, Attempts to induce sensitization in guinea pigs with nickel complexes, *Acta Derm Venereol* 55:478–480.
41. Moller, H., 1984, Attempts to induce contact allergy to nickel in the mouse, *Contact Dermatitis* 10:65–68. doi: http://dx.doi.org/10.1111/j.1600-0536.1984.tb00337.x
42. Rohold, A.E., Nielsen, G.D. and Andersen, K.E., 1991, Nickel-sulphate-induced dermatitis in the guinea pig maximization test: A dose-response study, *Contact Dermatitis* 24:35–39. doi: http://dx.doi.org/10.1111/j.1600-0536.1991.tb01627.x

43. Zissu, D., Cavelier, C. and De Ceaurriz, J., 1987, Experimental sensitization of guinea-pigs to nickel and patch testing with metal samples, *Food Chem Toxicol* 25:83–85. doi: http://dx.doi.org/10.1016/0278-6915(87)90309-7
44. Ikarashi, Y., Momma, J., Tsuchiya, T. and Nakamura, A., 1996, Evaluation of skin sensitization potential of nickel, chromium, titanium and zirconium salts using guinea-pigs and mice, *Biomaterials* 17:2103–2108. doi: http://dx.doi.org/10.1016/0142-9612(96)00038-5
45. Harzer, W., Schröter, A., Gedrange, T. and Muschter, F., 2001, Sensitivity of titanium brackets to the corrosive influence of fluoride-containing toothpaste and tea, *Angle Orthod* 71:318–323.
46. Ryhanen, J., Niemi, E., Serlo, W., Niemela, E., Sandvik, P., Pernu, H. and Salo, T., 1997, Biocompatibility of nickel titanium shape memory metal and its corrosion behavior in human cell cultures, *J Biomed Mater Res* 35:451–457. doi: http://dx.doi.org/10.1002/(SICI)1097-4636(19970615)35:4<451::AID-JBM5>3.0.CO;2-G
47. McKay, G.C., Macnair, R., MacDonald, C. and Grant, M.H., 1996, Interactions of orthopaedic metals with an immortalized rat osteoblast cell line, *Biomaterials* 17:1339–1344. doi: http://dx.doi.org/10.1016/0142-9612(96)88681-9
48. Kerosuo, H., Kullaa, A., Kerosuo, E., Kanerva, L. and Hensten-Ptterson, A., 1996, Nickel allergy in adolescents in relation to orthodontic treatment and piercing of ears, *Am J Orthod Dentofac Orthop* 109:148–154. doi: http://dx.doi.org/10.1016/S0889-5406(96)70175-0
49. Berger-Gorbet, M., Broxup, B., Rivard, C. and Yahia, L'H., 1996, Biocompatibility testing of NiTi screw using immune-histochemistry on sections containing metallic implants, *J Biomed Mater Res* 32:243–248. doi: http://dx.doi.org/10.1002/(SICI)1097-4636(199610)32:2<243::AID-JBM14>3.3.CO;2-5
50. Bass, J.K., Finem H, and Cisnero, G.J., 1993, Nickel hypersensitivity in the prosthodontics patient, *Am J Orthod Dentofac Orthop* 103:280–285. doi: http://dx.doi.org/10.1016/0889-5406(93)70009-D
51. Rogers, S.D., Howie, D.W., Graves, S.E., Pearcy, M.J. and Haynes, D.R., 1997, In vitro human monocyte response to wear particles of titanium alloy containing vanadium or niobium, *J Bone Joint Surg* 79B:311–315. doi: http://dx.doi.org/10.1302/0301-620X.79B2.7192
52. Horowitz, S.M., Luchetti, W.T., Gonzales, J.B. and Ritchie, C.K., 1998, The effects of cobalt chromium upon macrophages, *J Biomed Mater Res* 41:468–473. doi: http://dx.doi.org/10.1002/(SICI)1097-4636(19980905)41:3<468::AID-JBM17>3.0.CO;2-E
53. Schmalz, G., Schuster, U. and Schweikl, H., 1998, Influence of metals in IL-6 release in vitro, *Biomaterials* 19:1689–1694. doi: http://dx.doi.org/10.1016/S0142-9612(98)00075-1
54. Torgerson, S., Gjerdet, N.R., Erichsen, E.S. and Bang, G., 1995, Metal particle and tissue chang adjacent to miniplates. A retrieval study, *Acta Odontol Scand* 53:65–71. doi: http://dx.doi.org/10.3109/00016359509005948
55. Alpert, B. and Seligson, D., 1996, Removal of asymptomatic bone plates used for orthognathic surgery and facial fractures, *J Oral Maxillofac Surg* 54:618–621. doi: http://dx.doi.org/10.1016/S0278-2391(96)90645-X
56. Mjoberg, B., Hellquist, E., Mallmin, H. and Lindh, U., 1997, Aluminum, Alzheimer's disease and bone fragility, *Acta Orthop Scand* 68:511–514. doi: http://dx.doi.org/10.3109/17453679708999016
57. Boyce, B.F., Byars, J., McWilliams, S., Mocan, M.Z., Elder, H.Y., Boyle, I.T. and Junor, B.J., 1992, Histological and electron microprobe studies of mineralization in aluminum-related osteomalacia, *J Clin Pathol* 45:502–550. doi: http://dx.doi.org/10.1136/jcp.45.6.502
58. Zaffe, D., Bertoldi, C. and Consolo, U., 2004, Accumulation of aluminium in lamellar one after implantation of titanium plates, Ti-6Al-4V screws, hydroxyapatite granules, *Biomaterials* 25:3837–3844. doi: http://dx.doi.org/10.1016/j.biomaterials.2003.10.020

59. Takemoto, S., Yamamoto, T., Tsuru, K., Hayakawa, S., Osaka, A. and Takashima, S., 2004, Platelet adhesion on titanium oxide gels: Effect of surface oxidation, *Biomaterials* 25:3485–3492. doi: http://dx.doi.org/10.1016/j.biomaterials.2003.10.070
60. Huang, N., Yang, P., Leng, Y.X., Chen, J.Y., Sun, H., Wang, J., Wang, J.G., Ding, P.D., Xi, T.F. and Leng, Y., 2003, Hemocompatibility of titanium oxide films, *Biomaterials* 24:2177–2187. doi: http://dx.doi.org/10.1016/S0142-9612(03)00046-2
61. Dion, I., Baquey, C., Monties, J.R. and Havlik, P., 1993, Harmocompatibility of Ti6Al4V alloy, *Biomaterials* 14:122–126. doi: http://dx.doi.org/10.1016/0142-9612(93)90222-N
62. Eriksson, A.S., Bjursten, L.M., Ericson, L.E. and Thomsen, P., 1988, Hollow implants in soft tissue allowing quantitative studies of cells and fluid at the implant interface, *Biomaterials* 9:86–90. doi: http://dx.doi.org/10.1016/0142-9612(88)90076-2
63. Eriksson, A.S. and Thomsen, P., 1991, Leukotriene B4, interleukin 1 and leucocyte accumulation in titanium and PTFE chambers after implantation in the rat abdominal wall, *Biomaterials* 12:827–830. doi: http://dx.doi.org/10.1016/0142-9612(91)90069-M
64. Elwing, H., Tengvall, P., Askendal, A. and Lunstroem, I., 1991, Lens on surface: A versatile method for the investigation of plasma protein exchange reactions on solid surfaces, *J Biomater Sci Polmer Educ* 3:7–16. doi: http://dx.doi.org/10.1163/156856292X00042
65. Graham, T.R., Dasse, K., Coumbe, A., Salih, V., Marrinan, M.T., Frazier, O.H. and Lewis, C.T., 1990, Neo-intimal development on textured biomaterial surfaces during clinical use of an implantable left ventricular assist device, *Eur J Cardio-Thorac Surg* 4:182–190. doi: http://dx.doi.org/10.1016/1010-7940(90)90002-H
66. Ellingen, J.E., 1991, A study on the mechanism of protein adsorption to TiO_2, *Biomaterials* 12:593–596. doi: http://dx.doi.org/10.1016/0142-9612(91)90057-H
67. Sunny, M.C. and Sharma, C.P., Titanium–protein interaction changes with oxide layer thickness, *J Biomater Appl* 6:89–98. doi: http://dx.doi.org/10.1177/088532829100600107
68. Merritt, K., Edwards, C.R. and Brown, S.A., 1988, Use of an enzyme linked immunosorbent assay (ELISA) for quantification of proteins on the surface of materials, *J Biomed Mater Res* 22:99–109. doi: http://dx.doi.org/10.1002/jbm.820220203
69. Muramatsu, K., Uchida, M., Kim, H-M., Fujisawa, A. and Kokubo, T., 2003, Thromboresistance of alkali and heat-treated titanium metal formed with apatite, *J Biomed Mater Res A* 65:409–416. doi: http://dx.doi.org/10.1002/jbm.a.10494
70. Suska, F., Gretzer, C., Esposito, M., Tengvall, P. and Thomsen, P., 2005, Monocyte viability on titanium and copper coated titanium, *Biomaterials* 26:5942–5950. doi: http://dx.doi.org/10.1016/j.biomaterials.2005.03.017
71. Maitz, M.F. and Shevchenko, N., 2006, Plasma-immersion ion-implanted nitinol surface with depressed nickel concentration for implants in blood, *J Biomed Mater Res A* 76:356–365. doi: http://dx.doi.org/10.1002/jbm.a.30526
72. Martinesi, M., Bruni, S., Stio, M., Treves, C. and Borgioli, F., 2005, *In vitro* interaction between surface-treated Ti-6Al-4V titanium alloy and human peripheral blood mononuclear cells, *J Biomed Mater Res A* 74:197–207. doi: http://dx.doi.org/10.1002/jbm.a.30366
73. Thor, A., Rasmusson, L., Wennerberg, A., Thomsen, P., Hirsch, J.M., Nilsson, B. and Hong, J., 2007, The role of whole blood in thrombin in contact with various titanium surfaces, *Biomaterials* 28:966–974. doi: http://dx.doi.org/10.1016/j.biomaterials.2006.10.020
74. Li, Y., Wong, C., Xiong, J., Hodgson, P. and Wen, C., Cytotoxicity of titanium and titanium alloying elements, *J Dent Res* 89:493–497. doi: http://dx.doi.org/10.1177/0022034510363675
75. Kumazawa, R., Watari, F., Takashi, N., Tanimura, Y., Uo, M. and Totsuka, Y., 2002, Effects of Ti ions and particles on neutrophil function and morphology, *Biomaterials* 23:3757–3764. doi: http://dx.doi.org/10.1016/S0142-9612(02)00115-1

76. Harris, L.G., Patterson, L.M., Bacon, C., Gwynn, I. and Richards, R.G., 2005, Assessment of the cytocompatibility of different coated titanium surfaces to fibroblasts and osteoblasts, *J Biomed Mater Res A* 73:12–20. doi: http://dx.doi.org/10.1002/jbm.a.30276
77. Yamamoto, A., Honma, R. and Sumita, M., 1998, Cytotoxicity evaluation of 43 metal salts using murine fibroblasts and osteoblastic cells, *J Biomed Mater Res* 39:331–340. doi: http://dx.doi.org/10.1002/(SICI)1097-4636(199802)39:2<331::AID-JBM22>3.0.CO;2-E
78. Yamamoto, A., Honma, R., Tanaka, A. and Sumita, M., 1999, Generic tendency of metal salt cytotoxicity for six cell lines, *J Biomed Mater Res* 47:396–403. doi: http://dx.doi.org/10.1002/(SICI)1097-4636(19991205)47:3<396::AID-JBM15>3.0.CO;2-R
79. Yamamoto, A., Kobayashi, T., Sumita, M., Yamamoto, A. and Hanawa, T., 2002, Mutagenicity evaluation of forty-one metal salts by the *umu* tests, *J Biomed Mater Res* 59:176–183. doi: http://dx.doi.org/10.1002/jbm.1231
80. Okazaki, Y. and Gotoh, E., 2000, Effect of metal released from Ti alloy wear powder on cell viability, *Mater Trans JIM* 41:1247–1255.
81. Yamamoto, A., Honma, R., Sumita, M. and Hanawa, T., 2004, Cytotoxicity evaluation of ceramic particles of different sizes and shapes, *J Biomed Mater Res* 68A:244–256. doi: http://dx.doi.org/10.1002/jbm.a.20020
82. Mu, Y., Kohyama, Y. and Hanawa, T., 2000, Metal ion releases from titanium with active oxygen species generated by rat macrophages in vitro, *J Biomed Mater Res* 49:238–243. doi: http://dx.doi.org/10.1002/(SICI)1097-4636(200002)49:2<238::AID-JBM12>3.0.CO;2-J
83. Manceur, A., Chellat, F., Merhi, Y., Chumlyakov, Y. and Yahia, L'H., 2003, *In vitro* cytotoxicity evaluation of a 50.8% NiTi single crystal, *J Biomed Mater Res* 67A:641–646. doi: http://dx.doi.org/10.1002/jbm.a.10134
84. Bordji, K., Jouzeau, J.Y., Mainard, D., Payan, E., Netter, P., Rie, K.T., Stucky, T. and Hage-Ali, M., 1996, Cytocompatibility of Ti–6Al–4V and Ti–5Al–2.5Fe alloys according to three surface treatments, using human fibroblasts and osteoblasts, *Biomaterials* 17:929–940. doi: http://dx.doi.org/10.1016/0142-9612(96)83289-3
85. Wever, D.J., Veldhuizen, A.G., Sanders, M.M. and Schakenraad, J.M., 1997, Cytotoxic, allergic and genotoxic activity of a nickel–titanium alloy, *Biomaterials* 18:1115–1120. doi: http://dx.doi.org/10.1016/S0142-9612(97)00041-0
86. Yeung, K.W.K., Poon, J.W.Y., Liu, X.Y., Ho, J.P.Y., Chung, C.Y., Chu, P.K., Lu, W.W., Chan, D. and Cheung, K.M.C., 2005, Investigation of nickel suppression and cytocompatibility of surface-treated nickel-titanium shape memory alloys by using plasma immersion ion implantation, *J Biomed Mater Res A* 72:238–245. doi: http://dx.doi.org/10.1002/jbm.a.30201
87. Yeung, K.W.K., Poon, R.W.Y., Liu, X.Y., Ho, J.P.Y., Chung, C.Y., Chu, P.K., Lu, W.W., Chan, D. and Cheung, K.M.C., 2005, Corrosion resistance, surface mechanical properties, and cytocompatibility of plasma immersion ion implantation-treated nickel-titanium shape memory alloys, *J Biomed Mater Res A* 75:256–267. doi: http://dx.doi.org/10.1002/jbm.a.30413
88. Fukushima, O., Yoneyama, T., Doi, H. and Hanawa, T., 2006, Corrosion resistance and surface characterization of electrolyzed Ti–Ni alloy, *Dent Mater J* 25:151–160. doi: http://dx.doi.org/10.4012/dmj.25.151
89. Tada, H., Shibo, O., Kuroshima, K., Koyama, M. and Tsukamoto, K., 1986, An improved colorimetric assay for interleukin-2, *J Immunol Methods* 93:157–165.
90. Es-Souni, M., Es-Souni, M. and Brandies, H.F., 2001, On the transformation behavior, mechanical properties and biocompatibility of two NiTi-based shape memory alloys: $NiTi_{42}$ and $NiTi_{42}Cu_7$, *Biomaterials* 22:2153–2161. doi: http://dx.doi.org/10.1016/S0142-9612(00)00406-3

91. Niinomi, M., 2003, Fatigue performance and cytotoxicity of low rigidity titanium alloy, Ti-29Nb-13Ta-4.6Zr, *Biomaterials* 24:2673–2683. doi: http://dx.doi.org/10.1016/S0142-9612(03)00069-3
92. Borenfreund, E. and Purener, J.A., 1985, Toxicity determined in vitro by morphological alternations and neutral absorption, *Toxicol Lett* 24:119–124. doi: http://dx.doi.org/10.1016/0378-4274(85)90046-3
93. Mosman, T., 1983, Rapid colorimetric assay for cellular growth and survival, Application of proliferation and cytotoxicity assay, *J Immunol Methods* 65:55–63. doi: http://dx.doi.org/10.1016/0022–1759(83)90303-4
94. Spriano, S., Bosetti, M., Bronzoni, M., Vernè, E., Maina, G., Bergo, V. and Cannas, M., 2005, Surface properties and cell response of low metal ion release Ti-6Al-7Nb alloy after multi-step chemical and thermal treatments, *Biomaterials* 26:1219–1229. doi: http://dx.doi.org/10.1016/j.biomaterials.2004.04.026
95. Hou, X., Weiler, A., Winger, J.N., Morris, J.R. and Borke, J.L., 2009, Rat model for studying tissue changes induced by the mechanical environment surrounding titanium implants, *Int J Oral Maxillofac Implants* 24:800–807.
96. Kang, M.K., Moon, S.K., Kim, K.M. and Kim, K.N., 2011, Antibacterial effect and cytocompatibility of nano-structured TiO_2 film containing Cl, *Dent Mater J* 39:790–798. doi: http://dx.doi.org/10.4012/dmj.2011-021
97. Olmedo, D.G., Tasat, D.R, Guglielmotti, E.P. and Cabrini, R.L., 2008, Biological response of tissues with macrophagic activity to titanium dioxide, *J Biomed Mater Res A* 84:1087–1093. doi: http://dx.doi.org/10.1002/jbm.a.31514
98. Lim, Y.J., Oshida, Y., Barco, T. and Andres, C.J., 2001, Surface characterization of variously treated titanium materials, *Int J Oral Maxillofac Implants* 16:333–342.
99. Rupp, F., Scheideler, L., Eichler, M. and Geis-Gerstorfer, J., 2011, Wetting behavior of dental implants, *Int J Oral Maxillofac Implants* 26:1256–1266.
100. Eriksson, C., Lausmaa, J. and Nygren, H., 2001, Interactions between human whole blood and modified TiO_2-surfaces: Influence of surface topography and oxide thickness on leukocyte adhesion and activation, *Biomaterials* 22:1987–1996. doi: http://dx.doi.org/10.1016/S0142-9612(00)00382-3
101. Wen, X., Wang, X. and Zhang, N., 1996, Microsurface of metallic biomaterials: A literature review, *J Biomed Mater Eng* 6:173–189.
102. Keller, J.C., Dougherty, W.J., Grotendorst, G.R. and Wrightman, J.P., 1989, In vitro cell attachment to characterized cpTi surface, *J Adhesion* 28:115–133.
103. Keller, J.C., Wrightman, J.P. and Dougherty, W.J., 1989, Characterization of acid passivated cpTi surfaces, *J Dent Res* 68:872.
104. Keller, J.C., Draughn, R.A., Wrightman, J.P. and Dougherty, W.J., 1990, Characterization of sterilized CP titanium implant surfaces, *Int J Oral Maxillofac Implants* 5:360–369.
105. Schroeder, A., Van der Zypen, E., Stich, H. and Sutter, F., 1981, The reactions of bone, connective tissue and epithelium to endosteal implants with titanium sprayed surfaces, *J Maxillofac Surg* 9:15–25. doi: http://dx.doi.org/10.1016/S0301-0503(81)80007-0
106. Buser, D., Schenk, R.K., Steinemann, S., Fiorellinni, J.P., Fox, C.H. and Stich, H., 1991, Influence of surface characteristics on bone integration of titanium implants. A histomorpho-metric study in miniature pigs, *J Biomed Mater Res* 25:889–902. doi: http://dx.doi.org/10.1002/jbm.820250708
107. Rich, A. and Harris, A.K., 1981, Anomalous preferences of cultured macrophages for hydrophobic and roughended substrata, *J Cell Sci* 50:1–7.
108. Murray, D.W., Raem, T. and Rushton, N., 1989, The influence of the surface energy and roughness of implants on bone resorption, *J Bone Joint Surg* 71B:632–637.

109. Oshida, Y., 2000, Requirements for successful biofunctional implants. In: L'H.Yahia ed., *International Symposium on Advanced Biomaterials*, Montréal, Canada, p. 5.
110. Oshida, Y., 2007, *Bioscience and Bioengineering of Titanium Materials*, Elsevier, London, UK.
111. Cherhoudi, B., Gould, T.R. and Brunette, D.M., 1988, Effects of a grooved epoxy substratum on epithelial behavior in vivo and in vitro, *J Biomed Mater Res* 22:459–477. doi: http://dx.doi.org/10.1002/jbm.820220603
112. von Recum, A.F., 1990, New aspects of biocompatibility: Motion at the interface. In: G.Heimke, U.Soltesz, A.J.C.Lee, ed., *Clinical Implant Materials*. Elsevier Science Pub, Amsterdam, pp. 297–302.
113. Ratner, B.D., 1983, Surface characterization of biomaterials by electron spectroscopy for chemical analysis, *Ann Biomed Eng* 11:313–336. doi: http://dx.doi.org/10.1007/BF02363290
114. Baro, A.M., Garcia, N., Miranda, R., Vázquez, L., Aparicio, C., Olivé, J. and Lausmaa, J., 1986, Characterization of surface roughness in titanium dental implants measured with scanning tunneling microscopy at atmospheric pressure, *Biomaterials* 7:463–466. doi: http://dx.doi.org/10.1016/0142-9612(86)90036-0
115. Kasemo, B., 1983, Biocompatibility of titanium implants: Surface science aspects, *J Prosthet Dent* 49:832–837. doi: http://dx.doi.org/10.1016/0022-3913(83)90359-1
116. Moroni, A., Caja, V.L., Egger, E.L., Trinchese, L. and Chao, E.Y., 1994, Histomorphometry of hydroxylapatite coated and uncoated porous titanium bone implants, *Biomaterials* 15:926–930. doi: http://dx.doi.org/10.1016/0142-9612(94)90119-8
117. Keller, J.C., Young, F.A. and Natiella, J.R., 1987, Quantitative bone remolding resulting from the use of porous dental implants, *J Biomed Mater Res* 21:305–319. doi: http://dx.doi.org/10.1002/jbm.820210304
118. Pilliar, R., Deporter, D.A., Watson, P.A. and Valiquette, N., 1991, Dental implant design-effect on bone remodeling, *J Biomed Mater Res* 25:467–483. doi: http://dx.doi.org/10.1002/jbm.820250405
119. Gilbert, J.L. and Berkery, C.A., 1995, Electrochemical reaction to mechanical disruption of titanium oxide films, *J Dent Res* 74:92–96.
120. Brunette, D.M., 1988, The effects of implant surface topography on the behavior of cells, *Int J Oral Maxillofac Implants* 3:231–246.
121. Chehroudi, B., Gould, T.R.L. and Brunette, D.M., 1990, Titanium-coated micromachined grooves of different dimensions affect epithelial and connective tissue cells differently in vitro, *J Biomed Mater Res* 24:1206–1219. doi: http://dx.doi.org/10.1002/jbm.820240906
122. Chehroudi, B., Gould, T.R.L. and Brunette, D.M., 1990, Effects of a grooved titanium coated implant surface on epithelial cell behavior, in vitro and in vivo, *J Biomed Mater Res* 24:1067–1085.
123. Michaels, C.M., Keller, J.C., Stanford, C.M. and Solursh, M., 1989, In vitro cell attachment of osteblast-like cells to titanium, *J Dent Res* 68:276.
124. Keller, J.C., Stanford, C.M., Wightman, J.P., Draughn, R.A. and Zaharias, R., 1994, Characterizations of titanium implant surfaces (Pt. 3), *J Biomed Mater Res* 28:939–946. doi: http://dx.doi.org/10.1002/jbm.820280813
125. Oshida, Y., Hashem, A., Nishihara, T. and Yapchulay, M.V., 1994, Fractal dimension analysis of mandibular bones: Toward a morphological compatibility of implants, *J Biomed Mater Eng* 4:397–407.
126. Klokkevold, P.R., Nishimura, R.D., Adachi, M. and Caputo, A., 1997, Osseointegration enhanced by chemical etching of the titanium surface. A torque removal study in the rabbit, *Clin Oral Implants Res* 8:442–447. doi: http://dx.doi.org/10.1034/j.1600-0501.1997.080601.x

127. Mattila, R.H., Laurila, P., Rekola, J., Gunn, J., Lassila, L.V., Mäntylä, T., Aho, A.J. and Vallitu, P.K., 2009, Bone attachment to glass-fibre-reinforced composite implant with porous surface, *Acta Biomater* 5:1639–1646. doi: http://dx.doi.org/10.1016/j.actbio.2009.01.020
128. Chehroudi, B., Ghrebi, S., Murakami, H., Waterfield, J.D., Owen, G. and Brunette, D.M., 2010, Bone formation on rough, but not polished, subcutaneously implanted Ti surfaces is preceded by macrophage accumulation, *J Biomed Mater Res A* 93:724–737.
129. Bhola, R., Bhola, S.M., Brajendra Mishra, B., Ayers, R., Olson, D.L. and Ohno, T., 2011, Cellular response of titanium and its alloys as implants, *J Oral Implantol* 37:387–399. doi: http://dx.doi.org/10.1563/AAID-JOI-D-09-00075.1
130. Kasemo, B. and Lausmaa, J., 1986, Surfaces science aspects on inorganic biomaterials, *CRC Crit Rev Biocomp* 2:335–380.
131. http:www.medterms.com
132. http.alan.kennedy.name/crohns
133. Masuda, T., Salvi, G.E., Offenbacher, S., Fleton, D. and Cooper, L.F., 1997, Cell and matrix reactions at titanium implants in surgically prepared rat tibiae, *Int J Oral Maxillofac Implants* 1:472–485.
134. Rosengren, A., Johansson, B.R., Danielsen, N., Thomsen, P. and Ericson, L.E., 1996, Immuno-histochemical studies on the distribution of albumin, fibrinogen, fibronectin, IgG and collagen around PTFE and titanium implants, *Biomaterials* 17:1779–1786. doi: http://dx.doi.org/10.1016/0142-9612(95)00358-4
135. Chehroudi, B., McDonnel, D. and Brunette, D.M., 1997, The effects of micromachined surfaces on formation of bonelike tissue on subcutaneous implants as assessed by radiography and computer image processing, *J Biomed Mater Res* 34:279–290. doi: http://dx.doi.org/10.1002/(SICI)1097-4636(19970305)34:3<279::AID-JBM2>3.0.CO;2-H
136. Larsson, C., Thomsen, P., Lausmaa, J., Rodahl, M., Kasemo, B. and Ericson, L.E., 1994, Bone response to surface modified implants: Studies on electropolished implants with different oxide thickness and morphology, *Biomaterials* 15:1062–1074. doi: http://dx.doi.org/10.1016/0142-9612(94)90092-2
137. Wälivaara, B., Askendal, A., Lundström, I. and Tengvall, P., 1996, Blood protein interaction with titanium surfaces, *J Biomater Sci Polym Edn* 8:41–48.
138. Kanagaraja, S., Lundström, I., Nygren, H. and Tengvall, P., 1996, Platelet binding and protein adsorption to titanium and gold after short time exposure to heparinized plasma and whole blood, *Biomaterials* 17:2225–2232. doi: http://dx.doi.org/10.1016/0142-9612(95)00311-8
139. Nygren, H., Eriksson, C. and Lausmaa, J., 1997, Adhesion and activation of platelets and polymorpho-nuclear granulocyte cells at TiO_2 surfaces, *J Lab Clin Med* 129:35–46. doi: http://dx.doi.org/10.1016/S0022-2143(97)90159-1
140. Tan, P., Luscinskas, F.W. and Homer-Vanniasinkam, S., 1999, Cellular and molecular mechanisms of inflammation and thrombosis, *Eur J Vasc Endovasc Surg* 17:373–389. doi: http://dx.doi.org/10.1053/ejvs.1998.0759
141. Brown, K.K., Henson, P.M., Maclouf, J., Moyle, M., Ely, J.A. and Worthen, G.S., 1998, Neutrophil-platelet adhesion: Relative roles of platelet P-selection and neutrophil β2 (CD18) integrins, *Am J Respir Cell Mol Biol* 8:100–110. doi: http://dx.doi.org/10.1165/ajrcmb.18.1.2314
142. De La Cruz, C., Haimovich, B. and Greco, R.S., Immobilized IgG and fibrinogen differentially affect the cytoskeletal organization and bactericidal function of adherent neutrophils, *J Surg Res* 80:28–34. doi: http://dx.doi.org/10.1006/jsre.1998.5262
143. Berton, G., Yan, S.R., Fumagalli, L. and Lowell, C.A., 1996, Neutrophil activation by adhesion: Mechanisms and pathophysiological implications, *Int J Clin Lab Res* 26:160–177. doi: http://dx.doi.org/10.1007/BF02592978

144. Fröhlich, D., Spertini, O. and Moser, R., 1998, The Fcγ receptor-mediated respiratory burst of rolling neutrophils to cytokine-activated, immune complex-bearing endothelial cells depends on L-selection but not E-selection, *Blood* 91:2558–2568.
145. Hansson, H-A., Albreksson, T. and Brånemark, P-I., 1983, Structural aspects of the interface between tissue and titanium implants, *J Prosthet Dent* 50:108–113. doi: http://dx.doi.org/10.1016/0022-3913(83)90175-0
146. Albreksson, T., Brånemark, P-I., Hansson, H-A., Kasemo, B., Larsson, K., Lundström, I., McQueen, D.H. and Skalak, R., 1983, The interface zone of inorganic implants in vivo: Titanium implants in bone, *Ann Biomed Eng* 11:1–27. doi: http://dx.doi.org/10.1007/BF02363944
147. Linder, L., Albreksson, T., Bråemark, P-I., Hansson, H-A., Ivarsson, B., Jönsson, U. and Lundström, I., 1983, Electron microscopic analysis of the bone–titanium interface, *Acta Orthop Scand* 54:45–52. doi: http://dx.doi.org/10.3109/17453678308992868
148. Mwenifumbo, S., Li, M., Chen, J., Beye, A. and Soboyejo, W.J., 2007, Cell/surface interactions on laser micro-textured titanium-coated silicon surfaces, *J Mater Sci Mater Med* 18:9–23. doi: http://dx.doi.org/10.1007/s10856-006-0658-9
149. Albreksson, T. and Hansson, H-A., 1986, An ultrastructural characterization of the interface between bone and sputtered titanium or stainless steel surfaces, *Biomaterials* 7:201–205. doi: http://dx.doi.org/10.1016/0142-9612(86)90103-1
150. Kempien, B., Schulte, W., Kleineikenscheidt, H., Linder, K., Scareyka, R. and Heimke, G., 1978, Lichtoptische und rasterelectronen-mikroskopische Untersuchungen an der grenzfläche von Implantaten aus Aluminium-oxidkeramik im Unterkierferknochen von Hunden, *Dtsch Zahnärtzl Z* 33:332–340.
151. Albrektsson, T., Hansson, H-A. and Ivarsson, B., 1985, Interface analysis of titanium and zirconium bone implants, *Biomaterials* 6:97–101. doi: http://dx.doi.org/10.1016/0142-9612(85)90070-5
152. Parsegian, V.A., 1983, Molecular forces governing tight contact between cellular surfaces and substrates, *J Prosthet Dent* 49:838–842. doi: http://dx.doi.org/10.1016/0022-3913(83)90360-8
153. McQueen, D., Sundgren, J-E., Ivarsson, B., Lundstrøm, I., Ekenstam, B., Svensson, A., Brånemark, P-I. and Albreksson, T., 1982, Auger electroscopic studies of titanium implants, In: A.J.C. Lee AJC, T. Abreksson P-I. Brånemark ed., *Clinical Applications of Biomaterials*. John Wiley, Chichester, UK. pp. 179–185.
154. Abe, M., 1982, Oxides and hydrous oxides of multivalent metals as inorganic ion exchangers, In: A. Clearfield ed., *Inorganic Ion Exchange Materials*. CRC Press, Boca Raton, FL, pp. 161–273.
155. Luo, E., Liu, Z., Wei, S.C., Cai, X.X. and Hu, J., 2008, Osteoblast adhesion to clodronate-hydroxyapatite composite, *Appl Surf Sci* 255:308–311. doi: http://dx.doi.org/10.1016/j.apsusc.2008.06.090
156. Wu, J., Guo, Y-Q., Yin, G-F., Chen, H-Q. and Kang, Y., 2008, Induction of osteoconductivity by BMP-2 gene modification of mesenchymal stem cells combined with plasma-sprayed hydroxyapatite coating, *Appl Surf Sci* 255:336–339. doi: http://dx.doi.org/10.1016/j.apsusc.2008.06.160
157. Bernardi, G. and Kawasaki, T., 1968, Chromatography of polypeptides and proteins on hydroxylapatite columns, *Biochim Biophys Acta* 160:301–310. doi: http://dx.doi.org/10.1016/0005-2795(68)90203-1
158. Embery, G. and Rølla, G., 1980, Interaction between sulphated macromolcules and hydroxyapatite studied by infrared spectroscopy, *Acta Odontol Scand* 38:105–108. doi: http://dx.doi.org/10.3109/00016358009003486

159. Rosengren, A., Johansson, B.R., Thomsen, P. and Ericson, L.E., 1994, A method for immunolocalization of extracellular proteins in association with the implant–soft tissue interface, *Biomaterials* 15:17–24. doi: http://dx.doi.org/10.1016/0142-9612(94)90190-2
160. Röstlund, T., Thomsen, P., Bjursten, L.M. and Ericson, L.E., 1990, Difference in tissue response to nitrogen-ion implanted titanium and c.p. titanium in the abdominal wall of the rat, *J Biomed Mater* Res 24:847–860. doi: http://dx.doi.org/10.1002/jbm.820240705
161. Eriksson, A.S., Lindblad, R., Ericson, L.E. and Thomsen, P., 1994, Distribution of cells around implants in soft tissue in the rat, *J Mater Sci Mater Med* 5:269–278. doi: http://dx.doi.org/10.1007/BF00122396
162. Johansson, C.B., Albrektsson, T., Ericson, L.E. and Thomsen, P. A., 1992, Quantitative comparison of the cell response to commercially pure titanium and Ti6Al4V implants in the abdominal wall of the rat, *J Mater Sci Mater Med* 3:126–136. doi: http://dx.doi.org/10.1007/BF00705280
163. Anderson, J.M. and Miller, K.M., 1984, Biomaterial biocompatibility and the macrophase, *Biomaterials* 5:5–10. doi: http://dx.doi.org/10.1016/0142-9612(84)90060-7
164. Miller, K.M. and Anderson, J.M., 1989, In vitro stimulation of fibroblast activity by factors generated from human monocytes activated by biomedical polymers, *J Biomed Mater Res* 23:911–930. doi: http://dx.doi.org/10.1016/0142-9612(84)90060-7
165. Bonfield, T.L., Colton, E. and Anderson, J.M., 1989, Plasma protein adsorbed biomedical polymers: Activation of human monocytes and induction of interleukin, *J Biomed Mater Res* 23:535–548. doi: http://dx.doi.org/10.1002/jbm.820230602
166. Healy, K.E. and Ducheyne, P., 1992, Hydration and preferential molecular adsorption on titanium in vitro, *Biomaterials* 13:553–561. doi: http://dx.doi.org/10.1016/0142-9612(92)90108-Z
167. Zeng, H., Chittur, K.K. and Lacefield, W.R., 1999, Analysis of bovine serum albumin adsorption on calcium phosphate and titanium surfaces, *Biomaterials* 20:377–384. doi: http://dx.doi.org/10.1016/S0142-9612(98)00184-7
168. MacDonald, D.E., Deo, N., Msrkovic, B., Stranick, M. and Somasundaran, P., 2002, Adsorption and dissolution behavior of human plasma fibronectin on thermally and chemically modified titanium dioxide particles, *Biomaterials* 23:1269–1279. doi: http://dx.doi.org/10.1016/S0142-9612(01)00317-9
169. Deligianni, D.D., Katsala, N., Ladas, S., Sotiropoulou, D., Amedee, J. and Missirlis, Y.F., 2001, Effect of surface roughness of the titanium alloy Ti-6Al-4V on human bone marrow cell response and on protein adsorption, *Biomaterials* 22:1241–1251. doi: http://dx.doi.org/10.1016/S0142-9612(00)00274-X
170. Yang, Y., Cavin, R and Ong, L.J., 2003, Protein adsorption on titanium surfaces and their effect on osteoblast attachment, *J Biomed Mater Res* 67A:344–349. doi: http://dx.doi.org/10.1002/jbm.a.10578
171. Schenk, R.K. and Buser, D., 1998, Osseointegration: A reality, *Periodontol* 17:22–35. doi: http://dx.doi.org/10.1111/j.1600-0757.1998.tb00120.x
172. Larsson, C., Esposito, M., Liao, H. and Thomsen, P., 2001, The titanium–bone interface in vivo. In: D.M. Brunette, P. Tengvall, M. Textor, P. Thomsen ed.. *Titanium in Medicine: Materials Science, Surface Science, Engineering, Biological Responses, and Medical Applications*, Springer, New York, NY, pp. 587–648.
173. Masuda, T., Yliheikkaila, P.K., Fleton, D.A. and Cooper, L.F., 1998, Generalizations regarding the process and phenomenon of osseointegration. Part I. In vivo studies, *Int I Oral Maxillofac Implant* 13:17–29.
174. Oshida, Y., Sachdeva, R. and Miyazaki, S., 1992, Microanalytical characterization and surface modification of NiTi orthodontic archwires, *J Biomed Mater Eng* 2:51–69.

175. Zinger, O., Anselme, K., Denzer, A., Habersetzer, P., Wieland, M., Jeanfils, J., Hardouin, P. and Landolt, D., 2004, Time-dependent morphology and adhesion of osteoblastic cells on titanium model surfaces featuring scale-resolved topography, *Biomaterials* 25:2695–2711. doi: http://dx.doi.org/10.1016/j.biomaterials.2003.09.111
176. Leven, R.M., Virdi, A.S. and Sumner, D.R., 2004, Patterns of gene expression in rat bone marrow stromal cells cultured on titanium alloy discs of different roughness, *J Biomed Mater Res A* 70:391–401. doi: http://dx.doi.org/10.1002/jbm.a.30082
177. Li, J.P., Li, S.H., Van Blitterswijk, C.A. and de Groot, K., 2005, A novel porous Ti6Al4V: Characterization and cell attachment, *J Biomed Mater Res A* 73:223–233. doi: http://dx.doi.org/10.1002/jbm.a.30278
178. Müller, C., Lüders, A., Hoth-Hannig, W., Hannig, M. and Ziegler, C., 2010, Initial bioadhesion on dental materials as a function of contact time, pH, surface wettability, and isoelectric point, *Langmuir*, 26:4136–4141. doi: http://dx.doi.org/10.1016/j.apsusc.2008.06.112
179. Weng, Y.J., Qi, F., Huang, N., Wang, J., Cheng, J.Y. and Leng, Y.X., 2008, Photochemical immobilization of bovine serum albumin on Ti–O and evaluations in vitro and in vivo, *Appl Surf Sci* 255:489–493. doi: http://dx.doi.org/10.1016/0142-9612(96)83280-7
180. Wassell, D.T.H. and Embery, G., 1996, Adsorption of bovine serum albumin on to titanium powder, *Biomaterials* 17:859–864.
181. Webster, T.J., Ergun, C., Doremus, R.H. and Lanford, W.A., 2003, Increased osteoblast adhesion on titanium-coated hydroxylapatite that forms $CaTiO_3$, *J Biomed Mater Res A* 67: 975–980. doi: http://dx.doi.org/10.1002/jbm.a.10160
182. MacDonald, D.E., Rapuano, B.E., Deo, N., Stranick, M., Somasundaran, P. and Boskey, A.L., 2004, Thermal and chemical modification of titanium–aluminum–vanadium implant materials: Effects on surface properties, glycoprotein adsorption, and MG63 cell attachment, *Biomaterials* 25:3135–3146. doi: http://dx.doi.org/10.1016/j.biomaterials.2003.10.029
183. Oshida, Y., Sachdeva, R. and Miyazaki, S., 1992, Changes in contact angles as a function of time on some pre-oxidized biomaterials, *J Mater Sci Mater Med* 3:306–312. doi: http://dx.doi.org/10.1007/BF00705298
184. Webster, T.J. and Ejiofor, J.U., 2004, Increased osteoblast adhesion on nanophase metals: Ti, Ti6Al4V, and CoCrMo, *Biomaterials* 25:4731–4739. doi: http://dx.doi.org/10.1016/j.biomaterials.2003.12.002
185. Jain, R. and von Recum, A.F., 2004, Fibroblast attachment to smooth and microtextured PET and thin cp-Ti films, *J Biomed Mater Res A* 68:296–304. doi: http://dx.doi.org/10.1002/jbm.a.20045
186. Zhang, Y.M., Bataillon-Linez, P., Huang, P., Zhao, Y.M., Han, Y., Traisnel, M., Xu, K.W. and Hildebrand, H.F., 2004, Surface analyses of micro-arc oxidized and hydrothermally treated titanium and effect on osteoblast behavior, *J Biomed Mater Res A* 68:383–391. doi: http://dx.doi.org/10.1002/jbm.a.20063
187. Nayab, S.N., Jones, F.H. and Olsen, I., 2004, Human alveolar bone cell adhesion and growth on ion-implanted titanium, *J Biomed Mater Res A* 69:651–657. doi: http://dx.doi.org/10.1002/jbm.a.30032
188. Maitz, M.F., Poon, R.W.Y,, Liu, X.Y., Pham, M-T. and Chu, P.K., 2005, Bioactivity of titanium following sodium plasma immersion ion implantation and deposition, *Biomaterials* 26:5465–5473. doi: http://dx.doi.org/10.1016/j.biomaterials.2005.02.006
189. Muhonen, V., Heikkinen, R., Danilov, A., Jämsä, T., Ilvesaro, J. and Tuukkanen, J., 2005, The phase state of NiTi implant material affects osteoclastic attachment, *J Biomed Mater Res A* 75:681–688. doi: http://dx.doi.org/10.1002/jbm.a.30477
190. Walboomers, X.F., Elder, S.E., Bumgardner, J.D. and Jansen, J.A., 2006, Hydrodynamic compression of young and adult rat osteoblast-like cells on titanium fiber mesh, *J Biomed Mater Res A* 76:16–24.

191. Clem, W.C., Konovalov, V.K., Chowdhury, S., Vohra, Y.K., Catledge, S.A. and Bellis, S.L., 2006, Mesenchymal stem cell adhesion and spreading on microwave plasma-nitrided titanium alloy, *J Biomed Mater Res A* 76:279–287.
192. Advincula, M.C., Rahemtulla, F.G., Advincula, R.C., Ada, E.T., Lemons, J.E. and Bellis, S.L., 2006, Osteo-blast adhesion and matrix mineralization on sol-gel-derived titanium oxide, *Biomaterials* 27:2201–2212. doi: http://dx.doi.org/10.1016/j.biomaterials.2005.11.014
193. Kakehi, S., Takeda, S. and Nakamura, M., 2006, Effects of UV-O_3 irradiation on wettability and cell adhesion of titanium, *J Jpn Soc Dent Mater Devices* 25:475–478.
194. Wälivaara, B., Aronsson, B-O., Rodahl, M., Lausmaa, J. and Tengvall, P., 1994, Titanium with different oxides: In vitro studies of protein adsorption and contact activation, *Biomaterials* 15:827–834. doi: http://dx.doi.org/10.1016/0142-9612(94)90038-8
195. Meyle, J., Wolburg, H. and von Recum, A.F., 1993, Surface micromorphology and cellular interactions, *J Biomater Appl* 7:362–374. doi: http://dx.doi.org/10.1177/088532829300700404
196. Bowers, K.T., Keller, J.C., Randolph, B.A., Wick, D.G. and Michaels, C.M., 1992, Optimization of surface micromorphology for enhanced osteoblast responses in vitro, *Int J Oral Maxillofac Implants* 7:302–310.
197. Schwartz, Z., Martin, J.Y., Dean, D.D., Simpson, J., Cochran, D.L. and Boyan, B.D., 1996, Effect of titanium surface roughness on chondrocyte proliferation, matrix production, and differentiation depends on the state of cell maturation, *J Biomed Mater Res* 30:145- 155. doi: http://dx.doi.org/10.1002/(SICI)1097-4636(199602)30:2<145::AID-JBM3>3.0.CO;2-R
198. Ahmad, M., Gawronski, D., Blum, J., Goldberg, J. and Gronowicz, G., 1999, Differential response of human osteoblast-like cells to commercially pure (cp) titanium grades 1 and 4, *J Biomed Mater Res* 46:121–131. doi: http://dx.doi.org/10.1002/(SICI)1097-4636(199907)46:1<121::AID-JBM14>3.0.CO;2-P
199. Khakbaznejad, A., Chehroudi, B. and Brunette, D.M., 2004, Effects of titanium-coated micromachined grooved substrata on orienting layers of osteoblast-like cells and collagen fibers in culture, *J Biomed Mater Res* 70A:206–218. doi: http://dx.doi.org/10.1002/jbm.a.30058
200. Zhu, X., Chen, J., Scheideler, L., Reichl, R. and Geis-Gerstorfer, J., 2004, Effects of topography and composition of titanium surface oxides on osteoblast responses, *Biomaterials* 25:4087–4103. doi: http://dx.doi.org/10.1016/j.biomaterials.2003.11.011
201. Saldaña, L., Vilaboa, N., Vallés, G., González-Cabrero, J. and Munuera, L., 2005, Osteoblast response to thermally oxidized Ti6Al4V alloy, *J Biomed Mater Res A* 73:97–107.
202. Kim, H.J., Kim, S.H., Kim, M.S., Lee, E.J., Oh, H.G., Oh, W.M., Park, S.W., Kim, W.J., Lee, G.J., Choi, N.G., Koh, J.T., Dinh, D.B., Hardin, R.R., Johnson, K., Sylvia, V.L., Schmitz, J.P. and Dean, D.D., 2005, Varying Ti–6Al–4V surface roughness induces different early morphologic and molecular responses in MG63 osteoblast-like cells, *J Biomed Mater Res* 74A:366–373.
203. Meredith, D.S., Eschbach, L., Wood, M.A., Riehle, M.O., Curtis, A.S.G. and Richards, R.G., 2005, Human fibroblast reactions to standard and electropolished titanium and Ti-6Al-7Nb, and electropolished stainless steel, *J Biomed Mater Res A* 75:541–555.
204. Nayab, S.N., Jones, F.H. and Olsen, I., 2005, Effects of calcium ion implantation on human bone cell interaction with titanium, *Biomaterials* 26:4717–4727. doi: http://dx.doi.org/10.1016/j.biomaterials.2004.11.044
205. Feng, B., Chen, J. and Zhang, X., 2002, Interaction of calcium and phosphate in apatite coating on titanium with serum albumin, *Biomaterials* 23:2499–2597. doi: http://dx.doi.org/10.1016/S0142-9612(01)00384-2

206. Tetè, S., Mastrangelo, F., Bianchi, A., Zizzari, V. and Scarano, A., 2009, Collagen fiber orientation around machined titanium and zirconia dental implans necks: An animal study, *Int J Oral Maxillofac Implants* 24:52–58.
207. Salohoglu, U., Boynuegri, D., Engin, D., Duman, A.N., G□kalp, P. and Balos, K., 2011, Bacterial adhesion and clononization differences between zirconium oxide and titanium alloys: An in vivo human study, *Int J Oral Maxillofac Implants* 26:101–107.
208. Faghihi, S., Azari, F., Szpunar, J.A., Vali, H. and Tabrizian, M., 2009, Titanium crystal orientation as a tool for the improved and regulated cell attachment, *J Biomed Mater Res A* 91:656–662. doi: http://dx.doi.org/10.1002/jbm.a.32275
209. Kimura, Y., Matsuaka, K., Yoshinari, M. and Inoue, T., 2012, Initial attachment of human oral keratinocytes cultured on zirconia or titanium, *Dent Mater J* 31:346–353. doi: http://dx.doi.org/10.4012/dmj.2011-189
210. Pugdee, K., Shibata, Y., Yamamichi, N., Tsutsumi, H., Yoshinari, M., Abiko, Y. and Hayakawa, T., 2007, Gene expression of MC3T3-E1 cells on frobronectin-immobilized titanium using tresyl chloride activation technique, *Dent Mater J* 26:647–655. doi: http://dx.doi.org/10.4012/dmj.26.647
211. Ko, H.C., Han, J.S., Bächle, M., Jang, J.H., Shin, S.W. and Kim, D.J., 2007, Initial osteoblast-like cell response to pure titanium and zirconia/alumina ceramics, *Dent Mater* 23:1349–1355. doi: http://dx.doi.org/10.1016/j.dental.2006.11.023
212. Rosa, A.L., Crippa, G.E., de Oliveria, P.T., Taba, M., Lefebvre, L.P. and Beloti, M.M., 2009, Human alveolar bone cell proliferation, expression of osteoblastic phenotype, and matrix mineralization on porous titanium produced by powder metallurgy, *Clin Oral Implants Res* 20:472–481. doi: http://dx.doi.org/10.1111/j.1600-0501.2008.01662.x
213. Shapira, L., Klinger, A., Tadir, A., Wilensky, A. and Halabi, A., 2009, Effect of niobium-containing titanium alloy on osteoblast behavior in culture, *Clin Oral Implants Res* 20:578–582.
214. Lossdörfer, S., Schwartz, Z., Wang, L., Lohmann, C.H., Turner, J.D., Wieland, M., Cochran, D.L. and Boyan, B.D., 2004, Microrough implant surface topographies increase osteogenesis by reducing osteoclast formation and activity, *J Biomed Mater Res A* 70:361–369.
215. Hu, H., Lin, C., Lui, P.P.Y. and Leng, Y., 2003, Electrochemical deposition of hydroxyapatite with vinyl acetate on titanium implants, *J Biomed Mater Res A* 65:24–29.
216. Vehof, J.W.M., van den Dolder, J., de Ruijter, J.E., Spauwen, P.H.M. and Jansen, J.A., 2003, Bone formation in CaP-coated and noncoated titanium fiber mesh, *J Biomed Mater Res A* 64:417–426. doi: http://dx.doi.org/10.1002/jbm.a.10288
217. Spoerke, E.D. and Stupp, S.I., 2003, Colonization of organoapatite-titanium mesh by preosteoblastic cells, *J Biomed Mater Res A* 67:960–969.
218. Rodriguez, R., Kim, K. and Ong, J.L., 2003, *In vitro* osteoblast response to anodized titanium and anodized titanium followed by hydrothermal treatment, *J Biomed Mater Res A* 65:352–358.
219. Lu, X. and Leng, Y., 2003, Quantitative analysis of osteoblast behavior on microgrooved hydroxyapatite and titanium substrata, *J Biomed Mater Res A* 66:677–687.
220. Barrère, F., van der Valk, C.M., Dalmeijer, R.A.J., Meijer, G., van Blitterswijk, C.A., de Groot, K. and Layrolle, P., 2003, Osteogenecity of octacalcium phosphate coatings applied on porous metal implants, *J Biomed Mater Res A* 66:779–788.
221. Zhao, G., Schwartz, Z., Wieland, M., Rupp, F., Geis-Gerstorfer, J., Cochran, D.L. and Boyan, B.D., 2005, High surface energy enhances cell response to titanium substrate microstructure, *J Biomed Mater Res A* 74:49–58. doi: http://dx.doi.org/10.1002/jbm.a.30320

222. Takeuchi, K., Saruwatari, L., Nakamura, H.K., Yang, J-M. and Ogawa, T., 2005, Enhanced intrinsic biomechanical properties of osteoblastic mineralized tissue on roughened titanium surface, *J Biomed Mater Res A* 72:296–305. doi: http://dx.doi.org/10.1002/jbm.a.30227
223. Chiang, C.Y., Chiou, S.H., Yang, W.E., Hsu, M., Yung, M.C., Tsai, M.L., Chen, L.K. and Huang, H.H., 2009, Formation of TiO_2 nano-network on titanium surface increases the human cell growth, *Dent Mater* 25:1022–1029. doi: http://dx.doi.org/10.1016/j.dental.2009.03.001
224. Buser, D., Weber, H.P., Donath, K., Fiorellini, J.P., Paquette, D.W. and Williams, R.C., 1992, Soft tissue reactions to non-submerged unloaded titanium implants in beagle dogs, *J Periodontol* 63:225–235. doi: http://dx.doi.org/10.1902/jop.1992.63.3.225
225. Abrahamsson, I., Berglundh, T., Wennstrom, J. and Lindhe, J., 1996, The peri-implant hard and soft tissues at different implant systems. A comparative study in the dog, *Clin Oral Implants Res* 7:212–219. doi: http://dx.doi.org/10.1034/j.1600-0501.1996.070303.x
226. Gargiulo, A.W., Wentz, F.M. and Orban, B., 1961, Dimensions and relations of the dentogingival junction in humans, *J Periodontol* 32:261–267. doi: http://dx.doi.org/10.1902/jop.1961.32.3.261
227. Arvidson, K., Fartash, B., Hilliges, M. and Kondell, P.A., 1996, Histological characteristics of peri-implant mucosa around Branemark and single-crystal sapphire implants, *Clin Oral Implants Res* 7:1–10. doi: http://dx.doi.org/10.1034/j.1600-0501.1996.070101.x
228. Berglundh, T., Lindhe, J., Ericsson, I., Marinello, C.P., Liljenberg, B. and Thomsen, P., 1991, The soft tissue barrier at implants and teeth, *Clin Oral Implants Res* 2:81–90. doi: http://dx.doi.org/10.1034/j.1600-0501.1991.020206.x
229. Eisenbarth, E., Meyle, J., Nachtigall, W. and Breme, J., 1996, Influence of the surface structure of titanium materials on the adhesion of fibroblasts, *Biomaterials* 17:1399–1403. doi: http://dx.doi.org/10.1016/0142-9612(96)87281-4
230. Jansen, J.A., van der Waerden, J.P., van der Lubbe, H.B. and de Groot, K., 1990, Tissue response to percutaneous implants in rabbits, *J Biomed Mater Res* 24:295–307. doi: http://dx.doi.org/10.1002/jbm.820240303
231. Hormia, M., Kononen, M., Kivilahti, J. and Virtanen, I., 1991, Immunolocalization of proteins specific for adherens junctions in humans gingival epithelial cells growth on differently processed titanium surfaces, *J Periodontal Res* 26:491–497. doi: http://dx.doi.org/10.1111/j.1600-0765.1991.tb01800.x
232. Mustafa, K., Silva Lopez, B., Hultenby, K., Wennerberg, A. and Arvidson, K., 1998, Attachment and proliferation of human oral fibroblasts to titanium surfaces with TiO_2 particles. A scanning electron microscopic and histomorphometic analysis, *Clin Oral Implants Res* 9:195–207. doi: http://dx.doi.org/10.1034/j.1600-0501.1998.090307.x
233. Kononen, M., Hormia, M., Kivilahti, J., Hautaniemi, J. and Thesleff, I., 1992, Effect of surface processing on the attachment, orientation, and proliferation of human gingival fibroblasts on titanium, *J Biomed Mater Res* 26:1325–1341. doi: http://dx.doi.org/10.1002/jbm.820261006
234. Abrahamsson, I., Zitzmann, N.U., Bergundh, T., Linder, E., Wennerberg, A. and Lindhe, J., 2002, The mucosal attachment to titanium implants with different surface characteristics: An experimental study in dogs, *J Clin Periodotol* 29:448–455. doi: http://dx.doi.org/10.1034/j.1600-051X.2002.290510.x
235. Barboza, E.P., Caula, A.L. and Carvalho, W.R., 2002, Crestal bone loss around submerged and exposed unloaded dental implants: A radiograophic and microbiological descriptive study, *Implant Dent* 11:162–169. doi: http://dx.doi.org/10.1097/00008505-200204000-00018

236. Raghoebar, G.M., Friberg, B., Grunert, I., Hobkirk, J.A., Tepper, G. and Wendelhag, I., 2003, 3-year prospective multicenter study on one-stage implant surgery and early loading in the edentulous mandible, *Clin Implant Dent Relat Res* 5:39–46. doi: http://dx.doi.org/10.1111/j.1708-8208.2003.tb00180.x
237. Chou, L., Firth, J.D., Uitto, V.J. and Brunette, D.M., 1995, Substratum surface topography alters cell shape and regulates fibronectin mRNA level, mRNA stability, secretion and assembly in human fibroblasts, *J Cell Sci* 108:1563–1573.
238. Uo, M., Watari, F., Yokoyama, A., Matsuno, H. and Kawasaki, T., 2001, Tissue reaction around metal implant observed by X-ray scanning analytical microscopy, *Biomaterials* 22:677–685. doi: http://dx.doi.org/10.1016/S0142-9612(00)00230-1
239. Sundgren, J-E., Bodö, P. and Lundström, I., 1986, Auger electron spectroscopic studies of the interface between human tissue and implants of titanium and stainless steel, *J Collid Interf Sci* 110:9–20. doi: http://dx.doi.org/10.1016/0021-9797(86)90348-6
240. Voggenreiter, G., Leiting, S., Brauer, H., Leiting, P., Majetschak, M., Bardenheuer, M. and Obertacke, U., 2003, Immuno-inflammatory tissue reaction to stainless-steel and titanium plates used for internal fixation of long bones, *Biomaterials* 24:247–254. doi: http://dx.doi.org/10.1016/S0142-9612(02)00312-5
241. Deporter, D., Watson, P., Pharoah, M., Levy, D. and Todescan, R., 1999, Five- to six-year results of a prospective clinical trial using the ENDOPORE dental implant and a mandibular overdenture, *Clin Oral Implants Res* 10:95–102. doi: http://dx.doi.org/10.1034/j.1600-0501.1999.100203.x
242. Buser, D., Nydegger, T., Oxland, T., Cochran, D.L., Schenk, R.K., Hirt, H.P., Sneitivy, D. and Nolte, L.P., 1999, Interface shear strength of titanium implants with a sandblasted and acid-etched surface: A biomechanically study in the maxilla of miniature pigs, *J Biomed Mater Res* 45:75–83. doi: http://dx.doi.org/10.1002/(SICI)1097-4636(199905)45:2<75::AID-JBM1>3.0.CO;2-P
243. Palmer, R.M., Plamer, P.J. and Smith, B.J., 2000, A 5-year prospective study of Astra single tooth implants, *Clin Oral Implants Res* 11:179–182. doi: http://dx.doi.org/10.1111/j.1600-0501.2000.tb00012.x
244. Testori, T., Wiseman, L., Woolfe, S. and Porter, S.S., 2001, A prospective multicenter clinical study of the osseitite implant: Four-years interim report, *Int J Oral Maxillofac Implants* 16:193–200.
245. Sul, Y-T., 2003, The significance of the surface properties of oxidized titanium to the bone response: Special emphasis on potential biochemical bonding of oxidized titanium implant, *Biomaterials* 24:3893–3907. doi: http://dx.doi.org/10.1016/S0142-9612(03)00261-8
246. Ishizawa, H., Fujiino, M. and Ogino, M., 1995, Mechanical and histological investigation of hydrothermally treated and untreated anodic titanium oxide films containing Ca and P, *J Biomed Mater Res* 29:1459–1468. doi: http://dx.doi.org/10.1002/jbm.820291118
247. Larsson, C., Emanuelsson, L., Thomsen, P., Ericson, L., Aronsson, B., Rodahl, M., Kasemo, B. and Lausmaa, J., 1997, Bone response to surface-modified titanium implants: Studies on the tissue response after one year to machined and electropolished implants with different oxide thicknesses, *J Mater Sci Mater Med* 8:721–729. doi: http://dx.doi.org/10.1023/A:1018548225899
248. Skripitz, R. and Aspenberg, P., 1998, Tensile bond between bone and titanium, *Acta Orthop Scand* 69:2–6. doi: http://dx.doi.org/10.3109/17453679809000938
249. Fini, M., Cigada, A., Rondelli, G., Chiesa, R., Giardino, R., Giavaresi, G., Aldini, N., Torricelli, P. and Vicentini, B., 1999, In vitro and vivo behaviour of Ca and P-enriched anodized titanium, *Biomaterials* 20:1587–1594. doi: http://dx.doi.org/10.1016/S0142-9612(99)00060-5

250. Henry, P., Tan, A.E. and Allan, B.P., 2000, Removal torque comparison of TiUnite and turned implants in the Greyhound dog mandible, *Appl Osseointegration Res* 1: 15–17.
251. Sul, Y-T., Johansson, C.B., Jeong, Y., Wennerberg, A. and Albrektson, T., 2002, Resonance frequency and removal torque analysis of implants with turned and anodized surface oxide, *Clin Oral Implants Res* 13:252–259. doi: http://dx.doi.org/10.1034/j.1600-0501.2002.130304.x
252. Sul, Y-T., Johansson, C.B., Jeong, Y., Röser, K., Wennerberg, A. and Albreksson, T., 2001, Oxidized implants and their influence on the bone response, *J Mater Sci Mater Med* 12:1025–1031. doi: http://dx.doi.org/10.1023/A:1012837905910
253. Sul, Y-T., Johansson, C.B. and Albreksson, T., 2002, Oxidized titanium screws coated with calcium ions and their performance in rabbit bone, *Int J Oral Maxillofac Implants* 17:625–634.
254. Meachim, G. and Williams, D.F., 1973, Changes in nonosseous tissue adjacent to titanium implants, *J Biomed Mater Res* 7:555–571. doi: http://dx.doi.org/10.1002/jbm.820070607
255. Albrektsson, T. and Jacobsson, M., 1987, Bone–metal interface in osseointegration, *J Prosthet Dent* 57:5–10. doi: http://dx.doi.org/10.1016/0022-3913(87)90344-1
256. Lausmaa, J., 1986, Chemical composition and morphology of titanium surface oxides, *Mater Res Soc Symp Proc* 55:351–359.
257. Kohavi, D., Schwartz, Z., Amir, D., Muller Mai, C., Gross, U. and Sela, J., 1992, Effect of titanium implants on primary mineralization following 6 and 14 days of rat tibial healing, *Biomaterials* 13:255–260. doi: http://dx.doi.org/10.1016/0142-9612(92)90193-R
258. Jasty, M., Bragdon, C.R., Haire, T., Mulroy, R.D. and Harris, W.H., 1993, Comparison of bone ingrowth into cobalt chrome sphere and titanium fiber mesh porous coated cementless canine acetabular components, *J Biomed Mater Res* 27:639–644. doi: http://dx.doi.org/10.1002/jbm.820270511
259. Hazan, R., Brener, R. and Oron, U., 1993, Bone growth to metal implants is regulated by their surface chemical properties, *Biomaterials* 14:570–574. doi: http://dx.doi.org/10.1016/0142-9612(93)90172-X
260. http://www.teambone.com/wolff.html
261. Chang, Y.S., Oka, M., Kobayashi, M., Gu, H.O., Li, Z.L., Nakamura, T. and Ikada, Y., 1996, Significance of interstitial bone ingrowth under load-bearing conditions: A comparison between solid and porous implant materials, *Biomaterials* 17:1141–1148. doi: http://dx.doi.org/10.1016/0142-9612(96)85917-5
262. Piattelli, A., Corigliano, M. and Scarano, A., 1996, Microscopical observations of the osseous responses in early loaded human titanium implants: A report of two cases, *Biomaterials* 17:1333–1337. doi: http://dx.doi.org/10.1016/0142-9612(96)88680-7
263. Goodman, S. and Aspenberg, P., 1992, Effect of amplitude of micromotion on bone ongrowth into titanium chambers implanted in the rabbit tibia, *Biomaterials* 13:944–948. doi: http://dx.doi.org/10.1016/0142-9612(92)90118-8
264. Li, J., Liao, H., Fartash, B., Hermansson, L. and Johnsson, T., 1997, Surface-dimpled commercially pure titanium implant and bone ingrowth, *Biomaterials* 18:691–696. doi: http://dx.doi.org/10.1016/S0142-9612(96)00185-8
265. French, A.A., Bowles, C.Q., Parharn, P.L., Eick, J.D., Killoy, W.J. and Cobb, C.M., 1989, Comparison of peri-implant stresses transmitted by four commercially available osseointegrated implants, *Int J Periodont Rest Dent* 9:221–230.
266. Bidez, M.W. and Misch, C.E., 1992, Force transfer in implant dentistry. Basic concepts and principles, *J Oral Implantol* 18:264–274.

267. Adell, R., Lekholm, U., Rockler, B. and Brånemark, P-I., 1981, A 15-yeat study of osseointegrated implants in the treatment of the edentulous jaws, *Int J Oral Surg* 10:387–416. doi: http://dx.doi.org/10.1016/S0300-9785(81)80077-4
268. Schliephake, H., Scharnweber, D., Dard, M., Rößler, S., Sewing, A. and Hüttmann, C., 2003, Biological performance of biomimetic calcium phosphate coating of titanium implants in the dog mandible, *J Biomed Mater Res A* 64:225–234. doi: http://dx.doi.org/10.1002/jbm.a.10363
269. Groessner-Schreiber, B., Neubert, A., Müller, W-D., Hopp, M., Griepentrog, M. and Lange, K.P., 2003, Fibroblast growth on surface-modified dental implants: An *in vitro* study, *J Biomed Mater Res A* 64:591–599. doi: http://dx.doi.org/10.1002/jbm.a.10417
270. Vasudev, D.P., Ricci, J.L., Sabatino, C., Li, P. and Parsons, J.R., 2004, *In vivo* evaluation of a biomimetic apatite coating grown on titanium surfaces, *J Biomed Mater Res A* 69:629–636. doi: http://dx.doi.org/10.1002/jbm.a.30028
271. Knabe, C., Howlett, C.R., Klar, F. and Zreiqat, H., 2004, The effect of different titanium and hydroxyapatite-coated dental implant surfaces on phenotypic expression of human bone-derived cells, *J Biomed Mater Res A* 71:98–107. doi: http://dx.doi.org/10.1002/jbm.a.30130
272. Lu, X., Leng, Y., Zhang, X., Xu, J., Qin, L. and Chan, C-W., 2005, Comparative study of osteoconduction on micromachined and alkali-treated titanium alloy surfaces in vitro and in vivo, *Biomaterials* 26:1793–1801. doi: http://dx.doi.org/10.1016/j.biomaterials.2004.06.009
273. Elmengaard, B., Bechtold, J.E. and Søballe, K., 2005, *In vivo* effects of RGD-coated titanium implants inserted in two bone-gap models, *J Biomed Mater Res A* 75:249–255. doi: http://dx.doi.org/10.1002/jbm.a.30301
274. Elmengaard, B., Bechtold, J.E. and Søballe, K., 2005, In vivo study of the effect of RGD treatment on bone ongrowth on press-fit titanium alloy implants, *Biomaterials* 26:3521–3526. doi: http://dx.doi.org/10.1016/j.biomaterials.2004.09.039
275. Uo, M., Asakura, K., Yokoyama, A., Ishikawa, M., Tamura, K., Totsuka, Y., Akasaka, T. and Watari, F., 2007, X-ray absorption fine structure analysis of titanium-implanted soft tissue, *Dent Mater J* 26:268–273. doi: http://dx.doi.org/10.4012/dmj.26.268
276. Chen, G.J., Wang, Z., Bai, H., Li, J.M. and Cai, H., 2009, A preliminary study on investigating the attachment of soft tissue onto micro-arc oxidized titanium alloy implants, *Biomed Mater* 4:015017. doi: http://dx.doi.org/10.1088/1748-6041/4/1/015017
277. Davies, J.E., 2003, Understanding peri-implant endosseous healing, *J Dent Edu* 67:932–949.
278. Eriksson, C., Broberg, M., Nygren, H. and Öster, L., 2003, Novel *in vivo* method for evaluation of healing around implants in bone, *J Biomed Mater Res A* 66:662–668. doi: http://dx.doi.org/10.1002/jbm.a.10029
279. Osborn, J.F., Kovacs, E. and Kallenberger, A., 1980, Hydroxylapatit Keramik—Entwicklung lines neuen Bioverkstoffes und erste tierexperimentelle Ergebnisse, *Dtsch Zahnärztl Z* 5:54–56.
280. Steinemann, S. and Werkstoff, H., 1988, Titan: In: A.Schroeder, F.Sutter, G.Krekeler, ed., *Orale Implantologie*. Stuttgart, Thieme.
281. Sugarawa, A., 2005, Self-healing calcium phosphates—the properties and the applications for bone regeneration, *Jpn J Maxillo Facial Implants* 4:41–49.
282. Scarano, A., Piattelli, M., Vrespa, G., Petrone, G., Iezzi, G. and Piattelli, A., 2003, Bone healing around titanium and titanium nitride-coated dental implants with three surfaces: An experimental study in rats, *Clin Implant Dent Relat Res* 5:103–111. doi: http://dx.doi.org/10.1111/j.1708-8208.2003.tb00191.x

283. Lee, J.E., Heo, S.J., Koak, J.Y., Kim, S.K., Han, C.H. and Lee, S.J., 2009, Healing response of cortical and cancellous bone around titanium implants, *Int J Oral Maxillofac Implants* 24:655–662.
284. Franco, R.L., Chiesa, R., de Oliveira, P.T., Beloti, M.M. and Rosa, A.L., 2008, Bone response to a Ca- and P-enriched titanium surface obtained by anodization, *Braz Dent J* 19:15–20. doi: http://dx.doi.org/10.1590/S0103-64402008000100003
285. Colnot, C., Romero, D.M., Huang, S., Rahman, J., Currey, J.A., Nanci, A., Brunski, J.B. and Helms, J.A., 2007, Molecular analysis off healing at a bone–implant interface, *J Dent Res* 86:862–867. doi: http://dx.doi.org/10.1177/154405910708600911
286. Lin, D.J., Chuang, C.C., Cher Lin, J.H., Lee, J.W., Ju, C.P. and Yin, H.S., 2007, Bone formation at the surface of low modulus Ti-7.5Mo implants in rabbit femur, *Biomaterials* 28:2582–2589. doi: http://dx.doi.org/10.1016/j.biomaterials.2007.02.005
287. Sato, N., Kubo, K., Yamada, M., Hori, N., Suzuki, T., Maeda, H. and Ogawa, T., 2009, Osteoblast mechanoresponses on Ti with different surface topographies, *J Dent Res* 88:812–816. doi: http://dx.doi.org/10.1177/0022034509343101
288. Saito, S., Sugimoto, N.,Morohashi,T., Kurabayashi, H., Shimizu, H., Yamasaki, K., Shiba, A., Yamada, S. and Shibasaki, Y., 2000, Endosseous titanium implants as anchors for mesiodistal tooth movement in the beagle dog, *Am J Orthod Dentofac Orthop* 118:601–607. doi: http://dx.doi.org/10.1067/mod.2000.110636
289. Bothe, R.T., Beaton, L.E. and Davenport, H.A., 1940, Reaction of bone to multiple metallic implants, *Surg Gynecol Obstet* 71:598–602.
290. Brånemark, P-I., Hansson, B.O., Adell, R., Briene, U., Lindstrom, J., Hallen, O. and Ohman, A., 1977, Osseointegrated implants in the treatment of the edentulous jaw, Experience from a 10-year period, *Scand J Plast Reconstr Surg Suppl* 16:1–132.
291. Misch, C.E. and Misch, C.M., 1999, Generic root form component terminology. In: *Implant Dentistry*, C.E. Misch ed., *Mosby: An Affiliate of Elsevier*, pp.13–15.
292. Brånemark, R., Brånemark, P-I., Rydevik, B. and Myers, R.R., 2001, Osseointegration in skeletal reconstruction and rehabilitation, *J Rehabil Res Dev* 38:175–182.
293. Zaffe, D., Bacna, R.R., Rizzo, S., Brusotti, C., Soncini, M., Pietrabissa, R., Cavani, F. and Quaglini, V., 2003, Behavior of the bone–titanium interface after push-in testing: A morphological study, *J Biomed Mater Res A* 64:365–371. doi: http://dx.doi.org/10.1002/jbm.a.10366
294. Rønold, H.J., Lyngstadaas, S.P. and Ellingsen, J.E., 2003, A study on the effect of dual blasting with TiO_2 on titanium implant surfaces on functional attachment in bone, *J Biomed Mater Res A* 67:524–530.
295. Nishiguchi, S., Fujibayashi, S., Kim, H-M., Kokubo, T. and Nakamura, T., 2003, Biology of alkali- and heat-treated titanium implants, *J Biomed Mater Res A* 67:26–35.
296. Giavaresi, G., Fini, M., Cigada, A., Chiesa, R., Rondelli, G., Rimondini, L., Aldini, N.N., Martini, L. and Giardino, R., 2003, Histomorphometric and microhardness assessments of sheep cortical bone surrounding titanium implants with different surface treatments, *J Biomed Mater Res A* 67:112–120.
297. Fujibayashi, S., Neo, M., Kim, H.M., Kokubo, T. and Namamura, T., 2004, Osteoinduction of porous bioactive titanium metal, *Biomaterials* 25:443–450. doi: http://dx.doi.org/10.1016/S0142-9612(03)00551-9
298. Takemoto, M., Fujibayashi, S., Neo, M., Suzuki, J., Kokubo, T. and Nakamura, T., 2005, Mechanical properties and osteoinductivity of porous bioactive titanium, *Biomaterials* 26:6014–6023. doi: http://dx.doi.org/10.1016/j.biomaterials.2005.03.019
299. Takemoto, M., Fujibayashi, S., Neo, M., Suzuki, J., Matsushita, T., Kokubo, T. and Nakamura, T., 2006, Osteoinductive porous titanium implants: Effect of sodium removal by

dilute HCl treatment, *Biomaterials* 27;2682–2691. doi: http://dx.doi.org/10.1016/j.biomaterials.2005.12.014

300. Sul, Y-T., Johansson, C., Byon, E. and Albrektsson, T., 2005, The bone response of oxidized bioactive and non-bioactive titanium implants, *Biomaterials* 26:6720–6730. doi: http://dx.doi.org/10.1016/j.biomaterials.2005.04.058
301. Aebli, N., Krebs, J., Stich, H., Schawalder, P., Walton, M., Schwenke, D., Gruner, H., Gasser, B. and Theis, J-C., 2003, *In vivo* comparison of the osseointegration of vacuum plasma sprayed titanium- and hydroxyapatite-coated implants, *J Biomed Mater Res A* 66:356–363. doi: http://dx.doi.org/10.1002/jbm.a.10508
302. Stewart, M., Welter, J.F. and Goldberg, V.M., 2004, Effect of hydroxyapatite/tricalcium-phosphate coating on osseointegration of plasma-sprayed titanium alloy implants, *J Biomed Mater Res A* 69:1–10. doi: http://dx.doi.org/10.1002/jbm.a.20071
303. Habibovic, P., Li, J., van der Valk, C.M., Meijer, G., Layrolle, P., van Blitterswijk, C.A.C.A., de Groot, K., 2005, Biological performance of uncoated and octacalcium phosphate-coated Ti6Al4V, *Biomaterials* 26:23–36. doi: http://dx.doi.org/10.1016/j.biomaterials.2004.02.026
304. Stangl, R., Pries, A., Loos, B., Müller, M. and Erben, R.G., 2004, Influence of pores created by laser superfinishing on osseointegration of titanium alloy implants, *J Biomed Mater Res A* 69:444–453. doi: http://dx.doi.org/10.1002/jbm.a.30013
305. Götz, H.E., Müller, M., Emmel, A., Holzwarth, U., Erben, R.G. and Stangl, R., 2004, Effect of surface finish on the osseointegration of laser-treated titanium alloy implants, *Biomaterials* 25:4057–4064. doi: http://dx.doi.org/10.1016/j.biomaterials.2003.11.002
306. Giannuzzi, L.A., Phifer, D., Giannuzzi, N.J. and Capuano, M.J., 2007, Two-dimensional analysis of bone/dental implant interfaces with the use of focused ion beam and electron microscopy, *J Oral Maxillofac Surg* 65:737–747. doi: http://dx.doi.org/10.1016/j.joms.2006.10.025
307. Stenport, V.F. and Jphansson, C.B., 2008, Evaluations of bone tissue integration to pure and alloyed titanium implants, *Clin Implant Dent Relat Res* 10:191–199. doi: http://dx.doi.org/10.1111/j.1708-8208.2007.00077.x
308. Morinaga, K., Kido, H., Sato, A., Watazu, A. and Matsuura, M., 2009, Chronological changes in the ultrastructure of titanium–bone interfaces: Analysis by light microscopy, transmission electron microscopy, and micro-computed tomography, *Clin Implant Dent Relat Res* 11:59–68. doi: http://dx.doi.org/10.1111/j.1708-8208.2008.00093.x
309. Kerner, S., Mogonney, V., Pavon-Djavid, G., Helay, G., Sedel, L. and Anagnostou, F., 2010, Bone tissue response to titanium implant surfaces modified with carboxylate and sulfonate groups, *J Mater Sci Mater Med* 21:707–715. doi: http://dx.doi.org/10.1007/s10856-009-3928-5
310. Freeman, C.O. and Brook, I.M., 2006, Bone response to a titanium aluminium nitride coating on metallic implants, *J Mater Sci Mater Med* 17:465–470. doi: http://dx.doi.org/10.1007/s10856-006-8474-9
311. Cordero; J., Munuera, L. and Folgueira, M.D., 1994, Influence of metal implants on infection. An experimental study in rabbits, *J Bone Joint Surg Br* 76:717–720.
312. Mombelli, A., 1999, In vitro models of biological responses to implant microbiological models, *Adv Dent Res 13:*67–72. doi: http://dx.doi.org/10.1177/08959374990130011701
313. Omri, A., Anderson, M., Mugabe, C., Suntres, Z., Mozafari, M.R., Ali Azghani, A., 2007, Artificial implants—new developments and associated problems, In: M.R.Mozafari ed., *Nanomaterials and Nanosystems for Biomedical Applications*, Springer-Verlag, Berlin, Germany, pp.53–65. doi: http://dx.doi.org/10.1007/978-1-4020-6289-6_3
314. Trebše, R., 2012, Biomaterials in artificialjoint replacements, In: *Infected Total Joint Arthroplasty: The Algorithmic Approach*, Springer, Verlag, London.

315. Shtansky, D.V. and Roy, M., 2013, *Surface Engineering for Enhanced Performance Against Wear*, Springer, New York, NY, pp. 77–310.
316. Fujishiro, T., Nishikawa, T., Shibanuma, N., Akisue, T., Takikawa, S., Yamamoto, T., Yoshiya, S. and Kurosaka, M., 2004, Effect of cyclic mechanical stretch and titanium particles on prostagland in E_2 production by human macrophages *in vitro*, *J Biomed Mater Res A* 68:531–536. doi: http://dx.doi.org/10.1002/jbm.a.20098
317. Lin, H-Y. and Bumgardner, J.D., 2004, *In vitro* biocorrosion of Ti-6Al-4V implant alloy by a mouse macrophage cell line, *J Biomed Mater Res A* 68:717–724. doi: http://dx.doi.org/10.1002/jbm.a.20092
318. Sommer, B., Felix, R., Sprecher, C., Leunig, M., Ganz, R. and Hofstetter, W., 2005, Wear particles and surface topographies are modulators of osteoclastogenesis *in vitro*, *J Biomed Mater Res A* 72:67–76. doi: http://dx.doi.org/10.1002/jbm.a.30202
319. Yang, L. and Webster, T.J., 2012, Biological responses to and toxicity of nanoscale implant materials, In: N. Eliaz ed., *Degradation of Implant Materials*, Springer-Science, New York, NY, pp. 481–508. doi: http://dx.doi.org/10.1007/978-1-4614-3942-4_18
320. Tjellström, A., 1989, Osseointegrated systems and their applications in the head and neck, *Adv Otolaryyngol Head Neck Surg* 3:39–70.
321. Granström, G., 2005, Osseointegration in irradiated cancer patients. An analysis with respect to implant failures, *J Oral Maxillofac Surg* 63:579–585.

Chapter 4

Requirements for Successful Implant Systems

Examining published basic and clinical data, several important points can be found which can control the success, survival, and longevity of placed implants. These points should at least include biological compatibility, biomechanical compatibility, and morphological compatibility. As mentioned in previous chapters, a majority of implantable materials are not ready to be placed in their present conditions, rather they need further surface modifications to accommodate cytocompatibility. In this chapter, we will review three major compatibilities—biological, biomechanical, and morphological. To achieve these required compatibilities, the surface should be treated properly. As we will see later, for example, hydroxyapatite (HA) coating is originally done for biological compatibility since the chemistry of artificial HA resembles the main chemistry of vital receiving bone. But, as a hindsight, coated HA provides a proper level of surface morphology and also acts as a biomechanical buffering function between vital bone and implant material's core strength.

4.1. Introduction

The implantation of devices for the maintenance or restoration of a body function imposes extraordinary requirements on the construction materials. Foremost among these is the issue of biocompatibility. There can be interactions between the foreign material and the host's local and peripheral tissues, fluids, and blood elements. Some interactions are simply adaptive. Others constitute hazards, both short and long term, to the survival of the living organism [1,2]. There are mechanical and physical properties which the material must provide, and a structural nature which the system should exhibit. Some of these properties govern the ability of the device to perform its intended function, from an engineering viewpoint. Factors, such as tribology (specifically friction and wear), corrosion and mechanical compliance have a significant impact biocompatibility.

Human implantation applications impose more stringent requirements on reliability than any other engineering task. For example, in most applications, an implanted

DOI 10.5643/9781606506288/ch4

device is expected to function for the life of the patient. As the medical profession becomes more emboldened, a device's lifetime may be required to stretch to more than 30 years (if follow-up maintenance is carefully and thoroughly performed and excellent patient cooperation is obtained)—very few engineering devices have been designed to function for more than 30 years. It is necessary to think in terms of performance reliability and to establish a tolerable expectation of failure, perhaps no more than one in one thousand [2,3].

One of the many universal requirements of implants, wherever they may be used in the body, is the ability to form a suitably stable mechanical unit with the neighboring hard or soft tissues. A loose (or unstable) implant may function less efficiently or cease functioning completely, or it may induce an unintended and potentially harmful tissue response. In either case, it may cause the patient discomfort and pain. Numerous studies have experimented with altering the surface characteristics of implants in an effort to address and overcome some of the potential drawbacks of the implant therapy [4].

After extensive literature review, it was found that there are three major host tissue compatibility requirements for placed implants: biological compatibility (in short, biocompatibility), biomechanical compatibility, and morphological compatibility [5–7]. When these three criteria are met, an implant can exhibit biointegration with the receiving hard tissue and achieve biofunctionality thereafter. In this chapter, we will discuss how these factors contribute to the success (including survival and longevity) of placed implants.

4.2. Biological Compatibility

The saliva and bacteria found in the oral cavity pose a challenge to dental restorative materials because of their corrosive nature [8]. For chemical and biological evaluations, appropriate biological tests and standards have been developed over the past 10 to 15 years, and serve as the basis for recommending any dental restorative material.

Until a few years ago, almost all national and international dental standards and testing programs focused entirely on the physical and chemical properties of restorative dental materials. Today, biological testing is required as well. The science of dental materials now encompasses a broad knowledge and appreciation of certain biological considerations associated with the selection and use of materials designed for use in the oral cavity. Current standards require that before being evaluated clinically in humans, all dental materials should pass primary tests (cellular response screening), secondary tests (tissue response evaluation), and usage tests in animals.

Testing programs for dental materials are based on specifications or standards established by national or international standards organizations (ISO), such as the American National Standards Institute (ANSI) and ISO. The oldest and largest of these programs has been operated continuously by the American Dental Association (ADA) since the late 1920s. The evaluation of dental products for safety and efficacy has historically been the scope of both the ADA and the Food and Drug Administration (FDA). In accordance with these regulations (U.S. Medical Device Amendments, 1976), all dental materials are reviewed for safety and effectiveness, and classified by the FDA as Class I, II, or III. Class I materials are those considered to be of low risk in causing adverse reactions. Materials in Class II must satisfy the requirements outlined in the current ANSI/ADA specifications. The most extensive testing is required for Class III materials, which includes full safety and efficacy assessments prior to marketing. The FDA regulates the components of dental amalgam into Class II (special controls), whereas the United States Pharmacopoeia (USP) grade mercury into Class I (general controls) [9].

There are three ways to define the biocompatibility: (i) the ability of a material to perform a specific function that elicits an appropriate host response, (ii) the quality of not having toxic or injurious effects on biological systems, and (iii) comparison of the tissue response produced through the close association of the implanted candidate material to its implant site within the host animal to that tissue response recognized and established as suitable with control materials. All of these definitions focus on materials and not devices. This is a drawback since many medical devices are comprised of an aggregate of materials. Much of the preclinical testing of the materials is not conducted on the devices, but rather the material itself. At some point in time, biocompatibility testing will need to include examining devices, since their shape and geometry can affect the biocompatibility [10]. The biocompatibility of a long-term implantable medical device refers to the ability of the device to perform its intended function, with the desired degree of incorporation in the host, without eliciting any undesirable local or systemic effects from its host. This differs from the biocompatibility requirements of a short-term implant. For example, an implantable medical device that is placed within the cardiovascular system for transient diagnostic or therapeutic purposes is mainly required to carry out its intended function within flowing blood, to minimize interactions between itself and blood that could adversely affect device performance, and to avoid the inducing of uncontrolled activation of cellular or plasma protein cascades. Furthermore, in order for an engineered tissue product (such as a scaffold or matrix), to be deemed biocompatible it must meet additional engineering requirements. It must also act as a substrate that will support the appropriate cellular activity, including the facilitation of molecular and mechanical signaling systems, in order to optimize tissue regeneration. This too must be accomplished without eliciting any undesirable effects in those cells, or inducing any undesirable local or systemic responses in the target host.

The progress made in recent years in the areas of biotechnology, tissue engineering, biomaterials, cell and molecular biology, polymer science, and other related fields has resulted in numerous medical and pharmaceutical advances [11]. Of particular significance is the progress that has been made in the areas of implantable devices and drug/device combination products, such as drug-eluting stents [12–16], artificial organs [17–20], biosensors [21,22], catheters [23], scaffolds for tissue engineering [24–26], and heart valves [27,28]. Nevertheless, the biocompatibility of implantable devices remains a limiting factor for device longevity and functionality—particularly in the case of biosensors. Various natural, synthetic, and semisynthetic materials are currently utilized in the fabrication of implantable devices. Naturally occurring materials include collagen [29,30], chitosan [31–33], alginate [34], hyaluronan [35], and dextran [36,37]. Although all biomaterials (metals, polymers, ceramics, or composites) are normally considered to be relatively biocompatible, a number of studies have shown that devices made from these materials have biocompatibility issues [38]. In addition, it has been shown that biological reactions that are adverse for a material in one application may not be adverse for the same material in a different application; similarly, a material found to be safe in one application may not be safe in another [39].

There is research on Ti materials that focuses on biocompatibility evaluation. Compared to the (α + β) Ti alloys commonly used for medical applications, β–Ti alloys have many advantageous mechanical properties, an improved wear resistance, a high elasticity, and an excellent cold and hot formability. As a result there is increased reliance on β–Ti alloys as a material for orthopedic joint replacement. Not all elements with β-stabilizing properties in Ti alloys are suitable for biomaterial applications; corrosion and wear processes cause a release of these alloying elements (Nb, Ta, Ti, Zr, and Al) to the surrounding tissue. Eisenbarth et al. [40] evaluated the biological compatibility of the alloying elements of β–Ti and near β–Ti alloys in order to estimate their suitability as biomaterial components. CpTi (Grade II) and the implant steel (316L stainless steel) were used as reference materials. The investigation examined the corrosion properties of the elements, as well as their effect on cell proliferation and morphology, mitochondrial activity, and the size of MC3T3-E1 cells and GM7373 cells. They found a range of biocompatibility among the investigated metals. In an order of decreasing biocompatibility, this spectrum is: niobium (as a β-phase stabilizing element), tantalum (as a β-phase stabilizing element), titanium, zirconium (as an α-phase stabilizing element), aluminum (as an α-phase stabilizing element), 316L (Mo containing 18Cr–8Ni stainless steel with low carbon content), and molybdenum [40].

The biocompatibility of metallic implant surfaces is governed in large part by the interfacial kinetics associated with metal release and protein binding. The kinetics of metal release from, and protein binding to Co–Cr–Mo and Ti implants (CpTi and Ti–6Al–4V) in human serum were investigated. The studies [41] were carried out by (i) measuring the temporal release of Cr and Ti into serum from Co–Cr–Mo and Ti implants, (ii) examining the composition of human serum proteins adsorbed onto the surfaces of Co–Cr–Mo and Ti implants, and (iii) identifying the serum proteins associated with the binding of soluble Cr and Ti degradation products. It was reported that (i) Cr was released from Co–Cr–Mo implants at an order of magnitude higher than Ti was released from Ti implants, (ii) serum became saturated with soluble Cr and Ti at levels as high as 3,250 ng/ml Ti from CpTi, 3,750 ng/ml Ti from Ti–6Al–4V, and 35,400 ng/ml Cr from Co–Cr–Mo degradation, and (iii) both Cr and Ti released from Co–Cr–Mo and Ti materials exhibited a bimodal binding pattern to both low-molecular-weight serum protein(s) (<32 kDa), and to higher molecular weight protein(s) in the 180–250 kDa range. Based on these findings, it was concluded that identification of metal alloy-dependent biofilm compositions and dissolution products provides the basis for understanding the bioavailability and bioreactivity of these implant alloys and their degradation products [41].

The nanoscale wear response of the Co–Cr alloy (ASTM F-75) was investigated as a function of contact load and surface residual stress, in order to identify the mechanism governing the onset of surface damage in modular implants. A unique loading configuration was utilized to apply a range of known in-plane stress states to the specimen surface in order to simulate different residual stress levels. Using the tip of a scanning force microscope, controlled contact forces were applied to the specimen to mechanically stimulate the loaded surface. The volume of material removed was measured and used to characterize the wear rate as a function of the contact load and surface stress state. It was concluded that (i) a critical level of contact pressure is required to initiate wear of the Co–Cr surface and as expected, higher contact pressures accelerate the wear process, (ii) at a constant contact pressure, the wear rate is accelerated by compressive in-plane stress, while tensile in-plane stresses tend to suppress surface wear, and (iii) the surface damage mechanism is characterized by the successive damage/delamination of the native oxide covered surface, due to a single asperity contact and the repassivation of the exposed surface [42].

Krupa et al. [43] investigated the corrosion resistance and biocompatibility of titanium after surface modification by the separate implantation of calcium and phosphorus ions, and the simultaneous application of calcium + phosphorus ions. Calcium and phosphorus ions were implanted at a dose rate of 10^{17} ions/cm^2 at the ion beam energy of 25 keV. The corrosion resistance was examined by electrochemical methods in a simulated body fluid (SBF) at a temperature of 37 °C. Biocompatibility was evaluated *in vitro*. The results of the electrochemical examinations (Stern's method) indicated that (i) the calcium, phosphorus, and calcium + phosphorus implantation into the surface of titanium increases its corrosion resistance in stationary conditions after short- and long-term exposures in SBF, (ii) potentiodynamic tests showed that the calcium-implanted samples undergo pitting corrosion during anodic polarization, and (iii) the breakdown potentials measured were high (2.5–3 V) [43], which lie well outside of the reasonable range of intraoral potential (0–50 mV) (see Chapter 3). Nayab et al. [44] demonstrated that Ti surfaces implanted with Ca ions can enhance the expression of certain bone-associated components *in vitro* and suggest that this effect could be of potential benefit *in vivo*.

Sabetrasekh et al. [45] compared different commercial titanium dioxide powders in order to ascertain the most appropriate for scaffold production. X-ray photoelectron spectroscopy (XPS) analysis identified trace elements in the samples, mainly Al, Si, C, Ca, and P. Cellular response was measured by the cytotoxic effect, cell growth, and cytokine secretion from murine preosteoblasts (MC3T3-E1) *in vitro*. The XPS data substantiated that traces of carbon-based molecules, silicon, nitrogen, and aluminum in the powder were greatly reduced after cleaning in 1 M NaOH. It was found that the lessening of trace elements in the powders led to a reduction in cytotoxicity and inflammatory response, and that carbon contamination seemed to have only a minor effect on cellular response. Strong correlations were found between Al and Si contamination levels and the inflammatory response and cytotoxic effect; this suggests that the concentration of these elements should be reduced in order to enhance the scaffolds' biocompatibility [45].

Several methods have been proposed to enhance the biocompatibility of Ti materials. Li et al. [46] coated a thin HA layer on a micro-arc oxidized titanium substrate by means of the sol–gel method. The HA sol was aged fully to obtain a stable and phase-pure HA, and the sol concentration was varied to alter the coating thickness. Through the sol–gel HA coating, the Ca and P concentrations in the coating layer increased significantly. It was reported that (i) the microarc oxidation (anodizing) enhanced the biocompatibility of the Ti, and the bioactivity was improved further by the sol–gel HA coating on the anodized Ti, and (ii) the proliferation and alkaline phosphatase activity of the osteoblast-like cells on the microarc oxidized Ti/HA sol–gel treated Ti were significantly higher than those on the microarc oxidized Ti without the HA sol–gel treatment [46].

Schwarz et al. [47] evaluated the influence of plaque biofilm removal on the mitochondrial activity of human SaOs-2 osteoblasts grown on titanium surfaces. Volunteers wore acrylic splints with structured titanium discs for 72 hours to build up plaque biofilms. Specimens were randomly instrumented using either an ultrasonic system + chlorhexidine (CHX), or plastic curettes + CHX. Specimens were incubated with SaOs-2 cells for 6 days. Residual plaque biofilm/clean implant surface area (%), cellular mitochondrial activity (counts/second), and cell morphology were assessed. It was concluded that mitochondrial activity seemed to be impaired by the presence of residual plaque biofilm areas and that plaque removal alone may not be the crucial step in the re-establishment of the biocompatibility of titanium surfaces [47].

The nickel in NiTi is chemically joined to the titanium by a strong intermetallic bond, so the risk of a reaction, even in patients with nickel-sensitivity, is extremely low [48–51]. There are several studies that reveal that biocompatibility of NiTi is relatively low under certain conditions [52]. Surface preparation techniques have been shown to have a significant effect on the biocompatibility of the alloy [52]. Ion release measurements on NiTi (containing about 50 wt%Ni) alloy have shown that the initial rate of Ni ion release is high, but falls rapidly within 2 days, which is similar to that of Ni released from 316L stainless steel [53], although 316L stainless steel contains only 8 wt%. Armitage et al. [54] studied the influence of surface modifications on NiTi biocompatibility. They mechanically polished NiTi samples and followed this with a buff-polishing with the diamond paste. For another modification, surfaces were shot-peened with 160 μm spherical glass media, and electropolished in 30% HNO_3. The cytotoxicity and cytocompatibility studies with fibroblast and endothelial cells showed no differences in the biocompatibility of any of the NiTi surfaces; further, the cytotoxicity and cytocompatibility of all treated surfaces were favorable compared to the untreated controls. The hemolysis caused by the various NiTi surfaces was no different from that caused by polished 316L stainless steel or polished titanium surfaces. Heat treatment (by in-air oxidation at 400 °C for 30 minutes or 600 °C for 30 minutes) of NiTi was found to significantly reduce thrombogenicity to control levels. XPS results showed a significant decrease in the concentration of surface nickel with heat treatment and that the surface nickel was in an oxide state, rather than metallic. The surface contact angle of both pre-oxidized surfaces showed much lower (36.3° and 13.5° for 400 °C and 600 °C oxidation, respectively) than polished surfaces (64.6° for buff-polished and 42.5° for electro-polished) [54], indicating that pre-oxidation makes the Ti surface more active.

Filip et al. [55] characterized the surface and the bulk structure of NiTi implants by SEM (scanning electron microscope), TEM (transmission electron microscope), XPS (X-ray photoelectron spectroscopy), and scanning Auger electron microprobe analysis (AES). Reclaimed NiTi implants were compared with otherwise identically prepared nonimplanted specimens, sputter-cleaned and reoxidized samples. Nonimplanted and implanted samples had essentially the same surface topography and microstructure. Ti, O, and C were the dominant elements detected on the surface. Trace amounts (~1 at%) of Ni and Ca, N, Si, B, and S were also detected. Ti was present as TiO_2 on the surface, while nickel was present in the metallic form. A significant difference in Ni peak intensity was observed when retrieved or nonimplanted control samples (very low nickel content) were compared with sputter cleaned and reoxidized samples (well-detected Ni). It was, hence, concluded that the method of passivation has a great effect on the degree of Ni loosening. Also, no major changes occurred in the NiTi sample bulk structure or in the surface oxide during the implantation periods [55].

Early passive or active motion physical therapy programs have been shown to be extremely beneficial to patients' recovery after flexor tendon repair [56,57]. However, the application of early active motion increases the stress on the repair, leading to a significant number of repair ruptures [58]. It seems that two factors are involved in producing a strong mechanical repair: the technique used and the suture material. Stainless steel has better tensile strength and good knot-holding security but is difficult to use and is weakened by kinking [59–62]. The NiTi SME (shape memory effect) alloy has been introduced as a possible new suture material for flexor tendon surgery [63–65]. NiTi sutures were implanted for biocompatibility testing into the right medial gastrocnemiustendon in 15 rabbits for 2, 6, and 12 weeks. Additional NiTi sutures were implanted in subcutaneous tissue in order to determine the effect(s) of implantation on NiTi's strength properties. Braided polyester sutures of approximately the same diameter were used as control. It was found that (i) encapsulating membrane formation around the sutures was minimal in the case of both materials, (ii) the breaking load of NiTi was significantly greater compared to braided polyester, and (iii) implantation did not affect the strength properties of either material [66].

TiN coating has been demonstrated to improve the biocompatibility of bare NiTi alloys; however, essential biocompatibility differences between TiN coated and uncoated NiTi alloys are not yet known [67]. Lifeng et al. [67] compared the underlying biological mechanisms of biocompatibility differences between coated and uncoated samples, the changes of bare and TiN-coated NiTi alloys in surface chemical composition, morphology, hydrophilicity, Ni ions release, cytotoxicity, apoptosis, and gene expression profiles. It was found that, compared with the bare NiTi alloys, TiN coating significantly (i) decreased the Ni ion content on the surfaces of the NiTi alloys and reduced the release of Ni ions from the alloys, (ii) attenuated the inhibitory effect of Ni ions on the expression of genes associated with anti-inflammatory responses, and (iii) also suppressed the induction of apoptosis-related genes expression by Ni ions. Moreover, the TiN coating distinctly improved the hydrophilicity (in other words, enhancing wettability) and uniformity of the surfaces of the NiTi alloys and contributed to the expression of genes participating in cell adhesion and other physiological activities. It is, therefore, indicated that the TiN-coated NiTi alloys will help overcome the shortcomings of NiTi alloys currently used in clinical applications, and NiTi use as a replacement biomaterial will increase in the medical field and implant devices [67].

4.3. Biomechanical Compatibility

Biomaterials (especially implantable materials) must function under biomechanical environments. If the implanted biomaterials and the receiving host tissue are incompatible, the intended biofunctionality will not be realized. This is one of the three important compatibility requirements for successful biofunctional implant; the other two biocompatibility (in the previous section) and morphological compatibility will be discussed in the following section. Figure 4.1 shows a linear relationship between strength (in terms of yield strength) and rigidity (in terms of modulus of elasticity [MOE]) among various types of biomaterials, where **A**—alumina, **B**—bone, **CF**—carbon fiber, **D**—dentin, **E**—enamel, **HAP**—hydroxyapatite, **HSP**—high strength polymers (Kelvar, Kapton, PEEK, etc.), **MG**—magnesium materials, **P**—polymeric materials, **PSZ**—partially stabilized zirconia, **S**—surgical stainless steels (e.g., 304-series stainless steel), **TA**—titanium alloys (e.g., Ti–6Al–4V), **TCP**—tricalcium phosphate, **TI**—commercially pure titanium (all unalloyed grades), **TT**—tantalum materials, and **ZR**—Zirconium materials. When designing biomaterials, engineers need to consider physiological loads (axial rotation, flexion extension, and lateral bending); the implant should have sufficient structural integrity to withstand these forces [68]. In addition to these parameters, various mechanical properties (elastic modulus, tensile strength, ductility, fatigue life and strength, fretting fatigue life, and wear properties) [69] should be adjusted to suitable levels for implants used structural biomaterials. Hence, the biofunctionality of candidate materials should always be considered a crucial parameter.

Referring to Figure 4.1, we will discuss some mechanistic concerns related to the mechanical environment involved in the implantology, particularly in dental implantology. As described elsewhere, it is normal to employ titanium biomaterials as dental

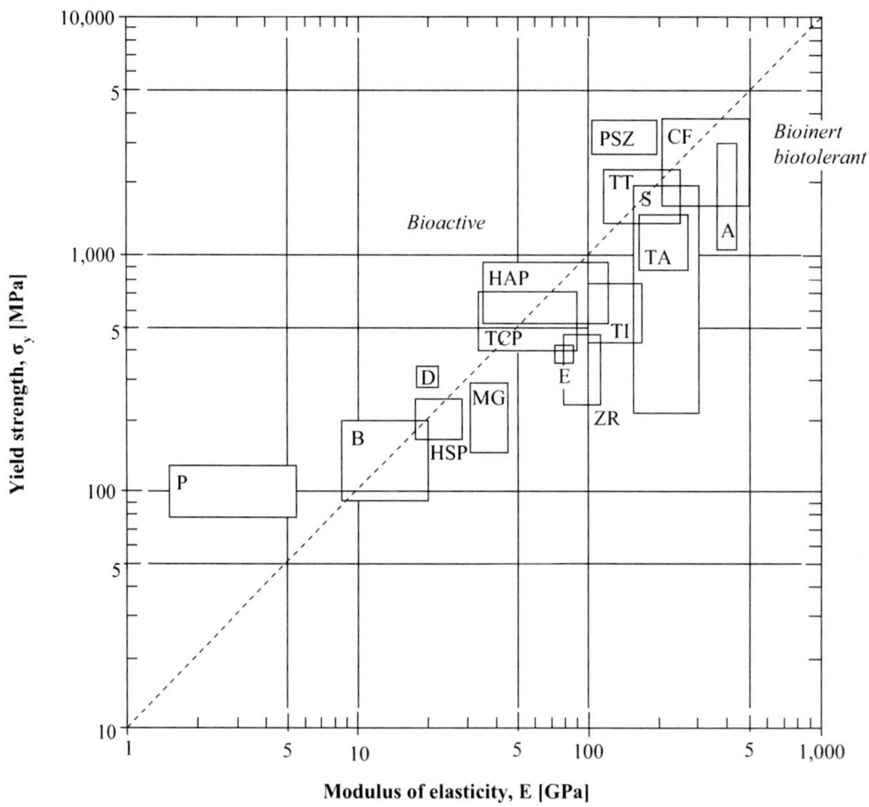

Figure 4.1. Linear relationship between strength and rigidity of various biomaterials in log–log plot.

and orthopedic implant materials. Following implantation, the implant's surface is expected to exhibit solid osseointegration with surrounding tissue over time. The resultant interface is comprised of the titanium implant and receiving bone's surfaces.

Now, imagine a dental implant that has a satisfactory level of osseointegration at its interface. Further, the composite structure of titanium implant and the bone is now ready to subject to a normal mastication (which has normally about 200 N force as a chewing force). Such a composite structure can, as a whole, deform elastically. This situation is described as "strain continuity." Even though each constituent of the composite (in this case, the titanium implant and bone) can bend with equal elasticity, each component should experience different stress levels because each possesses distinct values of MOE (as known as E). According to Figure 4.1, we can estimate that E for bone is around 15 G Pa, while that of titanium is around 150 GPa, of which the latter is an order of magnitude larger than the former. If we apply Hooke's law, we can describe the stress on titanium as $\sigma_T = E_T \times \varepsilon_T$, and $\sigma_B = E_B \times \varepsilon_B$, for bone. Since, as indicated before, the strain should be continuous, $\varepsilon_T = \varepsilon_B$, but because $E_T > E_B$, σ_T should be much larger than σ_B. This mechanistic situation is described as "discrete stress." The difference between these stresses can be expressed as $\Delta\sigma = \sigma_T—\sigma_B$. When the stress difference, $\Delta\sigma$, happens to be bigger than the interfacial bonding (or fused) strength of the implant (T) and bone structure (B), the interfacial bonding is subject to failure or debonding. Now, it is well documented that HA coating onto titanium implant substrates will promote and assist early stage of osseointegration, due to the similarity of their chemistries. But, once again referring to Figure 4.1, HAP (hydroxyapatite) is positioned between T and B materials, indicating that HAP material can play a role of mechanical buffering function. This is a good example of the hindsight. The application of HA onto implant surfaces is not limited only to dental implant systems, but orthopedic implant surfaces are also very often coated with HA, particularly after "cement disease" became a very critical issue. Polymethylmethacrylate (PMMA), which was dominantly employed as a bone cement for orthopedic implant systems (particularly total hip replacement and knee replacements) caused unwanted local heat due to an exothermic reaction during the polymerization process. Furthermore, the un-polymerized MMA monomer is toxic. Accordingly, as the prevention of cement disease was addressed, HA was extensively utilized. The positive effect of HA is twofold: the promotion of osseointegration and mechanical buffering function.

Further, ceramic materials are currently being used for implant fabrication: single crystal of alumina [70,71], polycrystal of zirconia [72–74], titania [75] or a combination of the latter two [76]. One remarkable advantage of these ceramic implants is their esthetic appearance of bright and white color. Again referring to Figure 4.1, we can identify these ceramics (PSZ and A) at further away from B than the T group, suggesting that the potential interfacial stress, $\Delta\sigma$, could be much higher than the previous $\Delta\sigma$ generated between T and B. It is crucial that this higher risk for interfacial debonding or even fracture of the ceramic implant or alveolar bone should be carefully taken into consideration when ceramic implants are placed.

As mentioned above, the main factors that reduce the *in vivo* lifespan of current load-bearing implants are the mismatch of MOE and the weak interfacial bond between bone and metallic implant materials. Additional limiting factors include wear-induced osteolysis and aseptic loosening of metal-on-polymer implants, and the absence of high recoverable strain as well as hysteresis in biocompatible metals, similar to natural bone [77]. An implant method that achieves a strong interfacial bond and also reduces modulus mismatch has been developed using porous metals. The use of porous metals can effectively reduce the MOE mismatch and provide pathways for bone in-growth through the pores for stable long-term anchorage or biological fixation of the implant. Interest is significant in patient-specific implants with the possibility of guided tissue regeneration, particularly for load-bearing implants. For such implants to succeed, novel design approaches and fabrication technologies that can achieve balanced mechanical and functional performances in the implants are necessary [77].

The lower premolars of six beagle dogs were extracted and the ridges were allowed to heal for 8 weeks [78]. Thirty-six implants were bilaterally placed and were left undisturbed *in situ* for either 1 or 3 weeks. The implant systems used are as follows: Group A: Ti–6Al–4V with a dual acid-etched surface with nanometer scale discrete crystalline deposition, Group B: Ti–6Al–4V with a titanium oxide-blasted fluoride-modified surface chemistry, and Group C: Ti–6Al–4V with a bioceramic microblasted surface. After 1 or 3 weeks, implants were torque-tested to the point of interface failure and histologically evaluated. It was reported that (i) torque values were significantly affected by time and implant types, and (ii) from highest to lowest order for the torque value was from Group C, Group B to Group A [78].

Metallic implantation materials having high yield strength, low elastic modulus, and noncytotoxic alloying elements would be advantageous for the long-term stability of implants [79]. The search for a suitable candidate has led to Ti–13Nb–13Zr. The ultra-fine-grained (0.3 μm) Ti–13Nb–13Zr was prepared by dynamic globularization without any severe deformation to assess the *in vitro* osteoconductivity. It was indicated that the dynamic globularized ultrafine grained Ti–13Nb–13Zr alloy was promising for load-bearing endosseous implant material because of excellent mechanical and biological compatibilities [79].

One important variable in the role of bone remodeling is the difference in MOE between bone and its replacement [80]. Normally the larger the difference, the more rapidly bone resorption takes place. Ti is particularly good in this regard because of its lower MOE. Sutherland et al. [81], however, pointed out that this is not true when the above mechanical environment is concerned. Medical grade titanium samples were examined using XPS before and after immersion in various proteins. Additionally, an implant removed from a patient following clinical failure was examined using scanning ion and electron microscopy. It was reported that (i) the surface of medical grade titanium samples was found to be mainly TiO_2, with contaminations of H_2O/OH^-, (ii) also calcium and nitrogen, which remained after autoclaving, (iii) the failed clinical sample was found to be partially fibrously encapsulated, with evidence of calcification, and (iv) small amounts of TiOOH were detected at the fibrous periphery [81], supporting the theory of Tengvall et al. [82,83].

The surface layer of implants should be biomechanically compatible with the mechanical properties of vital soft/hard tissues, as mentioned before. We have already discussed that coating of the implant material (with HAP or TCP) is a very effective method that accomplishes this specific aim. Another technique was introduced by Asaoka et al. [84] who prepared titanium powder with a granule diameter of 420–500 μm and fabricated porous titanium specimens made from this powder. The mechanical properties of these specimens were examined. It was reported that (i) the compressive strength and low cyclic compressive fatigue strength were 182 MPa and 40 MPa, respectively; (ii) the compressive strength of the porous-titanium-coated dental implants was 230 MPa, but fatigue strength was not improved; (iii) materials with MOE (70–200 GPa) have most frequently been used for dental implants, but porous titanium has a lower elastic modulus than this value; however (iv) a thick core with an ingrowth of tissue into void channels raises the elastic modulus of the material [84].

Once a biomechanical compatibility is established, the placed implant needs to bond with and incorporate firmly into the surrounding tissue structure. There are four basic methods to initially fix implants to bone. The first method is based on modifying the implant's surface form and texture to promote fixation by mechanical interlocking on the macro- or micro-scale. For example, plasma-sprayed coatings of metal or other materials (including ceramics) on the implant's surface promote macro-interlock and micro-interlock. The second basic method of bone-implant fixation involves the use to some type of "bioactive" biomaterials for the implant, either as a surface coating or as the bulk material, to promote stronger bone-implant attachment through the physical or chemical bonding, or both, between implant surface and tissue constituents. The third fixation concept is osseointegration, which indicates a direct structural and functional connection between vital bone and the surface of a load-carrying implant through the macro-interlocking as well as micro-interlocking. Over the last few years, the main advancements in implantology were achieved by creating optimal surface qualities of dental implants. New osteoinductive and osteoconductive surfaces have been developed [85–90]. The reason for working on an optimal surface was to achieve better osseointegration, and therefore better long-term stability of dental implants. To achieve a full osseointegration and good peri-implant gingival was the main task of much scientific work. Good peri-implant gingival has a protective function for the bone–implant interface [91,92]. The fourth fixation concept is "fibro-osseointegration" ("pseudo-periodontal ligament"). This is a connection of implant to tissue by means of a region of nonmineralized connective tissue which forms adjacent to the implant and attaches it to surrounding bone [93].

While it is known that the success of dental implants benefits from osseointegration, implants can still fail. In designing a successful dental implant, the main objective is to ensure that the implant can support biting forces and deliver them safely to interfacial tissues over the long term. The consideration of biomechanics is central in this design challenge. Key topics include: (i) the nature of the biting forces on the implants, (ii) how the biting forces are transferred to the interfacial tissues, and (iii) how the interfacial tissues react, biologically, to stress transfer conditions. For biting forces on dental implants, the basic problem is to determine the *in vivo* loading components on implants in various prosthetic situations, for example, for implants acting as single tooth replacements or as multiple supports of loaded bridgework. Significant progress has been made as several theoretical models have been presented for determining the partitioning of forces among dental implants supporting bridgework. Interfacial stress transfer and interfacial biology represent more difficult problems. While many engineering studies have shown that variables such as implant shape, elastic modulus, extent of bonding between implant, and bone can affect the stress transfer conditions, the unresolved question is whether there is any biological significance to such differences. Recent research suggests that the research for a more detailed hypothesis regarding the relationship between interface mechanics and biology should take into account basic bone physiology, for example, wound healing after implantations plus basic processes of bone modeling and remodeling [94]. The successful clinical results achieved with osseointegrated dental implants underscore the fact that such implants easily withstand considerable masticatory loads. In fact, one study showed that bite forces of patients with these implants were comparable to those in patients with natural dentitions. Studies of the interface between titanium implants and bone show that a close contact between a titanium implant and bone develops during the healing period. It is important to analyze macroscopic stress distribution and load transfer mechanisms where close apposition of bone to titanium implants is provided at the microscopic level. The close apposition of bone to the titanium implant is the essential feature that allows a transmission of stress from the implant to the bone without any appreciable relative motion or abrasion. The absence of any intermediate fibrotic layer allows stress to be transmitted without any progressive change in the bond or contact between the bone and implant. The osseointegrated implant provides a direct contact with bone, and therefore will transmit any stress waves or shocks applied to the fixtures. For this reason, it is advisable to use a shock-absorbing material such as acrylic resin in the form of acrylic resin artificial teeth in the fixed partial denture. This arrangement allows for the development of a stiff and strong substructure with adequate shock protection on its outer surface [93].

Since dental implants must withstand relatively large forces and moments in function, a better understanding of the *in vivo* bone response to loading would aid implant design. To this end, Brunski [95] pointed out that (i) theoretical models and experimental data are available for understanding implant loading as an aid to case planning, (ii) at least for several months after surgery, bone healing in gaps between implant and bone, as well as in pre-existing damaged bone, will determine interface structure and properties, (iii) an interfacial cement line exists between the implant surface and bone for titanium and HA, (iv) excessive interfacial micromotion early after implantation interferes with local bone healing and predisposes the implants to a fibrous tissue interface instead of osseointegration, and (v) large strains can damage bone. For implants that have healed *in situ* for several months before being loaded, data support the hypothesis that interfacial overload occurs if the strains are excessive in interfacial bone [95].

Beside the surface's qualities, there are other important factors for achieving perfect peri-implant bone and gingival conditions. In most cases eccentric forces, overloading of implants, and stress forces are the main reason for peri-implant bone loss in the crestal region, and therefore bad peri-implant results. So it is important to avoid large and eccentric force to prevent peri-implant bone damage. In some cases, it is not possible to avoid small tension forces caused by technical production of superstructures. This tension can only be minimized by bio-kinetic abutments positioned in the implant neck region. These intramobile elements were used in recent years as interpolated silicon shock-absorbing elements [94,96–98]. The silicon abutments were in direct contact to the peri-implant gingival, although this material is not suited as a bioinert implant material in this region. Therefore, it is necessary to develop a new implant system with good surface qualities in the intraosseous and trans-gingival region that includes a central shock-absorbing element without contact to the peri-implant region. It was reported that good functional properties are essential in dental implantology. The mobile implant (SIS Inc., Klagenfurt, Australia) is a self-cutting conical screw implant with an integrated bio-kinetic element. The shock absorber is a central part of the implant and a titanium ring encapsulates the shock-absorbing unit within the implant. The resilience of the implant was tested by axial and horizontal loading in a special testing unit. Furthermore, a survival test of the elastic titanium ring in the most exposed cervical part of the implant was performed. After the region was examined by electron microscopy after 122 million movements in the axial and horizontal direction, it was reported that (i) a progressive shock absorption was registered during horizontal and axial movements, (ii) the maximum movements were 0.06 mm in the axial and 0.16 mm in horizontal direction, and (iii) no signs of material destruction were observed in the electron microscopic analysis [99].

Recently, implant anchors such as titanium screws have been used for absolute anchorage during edgewise treatment. However, there have been few human studies reporting on the stability of implant anchors placed in the posterior region. Miyawaki et al. [100] investigated the success rates and factors associated with the stability of titanium screws placed into the buccal alveolar bone of the posterior region. Fifty-one patients with malocclusions, 134 titanium screws of three types, and 17 miniplates were retrospectively examined in relation to clinical characteristics. The 1-year success rate of screws with 1.0-mm diameter was significantly less than that of other screws with 1.5-mm or 2.3-mm diameter or than that of miniplates. Flap surgery was associated with the patient's discomfort. A high mandibular plane angle and inflammation of peri-implant tissue after implantation were risk factors for mobility of screws. It was reported that no significant association was detected between the success rate and the following variables: screw length, kind of placement surgery, immediate loading, location of implantation, age, gender, crowding of teeth, antero-posterior jaw base relationship, controlled periodontitis, and temporomandibular joint (TMJ) disorder symptoms. It was concluded that the diameter of a screw of 1.0 mm or less, inflammation of the peri-implant tissue, and a high mandibular plane angle (i.e., thin cortical bone), were associated with the mobility (i.e., failure) of the titanium screw placed into the buccal alveolar bone of the posterior region for orthodontic anchorage [100].

The noticeable difference between natural tooth and implant is the presence/absence of the periodontal membrane, as seen in Figure 4.2 [101]. The bottom half of the figure compares (force–displacement) diagrams under uniaxial compressive force. With the natural tooth, because it possesses periodontal membrane between tooth root and alveolar bone, the axial displacement under axial compression starts to increase linearly (due to Hook's elasticity), but, at and beyond a certain force, the compressive displacement plateaus. The left portion of the figure was obtained using a human first maxillary molar. With an artificial tooth root, since there is no mechanical buffering function between implant and alveolar bone, the force displacement should continuously increase—as seen on the right side of the figure. In order to compromise this difference and unique situation (though it might be a risky situation for a placed implant), there have been various ideas proposed and put into practice, including the coating of certain intermediate level of MOE value (such as HA), manipulating surface zone to make lower value of MOE (such as roughening or porous feature), or fabricating metal foams.

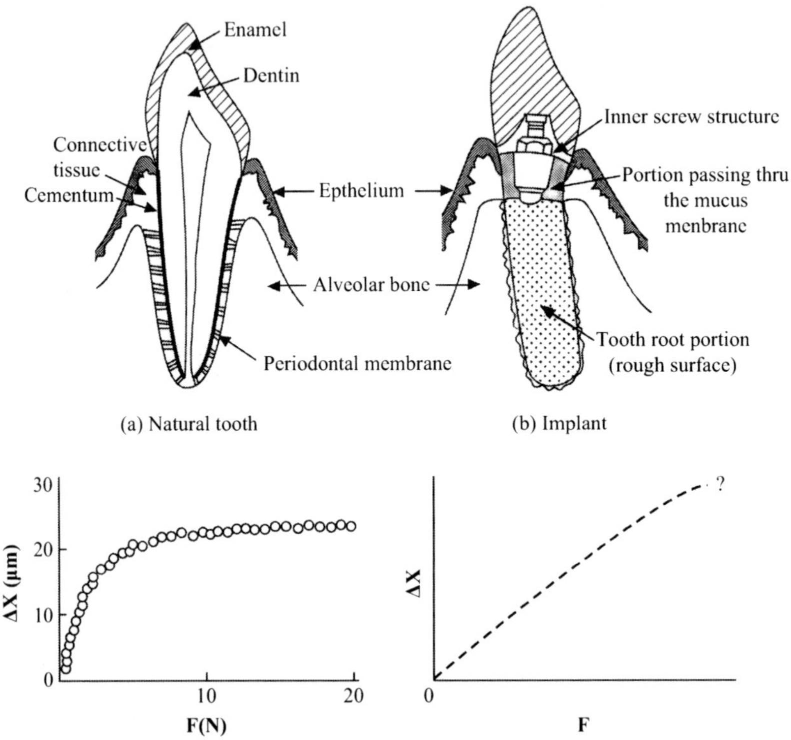

Figure 4.2. Schematic comparisons of anatomies and uniaxial compressive mechanical behaviors between natural tooth and implant tooth.

Lastly, due to the significant mechanical properties differences between a natural tooth and placed implant material at the interfaces, it has been emphasized how important it is to ensure mechanical compatibility at the interface between placed implant and the receiving hard tissue. This argument should not be limited to a single unit implant case, but should also be applied to clinical connecting implanted tooth and natural health tooth which would be more challenging.

4.4. Morphological Compatibility

Eriksson et al. [102] pointed out the importance of surface topography on cellular reactions. Surface plays a crucial role in biological interactions for four reasons. First, the surface of a biomaterial is the only part in contact with the bioenvironment. Second, the surface region of a biomaterial is almost always different in morphology and composition from the bulk. Differences arise from molecular rearrangement, surface reaction, and contamination. Third, for biomaterials that do not release nor leak biologically active or toxic substances, the characteristics of the surface govern the biological response. And fourth, some surface properties, such as topography, affect the mechanical stability of the implant/tissue interface and functionality of placed implants [103–105]. It has been reported that the rough-surfaced implants have significantly higher success rates compared with dental implants with smooth surfaces [106–109].

Biomaterials used in a living organism may come into contact with cells in the related tissue for long periods of time. For this reason, they should naturally be harmless to the organism, and their mechanical properties should be suited to the purpose and compatible with receiving tissue surfaces. Furthermore, they should possess a biological effect capable of providing circumstances favorable to the properties and functions of the cells at the implant site. For example, materials used in the construction of an artificial heart or heart valve must be anti-thrombogenic. In contrast, dental or bone implants must promote cell attachment because both the connective and epithelial cells (with which these materials mainly come into contact) are anchorage-dependent, and therefore need a scaffold in order for cell attachment, division, and differentiation to occur. It is therefore important to investigate the ability of local cells to attach to the materials used, which is one of the parameters in the evaluation of biomaterials. It has been shown that methods of implant surface preparation can significantly affect the resultant properties of the surface and subsequently the biological responses that occur at the surface [110–112]. Recent efforts have shown that the success or failure of dental implants can be related not only to the chemical properties of the implant surface, but also to its micromorphologic nature [113–115]. From an *in vitro* standpoint, the response of cells and tissues at implant interfaces can be affected by surface topography or geometry on a macroscopic basis [113,114], as well as by surface morphology or roughness on a microscopic level [115,116].

After analyzing published clinical reports on the success of placed implants, in terms of surface roughness, it was found that regardless of the type of implant materials used, if the surface roughness is manipulated to have a range from 1 to 10 μm, and an average pore size of 10–500 μm, the implant's survival rate is excellent [5]. This finding supports the importance of morphological compatibility, which is the third requirement for successful and biofunctional implant systems [6].

These characteristics undoubtedly affect how cells and tissues respond to various types of biomaterials. Of all the cellular responses, it has been suggested that cellular adhesion is considered as the most important response necessary for developing a rigid structural and functional integrity at the bone/implant interface [117]. Cellular adhesion alters the entire tissue response to biomaterials [118].

The bioactivity of titanium oxide [119] and porous Ti [120] was evaluated. Titanium oxide films were fabricated on titanium metal by electron-beam deposition techniques and in various oxygen partial pressures. The effect of oxygen content in titanium oxide on the bioactivity of the titanium implant was evaluated [119]. Raman spectra showed that the TiO_2 structure of titanium oxide films were oxygen deficient. It was concluded that the extent of hydroxyl group formation in SBF depends on the stoichiometry of TiO_2, which enhances the bioactivity of titanium [119]. Xue et al. [120], using the laser engineered net shaping (LENS) method, fabricated porous Ti implants. They reported their Ti preparation possessed a porosity in the range of 17–58 vol%, a pore size up to 800 μm, a mechanical strength of 24–463 MPa, and an elastic modulus of 2.6–44 GPa. It was further reported that (i) cells spread well on the surface of porous Ti and formed strong local adhesion, and the MTT assay indicated LENS processed porous Ti provides a preferential surface for bone cell proliferation, and (ii) porous Ti samples also stimulated faster osteoblast cell differentiation compared with polished Ti sheet, which could be due to the change in cell morphology within the pores of Ti samples. It was recommended that a critical pore size of 200 μm or higher is needed for cell ingrowth into the pores, below which osteoblast cells bridged the pore surface without any growth into the pores [120].

On a macroscopic level (roughness > 10 μm) roughness influences the mechanical properties of the titanium/bone interface, the mechanical interlocking of the interface, and the biocompatibility of the material [121,122]. Surface roughness in the range from 10 nm to 10 μm may also influence the interfacial biology, since it is the same order as the size of the cells and large biomolecules [123]. Microroughness at this level includes material defects, such as grain boundaries, steps and kinks, and vacancies that are active sites for adsorption, and therefore influence the bonding of biomolecules to the implant surface [124]. Microrough surfaces promote significantly better bone apposition than smooth surfaces, resulting in a higher percentage of bone in contact with the implant. Microrough surfaces may influence the mechanical properties of the interface, stress distribution, and bone remodeling [125]. Increased contact area and mechanical interlocking of bone to a microrough surface can decrease stress concentrations resulting in decreased bone resorption. Bone resorption takes place shortly after loading smooth surfaced implants [126], resulting in a fibrous connective tissue layer, whereas remodeling occurs on rough surfaces [127].

Rich and Harris [115] reported that macrophages exhibited rugophilia, or an affinity for rough surfaces, whereas fibroblasts failed to readily adhere to these same surfaces. This finding may complement previous work that indicates that rough surfaces promote inflammation via macrophage attraction, rather than wound healing by connective tissue [116]. Studies by Brunette [128] and Chehroudi at el. [129,130] have demonstrated that cells of differing origins can orient themselves in the grooves of differing micromachined surfaces. It was determined that epithelial cells were more likely to attach to grooves of specific dimension than to adjacent smooth surfaces. Michaels et al. [131] determined that a higher percentage of osteoblast-like cells attached to rough CpTi surfaces produced by sand-blasting than to smoother surfaces polished with 1 μm diamond paste. Keller et al. [132] later confirmed this.

In order to achieve morphological compatibility [4,5], titanium implant surfaces need to be modified. They can be treated by additive methods, such as the titanium beads plasma spray procedure, to increase the effective surface area. They have also been modified by subtractive methods such as acid pickling, acid etching, sand-blasting, and other small particle-blasting to change their texture, as well as to increase their surface area. The development and use of these surface modifications have been based on the idea that improved osseointegration can be achieved by increasing the topography or roughness of the implant surface [133]. In addition to the points discussed above, surface morphology can also be controlled and affected by porous coating, foam-forming, nanoscale structuring, or design alterations. Vasconcellos et al. [134] compared the fixation and the bone ingrowth at the interfaces of porous cylindrical implants (total porosity of 37% and average pores diameter of 480 μm), *in vivo* and rough cylindrical implants (R_a = 5.3 μm); both implant were constructed from commercially pure titanium, made by powder metallurgy. The implants were inserted into the tibias of 20 rabbits and the animals were sacrificed 4 and 8 weeks after surgery. The percentage of bone–implant contact (BIC) observed in porous implants was significantly larger than for rough implants for all sacrifice periods: 57% versus 46%

after 4 weeks, and 59% versus 50% after 8 weeks. The mechanical tests showed significantly higher shear strength for porous implants (14 and 20 MPa), as compared to rough implants (4 and 13 MPa) for the two periods analyzed, 4 and 8 weeks. Based on these results, it was suggested that (i) the porous implants improve the contact at the implant–bone interface and increase the fixation to the bone, thereby improving osseointegration and (ii), accordingly, the porous implant might be an alternative one to dental implant in less favorable conditions, and appear to be better fixed to bone, offering promising alternatives [134].

Implanted rough surfaces have long been associated with the accumulation of macrophages and other cells of monocytic lineage, such as foreign body giant cells and osteoclasts [135]. Chehroudi et al. [136] used a subcutaneous rat model to compare the interface events of implants possessing varied surface roughness topographies. Titanium-cast epoxy replicas were machined, etched, blasted, titanim-plasma-sprayed, sandblasted and etched, micromachined, and polished. Each type of replicas was implanted for up to 11 weeks. Based on their results, it was concluded that there appears to be two routes to bone-like tissue formation on Ti implants in the rat subcutaneous model: macrophage-mediated and macrophage-independent dense collagenous-matrix-associated [136].

Microrough Ti surfaces of dental implants have demonstrated more rapid and greater bone apposition when compared with machined Ti surfaces. Germanier et al. [137] further studied enhancement of osteoblastic activity and bone apposition by bio-functionalizing the implant surface with a monomolecular adsorbed layer of a co-polymer—that is, poly(L-lysine)-*graft*-poly(ethylene glycol) (PLL-*g*-PEG) and its derivatives (PLL-*g*-PEG/PEG-peptide) in terms of the early bone apposition to a modified sandblasted and acid-etched (SLA) surface coated with an Arg-Gly-Asp (RGD)-peptide-modified polymer (PLL-*g*-PEG/PEG–RGD) in the maxillae of miniature pigs. It was concluded that the (PLL-*g*-PEG/PEG–RGD) coatings may promote enhanced bone apposition during the early stages of bone regeneration [137].

Implant design features such as macro- and micro-design may influence overall implant success. Limited information is currently available. Abuhussein et al. [138] examined macro- and micro-design factors such as thread pitch, thread geometry, helix angle, thread depth and width as well as implant crestal module, which all may affect implant stability. It was shown that (i) the thread geometry affects the distribution of stress forces around the implant, (ii) a decreased thread pitch may positively influence implant stability, (iii) excessive helix angles, in spite of faster insertion rates, may jeopardize the ability of implants to sustain axial load, (iv) deeper threads seem to have an important effect on the stabilization in poorer bone quality situations, and (v) the addition of threads or micro-threads up to the crestal module of an implant might provide a potential positive contribution on bone-to to-implant contact as well as on the preservation of marginal bone; nonetheless this remains to be determined [138]. With regard to design parameters, a similar study was conducted by Petrie et al. [139], comparing the relative and interactive effects of implant diameter, length, and taper on calculated crestal bone strains. It was found that (i) increasing implant diameter resulted in as much as a 3.5-fold reduction in crestal strain, increasing length caused as much as a 1.65-fold reduction, whereas taper increased crestal strain, especially in narrow and short implants, where it increased 1.65-fold, (ii) diameter, length, and taper have to be considered together because of their interactive effects on crestal bone strain and (iii) if the objective is to minimize peri-implant strain in the crestal alveolar bone, a wide and relatively long, un-tapered implant appears to be the most favorable choice [139]. Kong et al. [140] applied a nonlinear finite element method to examine the effects of implant diameter (*D*) and length (*L*) on the maximum von Mises stresses in the jaw and to evaluate the maximum displacement of the implant-abutment complex in immediate-loading models. It was found that (i) the maximum von Mises stress in cortical bone was decreased by 65.8% under a bucco-lingual load with an increase in *D*, (ii) in cancellous bone, it was decreased by 71.5% under an axial load with an increase in *L*, (iii) the maximum displacement in the implant-abutment complex decreased by 64.8% under a bucco-lingual load with an increase in *D*, and (iv) the implant was found to be more sensitive to *L* than to *D* under axial loads, while *D* played a more important role in enhancing its stability under bucco-lingual loads. Based on these results, it was concluded that when *D* exceeded 4.0 mm and *L* exceeded 11.0 mm, both minimum stress and displacement were obtained; hence, these dimensions were the optimal biomechanical selections for immediate-loading implants in type B/2 bone [140].

Leonard et al. [141] compared the bone healing process around the plateau root from (PRF) and screw root from (SRF) titanium dental implants over the immediate 12-week healing period, post implant placement. The BIC and bone area fraction occupancy (BAFO) were made on the middle 5 mm portion of each 8 mm implant root length. It was reported that (i) although measurements of BIC and BAFO tended to be greater for the SRF implants at all four time points, the differences in measurements between implant types were not statistically significant, (ii) the effect of time on BIC and BAFO was found to be strongly significant for both implant types, thus indicating a statistically significant increase in BIC and BAFO overall with time, (iii) both PRF and SRF implants behaved similarly over time with measurements of BIC and BAFO progressing in parallel, and (iv) histomorphologic analysis of these sections demonstrated the prominent role of woven bone (callus) in the bone healing process around PRF implants. Although, from obtained results, a comparable development of secondary stability for both PRF and SRF implant designs can be indicated, as these parameters reflect the structural connection between implant and bone and not the functional properties of the bone to implant interface, they cannot be regarded as comprehensive measures of osseointegration [141]. Current trends in clinical dental implant therapy include the use of endosseous dental implant surfaces embellished with nanoscale topographies [142–144]. The common conclusion is that nanoscale modification of titanium endosseous implant surfaces can alter cellular and tissue responses that may benefit osseointegration and dental implant therapy.

Implant design and surface modification are independent conditions that can alter the implant-bone response. Aldosari et al. [145] compared the bone response to roughened tapered and cylindrical screw-type implants with and without HA surface coating in the femoral trabecular bone of rabbits. Their histomorphometric analysis revealed that the BIC values seemed to be higher for HA-coated tapered implants followed by cylindrical noncoated implants, and that all four types of implants showed a wide distribution of BIC with no statistical significance between different types of implants. It was concluded that under their experimental conditions, implant design and surface composition had little effect on the bone-to-implant interface [145].

Summarizing this discussion, we know three major compatibilities need to be met for placed implant systems to exhibit biofunctionality: biological, biomechanical, and morphological compatibility. Some systems already meet these requirements; however, the majority of implant systems do not. They should be reexamined because modifying their surface characteristics may help them gain lacking compatibilities. Effective surface modification technologies will be discussed in following two chapters.

References

1. Long, M. and Rack, H.J., 1998, Review: Titanium alloys in total joint replacement—A materials science perspective, *Biomaterials* 19:1621–1639. doi: http://dx.doi.org/10.1016/S0142-9612(97)00146-4
2. Brunski, J.B., Puleo, D.A. and Nanci, A., 2000, Biomaterials and biomechanics of oral and maxillofacial implants: Current status and future developments, *Int J Oral Maxillofac Implants* 15:15–46.
3. Bannon, B.P. and Mild, E.E., 1983, *Titanium Alloys in Surgical Implants, ASTM STP 796*, American Society for Testing and Materials; West Conshohocken, PA, pp. 7–15.
4. Oshida, Y. and Tuna, E.B., 2009, Science and technology integrated titanium dental implant systems, In: B. Basu, D.S. Katti, and A. Kumar, ed., *Advanced Biomaterials*, A John Wiley & Sons., pp. 143–177.
5. Oshida, Y., Hashem, A., Nishihara, T. and Yapchulay, M.V., 1994, Fractal dimension analysis of mandibular bones: Toward a morphological compatibility of implants, *Bio-Med Mater Eng* 4:397–407.
6. Oshida, Y., 2000, *Requirements for Successful Biofunctional Implants*, The 2nd Symposium International of Advanced Bio-Materials. Montreal, Canada, p. 5.
7. Oshida, Y., Tuna, E.B., Aktören, A. and Gençay, K., 2010, Dental implant systems. *Int J Mol Sci* 11:580–678. doi: http://dx.doi.org/10.3390/ijms11041580
8. Chang, J-C., Oshida, Y., Gregory, R.L., Andres, C.J., Barco, T.M. and Brown, D., 2003, Electrochemical study on microbiology-related corrosion of metallic materials, *Bio-Med Mater Eng* 13:281–295.
9. Anusavice, K.J., 2003, *Phillips' Science of Dental Materials*. Saunders: An Imprint of Elsevier, London, UK, pp. 185–196.
10. Williams, D.F., 2003, Revisiting the definition of biocompatibility, *Med Device Technol* 14:10–13.
11. Onuki, Y., Bhardwaj, U., Pharm., M., Papadimitrakopoulos, F. and Diane J. Burgess, D.J., 2008, A review of the biocompatibility of implantable devices: Current challenges to overcome foreign body response, *J Diabetes Sci Technol* 2:1003–1015.doi: http://dx.doi.org/10.1177/193229680800200610
12. Kipshidze, N.N., Tsapenko, M.V., Leon, M.B., Stone, G.W. and Moses, J.W., 2005, Update on drug-eluting coronary stents, *Expert Rev Cardiovasc Ther* 3:953–968. doi: http://dx.doi.org/10.1586/14779072.3.5.953
13. Moses, J.W., Kipshidze, N. and Leon, M.B., 2002, Perspectives of drug-eluting stents: The next revolution, *Am J Cardiovasc Drugs* 2:163–172. doi: http://dx.doi.org/10.2165/00129784-200202030-00004
14. Klonoff, D.C., Technological advances in the treatment of diabetes mellitus: Better bioengineering begets benefits in glucose measurement, the artificial pancreas, and insulin delivery, *Pediatr Endocrinol Rev* 1:94–100.

15. Frazier, O.H. and Jacob, L.P., Small pumps for ventricular assistance: Progress in mechanical circulatory support, *Cardiol Clin* 25:553–564. doi: http://dx.doi.org/10.1016/j.ccl.2007.09.001
16. Belverud, S., Mogilner, A. and Schulder, M., 2008, Intrathecal pumps, *Neurotherapeutics* 5:114–122. doi: http://dx.doi.org/10.1016/j.nurt.2007.10.070
17. Kizilel, S., Garfinkel, M. and Opara, E., 2005, The bioartificial pancreas: Progress and challenges, *Diabetes Technol Ther* 7:968–985. doi: http://dx.doi.org/10.1089/dia.2005.7.968
18. O'Connor, R.C., Lyon, M.B., Guralnick, M.L. and Bales, G.T., 2008, Long-term follow-up of single versus double cuff artificial urinary sphincter insertion for the treatment of severe postprostatectomy stress urinary incontinence, *Urology* 71:90–93. doi: http://dx.doi.org/10.1016/j.urology.2007.08.017
19. Fine, D.M. and Tobias, A.H., 2007, Cardiovascular device infections in dogs: Report of 8 cases and review of the literature, *J Vet Intern Med* 21:1265–1271. doi: http://dx.doi.org/10.1111/j.1939-1676.2007.tb01948.x
20. Prokop, A., 2001, Bioartificial organs in the twenty-first century: Nanobiological devices, *Ann N Y Acad Sci* 944:472–490. doi: http://dx.doi.org/10.1111/j.1749-6632.2001.tb03856.x
21. Wilson, G.S., Zhang, Y., Reach, G., Moatti-Sirat, D., Poitout, V., Thévenot, D.R., Lemonnier, F. and Klein, J.C., 1992, Progress toward the development of an implantable sensor for glucose, *Clin Chem* 38:1613–1617.
22. Koschwanez, H.E. and Reichert, W.M., 2007, In vitro, in vivo and post explantation testing of glucose-detecting biosensors: Current methods and recommendations, *Biomaterials* 28:3687–3703. doi: http://dx.doi.org/10.1016/j.biomaterials.2007.03.034
23. Callahan, T.D. and Natale, A., 2008, Catheter ablation of atrial fibrillation, *Med Clin North Am* 92:179–201. doi: http://dx.doi.org/10.1016/j.mcna.2007.09.001
24. Matsumoto, T., Okazaki, M., Nakahira, A., Sasaki, J., Egusa, H. and Sohmura, T., 2013, Modification of apatite materials for bone tissue engineering and drug delivery carriers, *Curr Med Chem* 14:2726–2733. doi: http://dx.doi.org/10.2174/092986707782023208
25. Salgado, A.J., Coutinho, O.P. and Reis, R.L., 2004, Bone tissue engineering: State of the art and future trends, *Macromol Biosci* 4:743–765. doi: http://dx.doi.org/10.1002/mabi.200400026
26. Abukawa, H., Papadaki, M., Abulikemu, M., Leaf, J., Vacanti, J.P., Kaban, L.B. and Troulis, M.J., 2006, The engineering of craniofacial tissues in the laboratory: A review of biomaterials for scaffolds and implant coatings. *Dent Clin North Am* 50;205–216. doi: http://dx.doi.org/10.1016/j.cden.2005.11.006
27. Nozyński, J.K., Religa, Z., Wszołek, J., Zembala-Nozyńska, E. and Rozentryt, P., 2001, Biological heart valve—an alternative to mechanical valve, *Med Sci Monit* 7:550–562.
28. Black, M.M. and Drury, P.J., 1994, Mechanical and other problems of artificial valves, *Curr Top Pathol* 86:127–59. doi: http://dx.doi.org/10.1007/978-3-642-76846-0_4
29. Sano, A., Hojo, T., Maeda, M. and Fujioka, K., 1998, Protein release from collagen matrices, *Adv Drug Deliv Rev* 31:247–266. doi: http://dx.doi.org/10.1016/S0169-409X(97)00119-1
30. Geiger, M., Li, R.H. and Friess, W., 2003, Collagen sponges for bone regeneration with rhBMP-2, *Adv Drug Deliv Rev* 55:1613–1629. doi: http://dx.doi.org/10.1016/j.addr.2003.08.010
31. Uchegbu, I.F., Schätzlein, A.G., Tetley, L., Gray, A.I., Sludden, J., Siddique, S. and Mosha, E., 1998, Polymeric chitosan-based vesicles for drug delivery, *J Pharm Pharmacol* 50:453–458. doi: http://dx.doi.org/10.1111/j.2042-7158.1998.tb06185.x

32. Khor, E. and Lim, L.Y., 2003, Implantable applications of chitin and chitosan, *Biomaterials* 24:2339–2349. doi: http://dx.doi.org/10.1016/S0142-9612(03)00026-7
33. Borchard, G. and Junginger, H.E., 2001, Modern drug delivery applications of chitosan, *Adv Drug Deliv Rev* 52:103–106. doi: http://dx.doi.org/10.1016/S0169-409X(01)00188-0
34. de Vos, P., Hoogmoed, C.G. and Busscher, H.J., 2002, Chemistry and biocompatibility of alginate-PLL capsules for immunoprotection of mammalian cells, *J Biomed Mater Res* 60:252–259. doi: http://dx.doi.org/10.1002/jbm.10060
35. Vercruysse, K.P. and Prestwich, G.D., 1998, Hyaluronate derivatives in drug delivery, *Crit Rev Ther Drug Carrier Syst* 15:513–555. doi: http://dx.doi.org/10.1615/CritRevTherDrugCarrierSyst.v15.i5.30
36. Cadée, J.A., Brouwer, L.A., den Otter, W., Hennink, W.E. and van Luyn, M.J., 2001, A comparative biocompatibility study of microspheres based on crosslinked dextran or poly(lactic-coglycolic)acid after subcutaneous injection in rats, *J Biomed Mater Res* 56:600–609. doi: http://dx.doi.org/10.1002/1097-4636(20010915)56:4<600::AID-JBM1133>3.0.CO;2-I
37. Draye, J.P., Delaey, B., Van de Voorde, A., Van Den Bulcke, A., De Reu, B. and Schacht, E., 1998, In vitro and in vivo biocompatibility of dextran dialdehyde cross-linked gelatin hydrogel films, *Biomaterials* 19:1677–1687. doi: http://dx.doi.org/10.1016/S0142-9612(98)00049-0
38. Mendes, S.C., Reis, R.L., Bovell, Y.P., Cunha, A.M., van Blitterswijk, C.A. and de Bruijn, J.D., 2001, Biocompatibility testing of novel starch-based materials with potential application in orthopaedic surgery: A preliminary study, *Biomaterials* 22:2057–2064. doi: http://dx.doi.org/10.1016/S0142-9612(00)00395-1
39. Anderson, J.M. and Langone, J.J., 1999, Issues and perspectives on the biocompatibility and immunotoxicity evaluation of implanted controlled release systems, *J Control Release* 57:107–113. doi: http://dx.doi.org/10.1016/S0168-3659(98)00178-3
40. Eisenbarth, E., Velten, D., Müller, M., Thull, R. and Breme, J., 2004, Biocompatibility of β-stabilizing elements of titanium alloys, *Biomaterials* 25:5705–5713. doi: http://dx.doi.org/10.1016/j.biomaterials.2004.01.021
41. Hallab, N.J., Skipor, A. and Jacobs, J.J., 2003, Interfacial kinetics of titanium- and cobalt-based implant alloys in human serum: Metal release and biofilm formation, *J Biomed Mater Res* 65A:311–318. doi: http://dx.doi.org/10.1002/jbm.a.10429
42. Mitchell, A. and Shrotriya, P., 2007, Onset of nanoscale wear of metallic implant materials: Influence of surface residual stresses and contact loads, *Wear* 263:1117–1123. doi: http://dx.doi.org/10.1016/j.wear.2007.01.068
43. Krupa, D., Baszkiewicz, J., Kozubowski, J.A., Lewandowska-Szumieł, M., Barcz, A., Sobczak, J.W., Biliński, A. and Rajchel, A., 2004, Effect of calcium and phosphorous ion implantation on the corrosion resistance and biocompatibility of titanium, *J Biomed Mater Eng* 14:525–536.
44. Nayab, S.N., Jones, F.H. and Olsen, I., 2007, Effects of calcium-implantation of titanium on bone cell function in vitro, *J Biomed Mater Res A* 83:296–302. doi: http://dx.doi.org/10.1002/jbm.a.31218
45. Sabetrasekh, R., Tiainen, H., Reseland, J.E., Will, J., Ellingsen, J.E., Lyngstadaas, S.P. and Haugen, H.J., 2010, Impact of trace elements on biocompatibility of titanium scaffolds, *Biomed Mater* 5:15003. doi: 10.1088/1748-6041/5/015003
46. Li, L-H., Kim, H-W., Lee, S-H., Kong, Y-M. and Kim, K-E., 2005, Biocompatibility of titanium implants modified by microarc oxidation and hydroxyapatite coating, *J Biomed Mater Res A* 73:48–54. doi: http://dx.doi.org/10.1002/jbm.a.30244
47. Schwarz, F., Papanicolau, P., Rothamel, D., Beck, B., Herten, M. and Becker, J., 2009, Influence of plaque biofilm removal on reestablishment of the biocompatibility of

contaminated titanium surfaces, *J Biomed Mater Res A* 77:437–444. doi: http://dx.doi.org/10.1002/jbm.a.30628

48. Shabalovskaya, S.A., 1996, On the nature of the biocompatibility and on medical applications of NiTi shape memory and superelastic alloys, *J Biomed Mater Eng* 6:267–289.
49. Oshida, Y. and Farzin-Nia, F., 2009, Chapter 6: Response of Ti-Ni alloys for dental biomaterials to conditions in the mouth, In: T.Yoneyama, S.Miyazakim ed., *Shape Memory Alloys for Biomedical Applications,* CRC Woodhead Pub., NY, pp. 101–149. doi: http://dx.doi.org/10.1533/9781845695248.1.101
50. Oshida, Y. and Miyazaki, S., 1991, Corrosion and biocompatibility of shape memory alloys, *Corr Eng* 40:1009–1025.
51. Castleman, L.S. and Motzkin, S.M., 1981, Biocompatibility of nitinol. In: D.F. Williams ed., *Biocompatibility of Clinical Implant Materials.* CRC Press. pp. 129–154.
52. Assad, M., Lomardi, S., Bernèche, S., DesRosiers, E.A., Yahia, L'H. and Rivard, C.H., 1994, Cytotoxicity testing of the nickel titanium shape memory alloy, *Ann Chir* 48:731–736.
53. Wever, D.J., Veldhuizen, A.G., deVries, J., Busscher, H.J., Uges, D.R.A. and van Horn, J.R., 1998, Electrochemical and surface characterization of a nickel titanium alloy, *Biomaterials* 19:761–766. doi: http://dx.doi.org/10.1016/S0142-9612(97)00210-X
54. Armitage, D.A., Parker, T.L. and Grant, D.M., 2003, Biocompatibility and hemocompatibility of surface-modified NiTi alloys, *J Biomed Mater Res A* 66:129–137. doi: http://dx.doi.org/10.1002/jbm.a.10549
55. Filip, P., Lausmaa, J., Musialek, J. and Mazanec, K., 2001, Structure and surface of NiTi human implants, *Biomaterials* 22:2131–2138. doi: http://dx.doi.org/10.1016/S0142-9612(00)00404-X
56. Elliot, D., Moiemen, N.S., Flemming, A.F., Harris, S.B. and Foster, A.J., 1994, The rupture rate of acute flexor tendon repairs mobilized by the controlled actions motion regimen, *J Hand Surg Eur Vol* 19:607–612. doi: http://dx.doi.org/10.1016/0266-7681(94)90126-0
57. Gelberman, R.H., Amifl, D., Gonsalves, M., Woo, S. and Akeson, W.H., 1981,The influence of protected passive mobilization on the healing of flexor tendons: A biochemical and minoangio-graphic study, *Hand* 13:120–128. doi: http://dx.doi.org/10.1016/S0072-968X(81)80051-4
58. Small, J.O., Brennen, M.D. and Colville, J., 1989, Early active mobilization following flexor tendon repair in zone 2, *J Hand Surg* 14B:383–391. doi: http://dx.doi.org/10.1016/0266-7681(89)90152-6
59. Trail, I.A., Powell, E.S. and Noble, J., 1989, An evaluation of suture materials used in tendon surgery, *J Hand Surg Eur Vol* 14:422–427. doi: http://dx.doi.org/10.1016/0266-7681(89)90160-5
60. Nystrom, B. and Holmlund, D., 1983, Separation of sutured tendon ends when different suture techniques and different suture materials are used: An experimental study in rabbits, *Scand J Plast Reconstr Surg* 17:19–23. doi: http://dx.doi.org/10.3109/02844318309007175
61. Silfrerskiod, K.I. and Anderssen, C.H., 1993, Two new methods tendon repair: An in vitro evaluation of tensile strength and gaps formation, *J Hand Surg Am* 18:58–65.
62. Aoki, A., Manske, P.R., Pruitt, D.L. and Larson, B.J., 1994, Tendon repair using flexor tendon splints: An experimental study, *J Hand Surg Am* 19:984–990.
63. Moneim, M.S., Firoozbakhsh, K., Mustapha, A.A., Larsen, K. and Shahinpoor, M., 2002, Flexor tendon repair using shape memory alloy suture: A biomechanical evaluation, *Clin Orthop* 402:251–259. doi: http://dx.doi.org/10.1097/00003086-200209000-00025
64. Miura, F., Mogi, M., Ohura, Y. and Hamanaka, H., 1986, The super-elastic property of the Japanese NiTi alloy wire for use in orthodontics, *Am J Orthod Dentofacial Orthop* 90:1–10. doi: http://dx.doi.org/10.1016/0889-5406(86)90021-1

65. Duerig, T.W., Pelton, A.P. and Stockel, D., 1996, The utility of superelasticity in medicine, *J Biomed Mater Eng* 6:255–266.
66. Kujala, S., Pajala, A., Kallioinen, M., Pramila, A., Tuukkanen, J. and Ryhänen, J., 2004, Biocompatibility and strength properties of nitinol shape memory alloy suture in rabbit tendon, *Biomaterials* 25:353–358. doi: http://dx.doi.org/10.1016/S0142-9612(03)00488-5
67. Lifeng, Z., Yan, H., Dayun, Y., Xiaoying, L., Tingfei, X., Deyuan, Z., Ying, H. and Yuan Jinfeng, Y., 2011, The underlying biological mechanisms of biocompatibility differences between bare and TiN-coated NiTi alloys, *Biomed Mater* 6:025012. doi: http://dx.doi.org/10.1088/1748-6041/6/2/025012
68. Zivić, F., Babić, M., Grujović, N. and Mitrović, S., 2010, Tribometry of materials for bioengineering applications, *Tribol Industry* 32:25–32.
69. Niinomi, M., 2008, Mechanical biocompatibility of titanium alloys for biomedical applications, *J Mech Bahav Biomed Mater* 1:30–42. doi: http://dx.doi.org/10.1016/j.jmbbm.2007.07.001
70. Treccani, L., Maiwald, M., Z llmer, V., Busse, M., Grathwohl, G. and Rezwan, K., 2009, Antibacterial and abrasion-resistant alumina micropatterns, *Adv Eng Mater* 11:B61–B66. doi: http://dx.doi.org/10.1002/adem.200800372
71. Lin, Y-S. and Burggraaf, A.J., 1991, Preparation and characterization of high-temperature thermally stable alumina composite membrane, *J Am Ceram Soc* 74:219–224. doi: http://dx.doi.org/10.1111/j.1151-2916.1991.tb07320.x
72. Liu, Y., Chen, O.Y., Wei, C.C. and Li, K., 2006, Preparation of yttria-stabilised zirconia (YSZ) hollow fibre membranes, *Desalination* 199:360–362. doi: http://dx.doi.org/10.1016/j.desal.2006.03.216
73. Wenz, H.J., Bartsch, J., Wolfart, S. and Kern, M., 2008, Osseointegration and clinical success of zirconia dental implants: A systematic review, *Int J Prosthodont* 21:27–36.
74. Femández-Fairén, M., Sala, P. and Gil, F.J., 2006, Failures of yttria-stabilised tetragonal zirconia: 52 retrieved ceramic femoral heads of total hip prostheses, *Biomed Mater Eng* 16:415–422.
75. Schincaglia, G.P., Marzola, R., Scapoli, C. and Scotti, R., 2007, Immediate loading of dental implants supporting fixed partial dentures in the posterior mandible: A randomized controlled split-mouth study: Machined versus titanium oxide implant surfaces, *Int J Oral Maxillofac Implants* 22:35–46.
76. Domanski, M., Winnubst, L., Luttge, R., Lamers, E., Walboomers, X.F., Jansen, J. and Gardeniers, H., 2012, Production and characterization of micro- and nano-features in biomedical alumina and zirconia ceramics using a tape casting route, *J Mater Sci Mater Med* 23:1637–1644. doi: http://dx.doi.org/10.1007/s10856-012-4635-1
77. Krishna, B.V., Xue, W., Bose, S. and Amit Bandyopadhyay, A., 2008, Engineered porous metals for implants, *JOM* 60:45–48.
78. Coelho, P.G., Granato, R, Marin, C., Bonfante, E.A., Freire, J.N., Janal, M.N., Gil, J.N. and Suzuki, M., 2010, Biomechanical evaluation of endosseous implants at early implantation times: A study in dogs, *Int Oral Maxillofac Surg* 68:1667–1675.
79. Park, C.H., Lee, C.S., Kim, Y.J., Jang, J.H., Suh, J.Y. and Park, J.W., 2011, Improved pre-osteblast response and mechanical compatibility of ultrafine-grained Ti–13Nb–13Zr alloy, *Clin Oral Impants Res* 22:735–742. doi: http://dx.doi.org/10.1111/j.1600-0501.2010.02053.x
80. Williams, D.F., 1986, The biological applications of titanium and titanium alloys, In: R.Kossowsky ed., *Materials Science and Implant Orthopedic Surgery*, Martinus Nijhoff, Dordrecht, Netherlands, pp. 107–116. doi: http://dx.doi.org/10.1007/978-94-009-4474-9_9

81. Sutherland, D.S., Forshaw, P.D., Allen, G.C., Brown, I.T. and Williams, K.R., 1993, Surface analysis of titanium implants, *Biomaterials* 14:893–899. doi: http://dx.doi.org/10.1016/0142-9612(93)90130-T
82. Tengvall, P., Lundstrom, I., Sjoqvist, L. and Elwing, H., 1989,Titanium-hydrogen peroxide interactions: Model studies of the influence of the inflammatory response on titanium implants, *Biomaterials* 10:166–175. doi: http://dx.doi.org/10.1016/0142-9612(89)90019-7
83. Tengvall, P. and Lundstrom, I., 1992, Physio-chemical considerations of titanium as a biomaterial, *Clin Mater* 9:115–134. doi: http://dx.doi.org/10.1016/0267-6605(92)90056-Y
84. Asaoka, K., Kuwayama, N., Okuno, O. and Miura, I., 1985, Mechanical properties and bio-mechanical compatibility of porous titanium for dental implants, *J Biomed Mater Res* 19:699–713. doi: http://dx.doi.org/10.1002/jbm.820190609
85. Cole, B.J., Bostrom, M.P., Pritchard, T.L., Summer, D.R., Tomin, E., Lane, J.M. and Weiland, A.J., 1997, Use of bone morphologentic protein 2 on ectopic porous coated implants in the rat, *Clin Orthop* 345:219–228. doi: http://dx.doi.org/10.1097/00003086-199712000-00032
86. Denissen, H., van Beek, E., van den Bos, T., de Blieck, J., Klein, C. and van den Hooff, A., 1997, Degradable biphosphonate-alkaline phosphatase-complexed hydroxyapatite implants in vitro, *J Bone Miner Res* 12:290–297. doi: http://dx.doi.org/10.1359/jbmr.1997.12.2.290
87. Piztelli, A., Scarano, A., Di Alberti, L. and Piatelli, M., 1997, Histological and histochemical analyses of acid and alkaline phosphatase around hydroxyapatite-coated implants: A time course study in rabbit, *Biomaterials* 8:1191–1194. doi: http://dx.doi.org/10.1016/S0142-9612(97)00055-0
88. Batzer, R., Liu, Y., Cochran, D.L., Szmuckler-Moncler, S., Dean, D.D., Buyan, B.D. and Schwartz, Z., 1998, Prostaglandins mediate the effects of titanium surface roughness on MG63 osteoblast-like cells and alter cell responsiveness to 1α,25-$(OH)_2D_3$, *J Biomed Mater Res* 41:489–496. doi: http://dx.doi.org/10.1002/(SICI)1097-4636(19980905)41:3<489::AID-JBM20>3.3.CO;2-K
89. Overgaard, S., Lindm, M., Glerup, H., Bunger, C. and Soballe, K., 1998, Porous-coated versus grit-blasted surface texture of hydroxyapatite-coated implants during controlled micromotion: Mechanical and histomorphological results, *J Arthrosplasty* 13:449–458. doi: http://dx.doi.org/10.1016/S0883-5403(98)90011-0
90. Wie, H., Hero, H. and Solheim, T., 1998, Hot isostatic pressing-processed hydroxyapatite-coated titanium implants: Light microscopic and scanning electron microscopic investigation. *Int J Oral Maxillofac Implants* 13:837–844.
91. Rohold, A.E., Nielsen, G.D. and Andersen, K.E., 1991, Nickel-sulphate-induced dermatitis in the guinea pig maximization test: A dose-response study, *Contact Dermatitis* 24:35–39. doi: http://dx.doi.org/10.1111/j.1600-0536.1991.tb01627.x
92. Kerosuo, H., Kullaa, A., Kerosuo, E., Kanerva, L. and Hensten-Ptterson, A., 1996, Nickel allergy in adolescents in relation to orthodontic treatment and piercing of ears, *Am J Orthod Dentofacial Orthop* 109:148–154. doi: http://dx.doi.org/10.1016/S0889-5406(96)70175-0
93. Skalak, R., 1983, Biomechanical considerations in osseointegrated prostheses, *J Prosthetic Dent* 49:843–848. doi: http://dx.doi.org/10.1016/0022-3913(83)90361-X
94. Kanth, L., 1971, The cast (intramobile) screw implant, *DDZ* 25:465–467.
95. Brunski, J.B., 1999, In vivo bone response to biomechanical loading at the bone/dental-implant interface, *Adv Dent Res* 13:99–119. doi: http://dx.doi.org/10.1177/08959374990130012301

96. Koch, W.L., 1976, 2-phasic endosseous implantation of intramobile cylindrical implants, *Quintessenz* 27:23–31.
97. Kanth, L., 1982, Titanium plasma coated intramobile conical implants, *ZWR* 91:42–46.
98. Kirsch, A., 1983, The two-phase implantation method using IMZ intramobile cylinder implants, *J Oral Implantol* 11:197–202.
99. Gaggl, A. and Schultes, G., 2001, Biomechnical properties in titanium implants with integrated maintenance free shock absorbing elements, *Biomaterials* 22:3061–3066. doi: http://dx.doi.org/10.1016/S0142-9612(01)00053-9
100. Miyawaki, S., Koyama, I., Inoue, M., Mishima, K., Sugahara, T. and Takano-Yamamoto, T., 2003, Factors associated with the stability of titanium screws placed in the posterior region for orthodontic anchorage, *Am J Orthod Dentofacial Orthop* 124:373–378. doi: http://dx.doi.org/10.1016/S0889-5406(03)00565-1
101. Oshida, Y., 2007, *Bioscience and Bioengineering of Titanium Materials*, Elsevier, London, UK, p. 232.
102. Eriksson, C., Lausmaa, J. and Nygren, H., 2001, Interactions between human whole blood and modified TiO_2-surfaces: Influence of surface topography and oxide thickness on leukocyte adhesion and activation, *Biomaterials* 22:1987–1996. doi: http://dx.doi.org/10.1016/S0142-9612(00)00382-3
103. Wen, X., Wang, X. and Zhang, N., 1996, Microsurface of metallic biomaterials: A literature review, *J Biomed Mater Eng* 6:173–189.
104. Niemczewska-Wójcik, M., 2011, The influence of the surface geometric structure on the functionality of implants, *Wear* 271:596–610. doi: http://dx.doi.org/10.1016/j.wear.2010.06.013
105. Smith, D.C., Pilliar, R.M. and Chernecky, C., 1991, Dental implant materials. I. Some effects of preparative procedures on surface topography, *J Biomed Mater Res* 25:1045–1068. doi: http://dx.doi.org/10.1002/jbm.820250903
106. Javed, F., Almas, K., Crespi, R. and Romanos, G.E., 2011, Implant surface morphology and primary stability: Is there a connection? *Implant Dent* 20:40–46. doi: http://dx.doi.org/10.1097/ID.0b013e31820867da
107. Fandridis, J. and Papadopoulos, T., 2008, Surface characterization of three titanium dental implants, *Implant Dent* 17:91–99. doi: http://dx.doi.org/10.1097/ID.0b013e318166d9ac
108. Iezzi, G., Aprile, G., Tripodi, D., Scarano, A., Piattelli, A. and Perrotti, V., 2011, Implant surface topographies analyzed using fractal dimension, *Implant Dent* 20:131–138. doi: http://dx.doi.org/10.1097/ID.0b013e31820fb171
109. Stanford, C.M., 2010, Surface modification of biomedical and dental implants and the processes of inflammation, wound healing and bone formation, *Int J Mol Sci* 11:354–369. doi: http://dx.doi.org/10.3390/ijms11010354
110. Keller, J.C., Dougherty, W.J., Grotendorst, G.R. and Wrightman, J.P., 1989, In vitro cell attachment to characterized cpTi surfaces, *A Adhesion* 28:115–133.
111. Keller, J.C., Wrightman, J.P. and Dougherty, W.J., 1989, Characterization of acid passivated cpTi surfaces, *J Dent Res* 68:872.
112. Keller, J.C., Draughn, R.A., Wrightman, J.P. and Dougherty, W.J., 1990, Characterization of sterilized CP titanium implant surfaces, *Int J Oral Maxillofac Implants* 5:360–369.
113. Schroeder, A., Van der Zypen, E., Stich, H. and Sutter, F., 1981, The reactions of bone, connective tissue and epithelium to endosteal implants with titanium sprayed surfaces. *J Maxillofac Surg* 9:15–25. doi: http://dx.doi.org/10.1016/S0301-0503(81)80007-0
114. Buser, D., Schenk, R.K., Steinemann, S., Fiorellinni, J.P., Fox, C.H. and Stich, H., 1991, Influence of surface characteristics on bone integration of titanium implants. A histomorphometric study in miniature pigs, *J Biomed Mater Res* 25:889–902. doi: http://dx.doi.org/10.1002/jbm.820250708

115. Rich, A. and Harris, A.K., 1981, Anomalous preferences of cultured macrophages for hydrophobic and roughended substrata, *J Cell Sci* 50:1–7.
116. Murray, D.W., Rae, T. and Rushton, N., 1989, The influence of the surface energy and roughness of implants on bone resorption, *J Bone Joint Surg Br* 71:632–637.
117. Cherhoudi, B., Gould, T.R.L. and Brunette, D.M., 1988, Effects of a grooved epoxy substratum on epithelial behavior in vivo and in vitro, *J Biomed Mater Res* 22:459–477. doi: http://dx.doi.org/10.1002/jbm.820220603
118. von Recum, A.F., 1990, New aspects of biocompatibility: Motion at the interface. In: G. Heimke, U. Soltesz, A.J.C. Lee, ed., *Clinical Implant Materials*. Elsevier Science Pub., Amsterdam, pp. 297–302.
119. Jeong, S.H., Park, Y.J., Kim, B.S. and Song, H.J., 2007, Effects of oxygen content on bioactivity of titanium oxide films fabricated on titanium by electron beam evaporation, *J Nanosci Nanotechnol* 7:3815–3818. doi: http://dx.doi.org/10.1166/jnn.2007.043
120. Xue, W., Krishna, B.V., Bandyopadhyyay, A. and Bose, S., 2007, Processing and biocompatibility evaluation of laser processed porous titanium, *Acta Biomater* 3:1007–1018. doi: http://dx.doi.org/10.1016/j.actbio.2007.05.009
121. Ratner, B.D., 1983, Surface characterization of biomaterials by electron spectroscopy for chemical analysis, *Ann Biomed Eng* 11:313–336. doi: http://dx.doi.org/10.1007/BF02363290
122. Baro, A.M., Garcia, N., Miranda, R., Vázquez, L., Aparicio, C., Olivé, J. and Lausmaa, J., 1986, Characterization of surface roughness in titanium dental implants measured with scanning tunneling microscopy at atmospheric pressure, *Biomaterials* 7:463–466. doi: http://dx.doi.org/10.1016/0142-9612(86)90036-0
123. Kasemo, B., 1983, Biocompatibility of titanium implants: Surface science aspects. *J Prosthet Dent* 49:832–837. doi: http://dx.doi.org/10.1016/0022-3913(83)90359-1
124. Moroni, A., Caja, V.L., Egger, E.L., Trinchese, L. and Chao, E.Y., 1994, Histomorphometry of hydroxyl–apatite coated and uncoated porous titanium bone implants, *Biomaterials* 15:926–930. doi: http://dx.doi.org/10.1016/0142-9612(94)90119-8
125. Keller, J.C., Young, F.A. and Natiella, J.R., 1987, Quantitative bone remolding resulting from the use of porous dental implants, *J Biomed Mater Res* 21:305–319. doi: http://dx.doi.org/10.1002/jbm.820210304
126. Pilliar, R., Deporter, D.A., Watson, P.A. and Valiquette, N., 1991, Dental implant design-effect on bone remodeling, *J Biomed Mater Res* 25:467–483. doi: http://dx.doi.org/10.1002/jbm.820250405
127. Gilbert, J.L. and Berkery, C.A., 1995, Electrochemical reaction to mechanical disruption of titanium oxide films, *J Dent Res* 74:92–96.
128. Brunette, D.M., 1988, The effects of implant surface topography on the behavior of cells. *Int J Oral Maxillofac Implants* 3:231–246.
129. Chehroudi, B., Gould, T.R.L, and Brunette, D.M., 1990, Tiatnium-coated micromachined grooves of different dimensions affect epithelial and connective tissue cells differently in vitro. *J Biomed Mater Res* 24:1206–1219. doi: http://dx.doi.org/10.1002/jbm.820240906
130. Chehroudi, B., Gould, T.R.L. and Brunette, D.M., 1990, Effects of a grooved titanium coated implant surface on epithelial cell behavior, in vitroand in vivo, *J Biomed Mater Res* 24:1067–1085.
131. Michaels, C.M., Keller, J.C., Stanford, C.M. and Solursh, M., 1989, Invitro cell attachment of osteblast-like cells to titanium, *J Dent Res* 68:276.
132. Keller, J.C., Stanford, C.M., Wightman, J.P., Draughn, R.A. and Zaharias, R., 1994, Characterizations of titanium implant surfaces (Pt. 3), *J Biomed Mater Res* 28:939–946. doi: http://dx.doi.org/10.1002/jbm.820280813

133. Klokkevold, P.R., Nishimura, R.D., Adachi, M. and Caputo, A., 1997, Osseointegration enhanced by chemical etching of the titanium surface. A torque removal study in the rabbit, *Clin Oral Implants Res* 8:442–447. doi: http://dx.doi.org/10.1034/j.1600-0501.1997.080601.x
134. Vasconcellos, L.M., Oliveira, M.V., Graça, M.L., Vasconcellos, L.G., Cairo, C.A. and Carvalho, Y.R., 2008, Design of dental implants, influence on the osteogenesis and fixation, *J Mater Sci Mater Med* 19:2851–2857. doi: http://dx.doi.org/10.1007/s10856-008-3421-6
135. Mattila, R.H., Laurila, P., Rekola, J., Gunn, J., Lassila, L.V., Mäntylä, T., Aho, A.J. and Vallitu, P.K., 2009, Bone attachment to glass-fibre-reinforced composite implant with potous surface, *Acta Biomater* 5:1639–1646. doi: http://dx.doi.org/10.1016/j.actbio.2009.01.020
136. Chehroudi, B., Ghrebi, S., Murakami, H., Waterfield, J.D., Owen, G. and Brunette, D.M., 2010, Bone formation on rough, but not polished, subcutaneously implanted Ti surfaces is preceded by macrophage accumulation, *J Biomed Mater Res A* 93:724–737.
137. Germanier, Y., Tosatti, S., Broggini, N., Textor, M. and Buser, D., 2006, Enhanced bone apposition around biofunctionalized sandblasted and acid-etched titanium implant surfaces—A histomorphometric study in miniature pigs, *Clin Oral Implants Res* 17:251–257. doi: http://dx.doi.org/10.1111/j.1600-0501.2005.01222.x
138. Abuhussein, H., Pagni, G., Rebaudi, A. and Wang, H-L., 2010, The effect of thread pattern upon implant osseointegration, *Clin Oral Implants Res* 21:129–136. doi: http://dx.doi.org/10.1111/j.1600-0501.2009.01800.x
139. Petrie, C.S. and Williams, J.L., 2005, Comparative evaluation of implant designs: Influence of diameter, length, and taper on strains in the alveolar crest—A three-dimensional finite-element analysis, *Clin Oral Implants Res* 16:486–494. doi: http://dx.doi.org/10.1111/j.1600-0501.2005.01132.x
140. Kong, L., Gu, Z., Li, T., Wu, J., Hu, K., Liu, Y., Zhou, H, and Baolin Liu, B., 2009, Biomechanical optimization of implant diameter and length for immediate loading: A nonlinear finite element analysis, *Int J Prosthodont* 22:607–615.
141. Leonard, G., Coelho, P., Polyzois, I., Stassen, L., Claffey, N., 2009, A study of the bone healing kinetics of plateau versus screw root design titanium dental implants, *Clin Oral Implants Res* 20:232–239. doi: http://dx.doi.org/10.1111/j.1600-0501.2008.01640.x
142. Mendonça, G., Mendonça, D.B.S., Aragão, F.J.L. and Cooper, L.F., 2008, Advancing dental implant surface technology—From micron- to nanotopography, *Biomaterials* 29:3822–3835. doi: http://dx.doi.org/10.1016/j.biomaterials.2008.05.012
143. Aljateeli, M. and Wang, H-L., 2013, Implant microdesigns and their impact on osseointegration, *Implant Dent* 22:127–132. doi: http://dx.doi.org/10.1097/ID.0b013e318278a90b
144. Tetè, S., Mastrangelo, F., Quaresima, R., Vinci, R., Sammartino, G., Stuppia, L. and Gherlone, E., 2010, Influence of novel nano-titanium implant surface on human osteoblast behavior and growth, *Implant Dent* 19:520–531. doi: http://dx.doi.org/10.1097/ID.0b013e3182002eac
145. Aldosari, A.A., Anil, S., Alasqah, M., Al Wazzan, K.A.A., Al Jetaily, S.A. and Jansen, J.A., 2013, The influence of implant geometry and surface composition on bone response, *Clin Oral Implants Res*. doi: http://dx.doi.org/10.1111/clr.12190

Chapter 5

Surface Modification

Although a material possesses excellent mechanical properties, if it does not meet requirements for an acceptable surface feature, the surface layer needs to be manipulated. In this chapter, nature and interface are first characterized, followed by a detailed discussion on surface modification technologies and preparation of coating materials.

5.1. Introduction

Some surfaces are already biocompatible *per se*; on the other hand, the other types of surfaces are required to modify the surface layer to show acceptable biocompatibility. The interaction between the implant surface and the living body will take place right after placing the implant into patient's body, and faster and earlier fixation or fusing to receiving hard tissue (in other words, osseointegration) [1–4] is expected. Among dental implant design alterations, surface modifications have been by far the most investigated topic. Regarding implant surface research, the lack of approaches relating *in vitro*, *in vivo*, clinical trials, and *ex vivo* analyses has hindered biomaterials scientists with clear informed rationale guidelines for the implant surface design [1]. Over the decade, surface texture, modifications, and functionalization, including novel nanotechnology-based fabrication processes have been the most utilized parameter for successful host-to-implant responses. Recently, dental implant surfaces utilizing reduced length scale physico/chemical features (atomic and nanometric) have shown the potential to synergistically use both texture and the inclusion of bioactive ceramic components on the surface. Although surface modifications have been shown to enhance osseointegration at early implantation times, information concerning its long-term benefit to peri-implant tissues is lacking due to the reduced number of controlled clinical trials [1]. To accommodate this faster and earlier osseointegration, there are several ideas and methods developed: surface roughening which is reflected to rugophilia of new-born bone cells [5–7], furthermore, chemical/physical modification of implant surfaces [8–15], manipulating surface energy status [16–20], and biomimetic coating [21–24] or biofunctionalizition [25,26].

Surfaces can be modified through various means including chemical, physical, thermal, mechanical, or combination of these to meet predetermined specific aims. From the

DOI 10.5643/9781606506288/ch5

different point of view, it can be said that surfaces can be treated by additive methods (for creating convex surfaces), such as the hydroxyapatite (HA) powder or titanium beads plasma spray coating, or they can also be modified by subtractive methods (for creating concave surfaces) such as acid pickling or acid etching, sandblasting, and other small particle-blasting to change the surface texture. In this chapter, conventional as well as newly developed surface modification technologies and methods will be discussed.

5.2. Nature of Surface and Interface

Before discussing surface modification in detail, it is worth reviewing briefly the nature of surface and interface. The surface of a material defines the boundary of an object and is not just a free end of a substance, but it is a contact and boundary zone with other substances (either in gaseous, liquid, or solid). A physical system which comprises of a homogeneous component such as solid, liquid, or gas and is clearly distinguishable from each other is called a phase, and a boundary at which two or three of these individual phases are in contact is called an interface. Surface and interface reactions include reactions with organic or inorganic materials, vital or nonvital species, hostile or friendly environments, and so forth. Surface activities may vary from mechanical actions (fatigue crack initiation and propagation, stress intensification, etc.), chemical action (discoloration, tarnishing, contamination, corrosion, oxidation, etc.), mechano-chemical action (corrosion fatigue, stress-corrosion cracking, etc.), thermo-mechanical action (thermal fatigue and creep), tribological and biotribological actions (wear and wear debris toxicity, friction, etc.) to physical and biophysical actions (surface contact and adhesion, adsorption, absorption, diffusion, cellular attachment, cell proliferation and differentiation, etc). Consequently, the properties of the surface determine the interaction of the second material [27,28]. The surface of an object determines various properties and reactivity (especially chemical); for example, in large objects with a small surface-area-to-volume ratio, the physical and chemical properties are primarily defined by the bulk, while in small objects with a large surface area to volume ratio, the properties are strongly influenced by the surface.

Coating is just a small portion of surface science and engineering. Structural elements beneath the surface function principally to support the surface and its characteristics determine not only esthetic appearance, but also interaction with the environment, including mechanical interactions, chemical interactions, optical and thermal interactions [29], and of course biological interactions. Accordingly, the longevity, safety, reliability, and structural integrity of dental and medical materials and devices are greatly governed by these surface phenomena, which can be detected, observed, characterized, and analyzed by virtue of various means of equipment and technologies [27,28,30,31].

5.3. Surface Modification Technologies

There are various reasons for a surface layer to receive alteration: for changing surface topology, for controlling surface energy, for managing hydrophilicity, for varying appearance, for enhancing surface chemistry and physics, for enriching surface elements or substances, and so forth. Methods for achieving such surface modification can be found in mechanical, chemical and electrochemical, physical, thermal, or combined techniques.

5.3.1. Mechanical Modification

Sandblasting, as well as shot-peening, possesses three purposes: (i) cleaning surface contaminants, (ii) roughening surfaces to increase the effective surface area, and (iii) producing beneficial surface compressive residual stress. As a result, such treated surfaces exhibit higher surface energy, indicating higher surface chemical and physical activities, and enhancing fatigue strength as well as fatigue life. Enhanced bond strength obtained in any possible bonding couples such as dentine bonding system, porcelain/Ti bonding or bone/Ti implant can be generally explained to a favorable result of having blasting (causing tons of small indentations on the surface layer) to increase the effective surface area, which is approximately doubled by mild sandblasting [32].

In order to obtain satisfactory fixation and biofunctionality of biotolerated and bioinert materials, some of the mechanical surface alternations such as threaded surface, grooved surface, pored surface, and rough surface have been produced that promote tissue and bone ingrowth. But so far, there is no report on suitable roughness to specific metallic biomaterials. In general, on the macroscopic level (>10 μm), roughness will influence the mechanical properties of the interface, the way stresses are distributed and transmitted, the mechanical interlocking of the interface, and the biocompatibility of biomaterials. On a smaller scale, surface roughness in the range from 10 nm to 10 μm may influence the interface biology, since it is of the same order in size as cells and large biomolecules. Topographic variations of the order of 10 nm and less may become important because microroughness consists of material defects such as grain boundaries, steps, and vacancies, which are known to be active sites for adsorption, and thus may influence the bonding of biomolecules to the implant surface. There is evidence that surface roughness on a micron scale allows cellular adhesion that alters the overall tissue response to biomaterials [33]. The microrough surface allows early better adhesion of mineral ions or atoms, biomolecules, and cells and forms stronger fixation of bone or connective tissue, resulting in a thinner tissue-reaction layer with inflammatory cells decreased or absent, and consequently microorganism adhesion and plaque accumulation can be prevented, when compared with the smooth surfaces [33].

Piattelli et al. [35] conducted a histological and histochemical evaluation in rabbits to study the presence of multinucleated giant cells (MGCs) at the interface with machined, sand-blasted (with 150 μm alumina media), and plasma-sprayed titanium implants. It was reported that (i) MGCs were not observed at any of the experimental times around machined and sand-blasted titanium surfaces, whereas (ii) MGCs were present at the interface with titanium plasma-sprayed implants at 2 weeks and at 2 months, (iii) at 4 and 8 weeks, these cells tended to decrease in number, and (iv) an inflammatory infiltrate was not present in connection with the MGCs [35]. Although alumina (Al_2O_3) or silica (SiO_2) particles are most frequently used as a blasting media, there are several different types of powder particles utilized as media. Surface roughness modulates the osseointegration of orthopedic and dental titanium implants. This process may cause the release of cytotoxic silicon or aluminum ions in the peri-implant tissue. To generate a biocompatible roughened titanium surface, an innovative grid-blasting process using biphasic calcium phosphate (BCP) particles was developed [36]. Ti–6Al–4V disks were either polished, BCP grid-blasted, or left as-machined. BCP grid-blasting created an average surface roughness of 1.57 μm compared to the original machined surface of 0.58 μm. X-ray photoelectron spectroscopy (XPS) indicated traces of calcium and phosphorus and relatively less aluminum on the BCP grid-blasted surface than on the initial titanium specimen. It was reported that (i) scanning electronic microscopy observations and measurement of mitochondrial activity (MTS assay) showed that osteoblastic MC3T3-E1 cells were viable in contact with the BCP grid-blasted titanium surface, (ii) MC3T3-E1 cells expressed alkaline phosphate (ALP) activity and conserved their responsiveness to bone morphogenetic protein BMP-2, and (iii) the calcium phosphate grid-blasting technique increased the roughness of titanium implants and provided a noncytotoxic surface with regard to mouse osteoblasts [36].

Although the recent development of investment materials and casting machines has enabled clinical applications of titanium in dentistry, there remain several problems to be solved. First of all, efficient finishing techniques are required. Titanium is known to be difficult to grind because of its plasticity, stickiness, low heat conductivity, and chemical reactivity at high temperatures [36,37]. Although blasting shows several advantages, there is evidence of adverse effects: (i) surface contamination, depending on the type of blasting media, and (ii) distortion of blasted workpiece, depending on blasting manner and intensity. Miyakawa et al. [38] studied the surface contamination of abraded titanium. Despite low grinding speeds and water cooling, the abraded surfaces were found to be contaminated by abrasive constituent elements. Element analysis and chemical bond state analysis of the contaminants were performed using an electron probe microanalyzer. X-ray diffraction (XRD) of the abraded surface was performed to identify the contaminants. It was reported that (i) the contamination of titanium is related to its reactivity as well as its hardness, (ii) in spite of water cooling and slow-speed abrading, titanium surfaces were obviously contaminated, (iii) contaminant deposits with dimensions ranging from about 10 to 30 μm occurred throughout the surfaces, and (iv) the contaminant of titanium, although related also to the hardness, resulted primarily from a reaction with abrasive materials, and such contamination could negatively influence titanium's resistance to corrosion and its bio-compatibility [38].

Normally, fine alumina particles (50 μm Al_2O_3) are recycled within the sandblasting machine. Ceramics such as alumina are brittle in nature; therefore some portions of recycled alumina might be brittle-fractured. If fractured sandblasting particles are involved in the recycling media, it might result in irregular surfaces, as well as potential contamination. Balza et al. [39] analyzed a sandblasting process using alumina abrasive particles on Ti–6Al–4V surfaces. The metallic samples were first characterized by optical microscopy, revealing an $\alpha + \beta$ microstructure with a Widmanstätten morphology. Topography of the samples was assessed by scanning electron microscopy (SEM), before and after sandblasting. The Al_2O_3 particles used had a granulometric distribution between 420 and 850 μm, with a median particle size (d50) of 670 μm, which decreased to 420 μm after sandblasting for 10 seconds. It was reported that this change in the size of the particles generated a loss on particle kinetic energy by a factor of 3.5.

Such variation on processing conditions induced a progressive increase on average roughness (R_a) of the Ti–6Al–4V surfaces, until the first 7 seconds were reached. From that point on, a reverse process was observed, exerting a polishing effect on the surface of the Ti–6Al–4V alloy [39]. Using fractal dimension analysis [40–42], a sample plate surface was weekly analyzed in terms of topographic changes, as well as chemical analysis of sampled recycled Al_2O_3 particles. It was found that after accumulated use time exceeded 30 minutes, the fractal dimension (D_F) [40] remained a constant value of about 1.4, prior to that it continuously increased from 1.25 to 1.4. By the electron probe microanalysis on collected blasting particles, unused Al_2O_3 contains 100% Al, whereas used (accumulated usage time was about 2,400 seconds) particles contained Al (83.32 wt%), Ti (5.48), Ca (1.68), Ni (1.36), Mo (1.31), S (1.02), Si (0.65), P (0.55), Mn (0.49), K (0.29), Cl (0.26), and V (0.08), strongly indicating that used alumina powder was heavily contaminated, and a high risk for the next material surface to be contaminated. Such contaminants are from previously blasted materials having various chemical compositions, and investing materials as well [43].

There are several evidences of surface contamination due to mechanical abrasive actions. As a metallographic preparation, the surface needs to be mechanically polished with a metallographic paper (which is normally SiC-adhered paper) under running water [44,45]. It is worth mentioning here that polishing paper should be changed between different types of materials, and particularly when a dissimilar metal-couple is used for galvanic corrosion tests, such couple should not be polished prior to corrosion testing because both materials could become cross-contaminated [45]. Hence, there are attempts to use TiO_2 powder for blasting onto titanium material surfaces. It was reported that titanium surfaces were sand-blasted using TiO_2 powder (particle size ranging from 45 μm, 45–63 μm, and 63–90 μm) to produce the different surface textures prior to fibroblast cell attachment [46].

In the rabbit tibia, CpTi implants, which were sand-blasted with 25 μm Al_2O_3 and TiO_2 particles, were inserted in the rabbit tibia for 12 weeks. Even though the amount of Al on the implant surface was higher than for the Al_2O_3-blasted implants compared to implants not blasted with Al_2O_3, any negative effects of the Al element were not detected [47], which is in contrast to those reported by Johansson et al. [48], who reported that Al release from Ti–6Al–4V implants was found to coincide with a poorer bone-to-implant over a 3 month period. It is possible that the lack of differences between TiO_2-blasted and the Al_2O_3-blasted implants depends on lower surface concentrations of toxic Al ions than those reported by Johansson et al. [48]. Wang [49] investigated the effects of various surface modifications on porcelain bond strengths. Such modifications included Al_2O_3 blasting, TiO_2 blasting, $HNO_3 + HF + H_2O$ treatment, H_2O_2 treatment, and pre-oxidation in air at 600 °C for 10 min. Ti-porcelain couples were subjected to 3-point bending tests. It was concluded that TiO_2 air abrasion showed the highest bond strength, which was significantly different from other surface treatments.

Recently, it was reported that sandblasting using alumina as a media caused a remarkable distortion on a Co–Cr alloy and a noble alloy [50,51]. It was estimated that the stress causing the deflection exceeded the yield strength of tested materials. It was also suggested that the sandblasting should be done using the lowest air pressure, duration of blasting period, and particle size alumina in order to minimize distortion of crowns and frameworks. To measure distortion, Co–Cr alloy plates (25 mm long,

5 mm wide, and 0.7 mm thick) were sand-blasted with Al_2O_3 of 125 μm. Distortion was determined as the deflection of the plates as a distance of 20 mm from the surface. It was reported that (i) the mean deflections varied between 0.37 and 1.72 mm, and (ii) deflection increased by an increase in duration of the blasting, pressure, particle size, and by a decrease in plate thickness [50]. All these parameters are related to cumulative input energy of the media.

Shot peening (which is a similar process to sandblasting, but has more controlled peening power, intensity, and direction) is a cold-working process in which the surface of a part is bombarded with small spherical media called shot. Each piece of shot striking the material acts as a tiny hammer, imparting to the surface small indentations or dimples. In order for the dimple to be created, the surface fibers of the material must be yielded in tension. Below the surface, the fibers try to restore the surface to its original shape, thereby producing below the dimple a hemisphere of cold-worked material highly stressed in compression. Overlapping dimples (which are sometimes called forged dimples) develop an even layer of metal in residual compressive stress. It is well known that cracks will not initiate or propagate in a compressively stressed zone due to a tendency of crack-closure phenomenon. Since nearly all fatigue and stress corrosion cracking failures originate at the surface of a part, compressive surface residual stresses induced by shot peening provide considerable increases in part life, since advancing crack-opening is suppressed by pre-existing compressive residual stress. The maximum compressive residual stress produced at or under the surface of a part by shot peening is at least as great as half the yield strength of the material being peened. Many materials will also increase in surface hardness due to the cold working effect of shot peening [52,53]. Both compressive stresses and cold working effects are used in the application of shot peening in forming metal parts, called "shot forming" [53]. Oshida investigated the compressive residual stress distribution in depth underneath the surface of the Ti–6Al–4V alloy using the XRD. It was found that the compressive residual stress at the surface was –50 MPa, followed by the maximum compressive residual stress of –80 MPa at 20 μm below the surface. Then, the compressive residual stress starts to decrease to show almost zero stress at about 50 μm underneath the surface [54]. It was also shown that shot-peening resulted in better bonding strengths between the titanium substrate and porcelain than sandblasting [45].

Recent advances in biomaterials' research suggest that electrical charges on a dental implant surface significantly improve its osseointegration to living bone, as a result of selective osteoblast activation and fibroblast inhibition. Guo et al. [55] investigated the possibility of using sandblasting to modify the electrical charges on the surface of titanium materials, using Al_2O_3 grits on CpTi (grade II) plates, for durations between 3 and 30 seconds. After sandblasting, Ti surfaces were measured for their electrostatic voltage. The results indicate a novel finding, that is negative static charges are generated on the titanium surface, which may stimulate osteoblast activity to promote osseointegration around the dental implant surface. This finding may at least partially explain the good osseointegration results of sandblasted titanium dental implants, in addition to other known reasons, such as topological changes on the implant's surface. However, the static charges accumulated on the titanium surface during sandblasting decayed to a lower level with time. It remains a challenging task to seek ways to retain these charges after the quantification of a desired level of negative charges needed to promote osteoblast activity for osseointegration around dental implants [55].

The laser peening technology is recently developed, claiming a noncontact, no-media, and contamination-free peening method. Before treatment, the workpiece is covered with a protective ablative layer (paint or tape) and a thin layer of water. High-intensity (5–15 GW/cm^2) nanosecond pulses (10–30 ns) of laser light beam (3–5 mm width) striking the ablative layer generate a short-lived plasma which causes a shock wave to travel into the workpiece. The shock wave induces compressive residual stress that penetrates beneath the surface and strengthens the workpiece [56–59], resulting in improvements in fatigue life and retarding in stress corrosion cracking occurrence. Cho et al. [60] laser-treated CpTi screws and inserted in right tibia metaphysics of white rabbits for 8 weeks. It was reported that (i) SEM of laser-treated implants demonstrated a deep and regular honeycomb pattern with small pores, and (ii) after 8-week implantation, the removal torque was 23.58 N cm for control machined and 62.57 N cm for laser-treated implants. Gaggl et al. [61] reported that (i) surfaces of laser-treated Ti implants showed a high purity with enough roughness for good osseointegration, and (ii) the laser-treated Ti had regular patterns of micropore with an interval of 10–12 μm, diameter of 25 μm, and depth of 20 μm [61].

Jindal et al. [62] studied the effect of a novel process of surface modification, surface nano structuring by ultrasonic shot peening, on osteoblast proliferation and corrosion behavior of CpTi, in simulated body fluid (SBF). A mechanically polished disc of CpTi was subjected to ultrasonic shot peening with stainless steel balls, to create a nanostructure at the surface. A nanostructure (<20 nm), with inhomogeneous distribution, was revealed by atomic force and SEM. There was an increase of ~10% in cell proliferation, but there was drastic fall in corrosion resistance. The corrosion rate was increased by 327%, in the shot peened condition. In order to examine the role of residual stresses, a part of the shot peened specimen was annealed at 400 °C for 1 hour. It was found that (i) the surface nanostructure was much prominent, with increased number density and sharper grain boundaries, (ii) cell proliferation was enhanced to ~50%, and the corrosion rate was reduced by 86.2% and 41%, as compared with that of the shot peened and the as-received conditions treated conditions, respectively, (iii) the highly significant improvement in cell proliferation, resulting from annealing of the shot peened specimen, was attributed to increased volume fraction of stabilized nanostructure, stress recovery, and crystallization of the oxide film, and (iv) increase in corrosion resistance, from annealing of shot peened material, was related to more effective passivation. Thus, the surface of CpTi, modified by this novel process, possessed unique quality of enhancing cell proliferation as well as the corrosion resistance. It could be highly effective in reducing treatment time of patients adopting dental and orthopedic implants of titanium and its alloys [62].

Electric discharge machining (EDM) can alter the surface energy status [63,64]. Hercuba et al. [63] investigated the properties of the Ti–6Al–4V alloy after surface treatment by the EDM process. The EDM process with high peak currents proved to induce surface macro-roughness and to cause chemical changes to the surface. Evaluations were made of the mechanical properties by means of tensile tests, and of surface roughness for different peak currents of the EDM process. The EDM process with peak current of 29 A was found to induce sufficient surface roughness and to have a low adverse effect on tensile properties. The chemical changes were studied by SEM equipped with an energy dispersive X-ray analyser (EDX). The surface of the benchmark samples was obtained by plasma-spraying a titanium dioxide (TiO_2) coating. An investigation of the biocompatibility of the surface-treated Ti–6Al–4V samples in cultures of human osteoblast-like MG 63 cells revealed that the samples modified by EDM provided better substrates for the adhesion, growth, and viability of MG 63 cells than the TiO_2-coated surface. Thus, it was reported that EDM treatment can be considered as a promising surface modification to orthopedic implants, in which good integration with the surrounding bone tissue is required [63].

Plastic deformation can also change the surface conditions [65,66]. The processes of equal-channel angular pressing and high-pressure torsion are now established for the fabrication of ultrafine-grained metals having superior properties by comparison with their coarse-grained counterparts. Although titanium and zirconium alloys are considered to be promising materials for orthopedics because of their biocompatibility with tissues, their main drawbacks for application as implants have generally been considered to be insufficient levels of mechanical and tribological properties. The influence of equal channel angular pressing and nitrogen ion implantation on the structure and properties of Ti and Zr alloys has been investigated to ensure the optimum combination of the bulk material and surface layer properties [66]. The data obtained showed that the equal channel angular pressing and nitrogen ion implantation can be efficiently used to improve bulk and surface properties of Ti- and Zr-based implants [66].

At the end of this section, it is necessary to summarize various techniques to measure and characterize the surface roughness. They include that (i) surface roughness can be measured using a profilometer with sharp edge stylus, which is a contact method, (ii) atomic force microscopy can provide noncontact surface topography from which the surface roughness can be indirectly measured, and (iii) fractal dimension analysis can be used to present the surface roughness in non-Euclidian dimension [40–43]. Recently, Hansson et al. [67] employed computer simulations to measure surface roughness. The lateral resolution was defined as the pixel size of a profiling system. A surface roughness was simulated by a trigonometric function with random periodicity and amplitude. The function was divided into an array of pixels simulating the pixels of the profiling system. The mean height value for each pixel was used to calculate the surface roughness parameters. It was found that the accuracy of all the surface roughness parameters investigated decreased with increasing pixel size. This tendency was most pronounced for mean slope and developed length ratio, amounting to about 80% of their true values for a pixel size of 20% of the true mean high-spot spacing. It was concluded that the lateral resolution of an instrument/method severely compromises the precision of surface roughness parameters which are measured for roughness features with a mean high-spot spacing less than five times the lateral resolution [67].

5.3.2. Chemical and Electrochemical Modifications

In general speaking, the chemical method has been adopted for (i) forming a stable oxide film and (ii) resulting surface having an appropriate level of surface roughness, on the other hand, the electrochemical method possesses also twofold purposes;

(i) forming a stable oxide film, and (ii) through an electrochemical reaction to deposit target substance(s) onto the substrate surface [68]. In either method, enhanced biocompatibility of implants (in particular, titanium implants) highly depends on the possibility of achieving high degrees of surface functionalization for an enhanced mineralization of bioactive minerals (e.g., HA) [69].

In chemical treatment, there found a variety of acid and alkali agents. Variola et al. [70] used a mixture of H_2SO_4 and H_2O_2 on Ti–6Al–4V surfaces having both a microtexture and a nanotexture to promote cell activity at the surface of implants. It was reported that the resulting new surfaces selectively promote the growth of osteoblasts while inhibiting the growth of fibroblasts, making them promising tools for regulating the activities of cells in biological environments [70]. A mixture of H_2SO_4 and H_2O_2 and H_2O_2 [69,71], a mixture of H_2SO_4 and HCl [72], and 3% H_2O_2 in hydrothermal [73], in common, can promote easy deposition bioactive substance and further adhesion of biomimetic pieces. Grit-blasted (with alumina particles) titanium was treated in hydrofluoric acid (HF) to evaluate the osseointegration in ovariectomized rats [74]. It was found that, 12 weeks after implant insertion, (i) the fluoride-modified implants showed improved osseointegration compared to control, with the bone area ratio and bone-to-implant contact (BIC) increased by 0.9- and 1.4-fold in histomorphometry, (ii) the bone volume ratio and percent osseointegration by 0.8- and 1.3-fold, and (iii) the maximal push-out force and ultimate shear strength by 1.2- and 2.0-fold in the biomechanical test. It was then concluded that HF treatment of the Ti surface improved implant osseointegration in rats and suggested the feasibility of using fluoride modification to improve Ti implant osseointegration in osteoporotic bone [74]. To enhance the bone bonding and osteoblast response, H_3PO_4 was used for titanium surface treatment [75–77]. Acid etching is a popular method to texture the surface of dental implants. During etching, the titanium oxide protective layer is dissolved and small native hydrogen ions diffuse into the unprotected implant surface. They enrich the implant surface with hydrogen and precipitate into titanium hydride (TiH). Szmukler-Moncler et al. [78] measured the concentration of TiH at the implant surface and the total concentration of hydrogen at five commercially available implant systems, made of either CpTi or titanium alloy. XRD was conducted on each implant system to determine the compounds present at the implant surface. Following a TiH_2/Ti calibration curve, the concentration of TiH was determined. The concentration of hydrogen in the implants was measured by the inert gas fusion thermal conductivity/infrared detection method. It was found that (i) XRD data showed that TiH was present on all CpTi implants but not on the alloyed implants, (ii) TiH concentration varied between 5% and 37%, and hydrogen concentration varied between 43 and 108 ppm, no difference in uptake was found between CpTi and alloyed implants, (iii) low solubility of hydrogen in α-titanium is responsible for precipitation into TiH, and (iv) stronger etching conditions led to higher concentration of TiH2-*x*. Based on these results, it was concluded that high solubility of hydrogen in the β-phase of the alloy is preventing hydrogen from precipitating into TiH. All implants, even those lacking TiH at the surface, were enriched with hydrogen, and in all implants, hydrogen concentration was within the normative limit of 130 ppm [78].

Sodium hydroxide (NaOH) was equally employed as pre-treatment for subsequent depositing bioactive materials [71,77,79,80]. Alkali treatment of the Ti–6Al–7Nb alloys with subsequent heat treatment has been adopted as an important surface treatment procedure for apatite formation in dental implants. Park et al. [81] examined the effects of alkali treatment on the precipitation of apatite on a Ti–6Al–7Nb alloy. All samples were immersed in a Hanks' balanced salts solution (SBF) at pH 7.4 and 36.5 °C for 15 days. The surface structural changes of samples due to the alkali treatment and immersing in SBF were analyzed by XRD, SEM, and XPS. The cell toxicity was evaluated based on the optical density of the surviving cells. The samples were implanted into the abdominal connective tissue of mice for 4 weeks. A sodium titanate hydrogel layer was formed after immersion in an NaOH solution. A dense and uniform bone-like apatite layer was precipitated on the alkali and heat-treated Ti–6Al–7Nb alloy in the SBF. There was a significant difference in cell toxicity between the treated and untreated Ti–6Al–7Nb. The thickness of the fibrous capsule formed around the implant body was decreased significantly by the alkali and heat treatment. It was, hence, concluded that the alkali treatment samples showed a better biocompatibility than the untreated commercial metal samples [81].

Among the many methods of titanium surface modification, electrochemical techniques are simple and cheap. Anodic oxidation is the anodic electrochemical technique while electrophoretic and cathodic depositions are the cathodic electrochemical techniques. By anodic oxidation, it is possible to obtain desired roughness, porosity, and chemical composition of the oxide.

Electrochemistry deals with charge transfer across interfaces. One of the first applications of electrochemistry was for coating conducting surfaces with either metal, for example, electroplating, or by inorganic or organic substances, such as oxides and polymers. Coatings ranging from a monoatomic layers (e.g., via under potential deposition, to microns thick have been carried out), which affected the physical and chemical properties of the coated surface. Hence, electrochemically deposited films have been used to inhibit corrosion, accommodate enzymes and biosensors, control optical properties, and in numerous others applications [82]. Anodizing in the electrochemical reaction can control the thickness of oxide films formed on the substrate, depending on used electrolyte [83–85]. Xiao et al. fabricated titania nanotubes by the anodization method using an electrolyte dimethyl sulfoxide electrolyte containing 1 wt% HF solution at above 50 °C and reported that the formed oxide was anatase type TiO_2 [86]. Major purpose of HA coating can be found for better implant-bone fixation in dental and orthopedic implants under load-bearing conditions. In recent works, it has been demonstrated that an *in vitro*, chemically deposited, bone-like apatite layer with bone-bonding ability could be induced on a titanium surface. By reproducing that the chemical procedure, a dense bone-like apatite layer can be formed on the surface of the titanium in SBF. For the last decade, different surface modifications have been investigated to provide these implants with bone-bonding ability. The main attempts consisted of physical coating processes on the metals, involving ceramic materials such as Bioglass (US Biomaterials, Gainesville, FL) and Cerabone A/W glass-ceramic (Nippon Electric Co., Yokohama, Japan). They are commonly coated with a plasma-sprayed HA layer to give their surfaces bioactive properties. However, the plasma-spray technique does not allow an accurate control of the chemical composition, the crystallographic structure, and the crystallinity of the coating. As a result, the HA layer can be mechanically and chemically unstable [21]. Most of the problems that have been associated with HA-coated implants are caused by the electrochemical deposition method. Due to the high temperatures that occur during the plasma spraying process, the resulting coatings do not have an exactly defined phase composition. Additionally, layers produced by this method have a rather high thickness, resulting in insufficient adhesion strength. When the selected electrolyte contains Ca and P ions as major constituents, it is highly expected to see bone-like compound be deposited onto substrates [87–89]. For example, Simka et al. used mixed electrolytes NaH_2PO_2 in 4.3 M H_3PO_4 and $Ca(H_2PO_2)_2$ in 4.3 M H_3PO_4 [90], and $Ca(H_2PO_2)_2$, H_3PO_4, or $(HCOO)_2Ca$ [91]. Sharma et al. [92] investigated the influence of synthesis parameters like pH of suspension and current density. It was found that (i) the addition of chitosan increased the adhesive strength of the composite coating, (ii) modulus of elasticity of the coating was found to be 9.23 GPa, and (iii) in the presence of chitosan, the dense negatively charged surface with homogenous nucleation was the primary factor for sheet-like evolution of apatite layer. Based on these findings, it was suggested that incorporation of chitosan with apatite-wollastonite in composite coating could provide excellent *in vitro* bioactivity with enhanced mechanical properties [92]. Similarly, using the electrochemical reaction, deposition of biocompatible platinum foil (Pt) onto the TiN substrate [93], conductive polymer, poly(3,4-ethylenedioxythiophene) film onto the biodegradable Mg substrate [94], and (Ti,Al)N onto the Ni–Cr dental base-alloy [95] have been reported.

Anodic oxidation at high voltages can improve the crystallinity of the oxide. The chief advantage of this technique is doping of the coating of the bath constituents and incorporation of these elements improves the properties of the oxide. Electrophoretic deposition (EPD) uses HA powders dispersed in a suitable solvent at a particular pH. Under these operating conditions, these particles acquire positive charge and coatings are obtained on the cathodic titanium by applying an external electric field. These coatings require a post-sintering treatment to improve the coating properties. Cathodic deposition is another type of electrochemical method where HA is formed *in situ* from an electrolyte containing calcium and phosphate ions. It is also possible to alter structure or chemistry, or both, of the obtained deposit. Nano-grained HA has higher surface energy and greater biological activity and therefore emphasis is being laid to produce these coatings by cathodic deposition [96]. Titanium surface characteristics determine the degree of success of permanent implants. The topography, morphology of the surface in micro and nano scales, the impurities present and other characteristics are main concerns, and therefore a multitechnique approach is required in order to evaluate modification process effects on the surface. Surface modification of titanium in the nanometrical range was performed by means of anodization in phosphoric with the aim of improving both the biocompatibility and the corrosion resistance in the biological media. Sanchez et al. [97] investigated biocompatible characteristics of the modified titanium surface, as the presence of anatase in the oxide film and the incorporation of phosphate to the surface. It was reported that the increase in the film thickness from 3 to 42 nm was estimated from EIS (Electrochemical Impedance Spectroscopy) results when anodizing potentials from 0 to 30 V were applied, whereas a bi-layer structure of the protective oxides formed was determined [97].

It may be worth to review the types of oxides formed on titanium. TiO_2 possesses three crystalline structures: anatase, rutile, and brookite. Anatase-type TiO_2 is a tetragonal crystalline system with a_0 = 3.78Å and c_0 = 9.50 Å; the rutile-type TiO_2 is also a tetragonal structure, but the lattice constants are quite different from those of anatase-type (i.e., a_0 = 4.58 Å and c_0 = 2.98 Å). The third type is brookite-type and has an orthorhombic crystalline structure with a_0 = 9.17Å, b_0 = 5.43 Å, and c_0 = 5.13 Å. Among these oxides, rutile is known to be the most stable phase [98].

Lee et al. [99] examined the effect of electrolyte temperature on the surface characteristics of anodized pure titanium in DL-α-glycerophosphate and calcium acetate. It was reported that (i) the anodic oxide films contained a large proportion of anatase with some rutile, (ii) the relative intensity of the anatase peaks and the surface roughness increased with increasing electrolyte temperature, and (iii) as the electrolyte temperature was increased, the pore size increased to 1–4 μm, and the apatite crystals became coarser and denser [99].

There are several techniques for the deposition of coatings on metals, including physical vapor deposition (PVD), chemical vapor deposition (CVD), electrochemical deposition, plasma spraying, and sol–gel process. The sol–gel coating process possesses unique advantages as follows: (i) excellent chemical stability, oxidation control, and enhanced corrosion resistance for metal substrates [100,101]; (ii) it is an environmentally friendly technique of surface protection and had showed the potential for the replacement of toxic pretreatments and coatings which have traditionally been used for increasing corrosion resistance of metals [102,103]; (iii) the processing temperature generally is low, frequently close to room temperature; thus thermal volatilization and degradation of entrapped species, such as organic inhibitors, is minimized [102]; (iv) since liquid precursors are used, it is possible to cast coatings in complex shapes and to produce thin films without the need for machining or melting, and (v) the sol–gel films are formed by "green" coating technologies [102].

Velu et al. used single-phase calcium HA to synthesize by a sol–gel route using a calcium nitrate solution and ammonium dihydrogen phosphate solution as Ca and P sources and alginic acid as a chelating agent and found that the development of hexagonal-shaped nanoparticles was developed with the average particle size in the range of 50–100 nm [104]. Similarly, HA was deposited by this technique by Ben-Nissan et al. [105]. Although metallic materials are the most used materials as orthopedic or dental implants for their excellent mechanical properties, they are not able to create a natural bonding with the mineralized bone and they could release metallic particles that could finally end in the removal of the implant. One way to avoid these effects is to protect the metallic implant with a biocompatible coating. Ballarre et al. [106] employed the sol–gel method to deposit amorphous HA surgical stainless steel substrate. It was further reported that $CaTiO_3$ (perovskite) was deposited onto the titanium substrate [107]. Although the crystalline structure was not clearly identified as to whether it is the anatase type or the rutile type, TiO_2 was deposited through the sol–gel method [107–109].

It was reported that adhesive biodegradable polymer, poly(vinyl acetate) (PVA) was coated by the dip processing onto the biodegradable Mg alloy for purpose to control the degradation rate and enhance the biocompatibility of magnesium alloys [110]. Using the powder slurry method, Kim et al. [111] coated an HA/fluorapatite double layer onto the ZrO_2 substrate and it was reported that the osteoblast-like cells cultured on the HA/fluorapatite coating layer spread and proliferated favorably, having a cell proliferation rate comparable to that of a plastic control and HA bulk ceramic [111].

Kado et al. [112] developed a simple chemical modification method to immobilize cell-adhesive molecules on a titanium surface to improve its compatibility with human periodontal ligament cells (HPDLCs).The polished titanium disk was immersed in 1% *p*-vinylbenzoic acid solution for 2 hours to introduce carboxyl groups onto the surface. After rinsing with distilled de-ionized water, the titanium disk was dipped into a 1.47% 1-ethyl-3-(3-dimethylaminopropyl) carbodiimide solution containing 0.1 mg/ml Gly-Arg-Gly-Asp-Ser (GRGDS), human plasma fibronectin (pFN), or type I collagen from calf skin (Col) to covalently immobilize the cell-adhesive molecules on the titanium surface via the formation of peptide bonds. XPS analyses revealed that cell-adhesive molecules were successfully immobilized on the titanium surfaces. The Col-immobilized titanium surface revealed higher values regarding nano rough characteristics than the as-polished titanium surface under scanning probe microscopy. It was reported that (i) the number of HPDLCs attached to both the pFN- and Col-immobilized titanium surfaces was twice that attached to the as-polished titanium surfaces, (ii) the cells were larger with the cellular processes that stretched to a greater extent on the pFN- and Col-immobilized titanium surfaces than on the as-polished titanium surface, and (iii) HPDLCs on the Col-immobilized titanium surfaces showed more extensive expression of vinculin at the tips of cell projections and more contiguously along the cell outline than on the as-polished, GRGDS-immobilized and pFN-immobilized titanium surfaces. It was, hence, concluded that cell-adhesive molecules successfully immobilized on the titanium surface and improved the compatibility of the surface with HPDLCs, suggesting that the Col-immobilized titanium surface could be used for forming ligament-like tissues around titanium dental implants [112].

Reis et al. [113] assessed possible morphological and chemical changes, using SEM and energy dispersive X-ray detector (EDS (energy dispersive X-ray spectroscopy), after performing double insertion and pull-out tests of implants of different shapes and surface treatments. Different types of screw implants were prepared: cylindrical machined-surface implants, cylindrical double-surface treated porous implants, cylindrical surface-treated porous implants, surface-treated porous implants, and tapered surface-treated porous implants. The implants were inserted into synthetic bone femurs, before performing each insertion with standardized torque, and after each pullout the implants were analyzed by SEM and EDS. It was concluded that (i) implants with surface acid treatment undergo greater superficial change regarding the chemical composition than the machined implants (namely, the greater the contact area of the implant with the substrate, the greater the oxide layer change), and (ii) prior manipulation can alter the chemical composition in the implants and to a greater degree in surface-treated implants [113].

Lee et al. [114] examined the gelatin nano gold (GnG) composite for surface modification of titanium in addition to insure biocompatibility on dental implants or biomaterials. The GnG composite was constructed by gelatin and hydrogen tetrachloroaurate in the presence of reducing agent, sodium borohydrate ($NabH_4$). A dipping method was used to modify the titanium surface by GnG composite. The MC-3T3 E1 cell viability was assessed by trypan blue and the expression of proteins to biocompatibility was analyzed by Western blotting. It was reported that (i) the GnG composite showed well-dispersed character, the strong absorption at 530 nm, roughness, regular crystal, and clear C, Na, Cl, P, and Au signals onto titanium, and (ii) further, this composite allowed

MC-3T3 E1 growth and viability compared to gelatin and pure titanium, indicating that GnG composite-coated titanium surfaces have a good biocompatibility for osteoblast growth and attachment than in intact by a simple and versatile dipping method [114].

5.3.3. Physical Modification

In this section, we will discuss the microarc oxidation (MAO), ion implantation including Plasma Immersion Ion Implantation (PIII), other plasma treatments, and laser technologies.

Wu et al. [115], using the Ti–24Nb–4Zr–7.9Sn alloy (which is a newly developed β-titanium alloy having a low value of modulus of elasticity), evaluated the effects of MAO treatment on biological performance and characterized treated surface and reported that MAO treatment helps to form a porous surface with a biologically active bone-like apatite layer on the Ti alloy [115]. Since the TiO_2 surface possesses high apatite-forming ability, porous Ti was MAO processed to form the TiO_2 thin layer [116], and CpTi was subjected to MAO treatment to form porous TiO_2, indicating that the cortex-like coating was conducive to cell retention and implant stabilization [117]. Most of MAO application can be found in depositing bioactive or biocompatible substances onto biomaterials. The Ca- and P-containing coating electrolyte (α-$Ca(PO_3)_2$, or $CaTiO_3$) was coated on Ti–6Al–4V [118], and on Mg [119]. HA was MAO processed on the titanium substrate and a mixture of HA and TiO_2 was detected [120]. Song et al. [121] treated MAO processed CpTi surface (which has porous TiO_2) with an electrolyte containing Ca and P ions by hydrothermal treatment. It was reported that (i) a small number of micro-sized HA crystallites and a thin layer composed of nano-sized HA were formed on the MAO processed Ti followed by treatment in the alkaline aqueous solution, (ii) whereas a large number of micro-sized HA crystallites and dense anatase TiO_2nanorods were formed on the MAO processed Ti followed by treatment in the phosphorous-containing alkaline solution, and (iii) the layer of bone-like apatite that formed on the surface of the treated sample in the phosphorous-containing alkaline solution after soaking in a modified SBF was thicker than that on the treated samples in the alkaline aqueous solution [121]. A composite of potassium titanate ($K_2Ti_6O_{13}$) was also coated on the titanium surface and it was indicated that the potassium/TiO_2 bio-ceramic coatings possess excellent capability of including bone-like apatite to deposit [122].

A comparative study was performed on the behavior of titanium electrode in a sulfuric acid solution with and without Ti^{+3} during MAO under the constant current density control regime. The composition and microstructure of the obtained microarc films were analyzed using SEM, glancing-angle X-ray diffractometry, Raman and energy-dispersive X-ray spectroscopies. Galevičius et al. [123] have shown that the addition of a Ti^{+3}salt extends the region of current densities can be used for MAO of Ti and results in an obvious change of sparking behavior from extensive, large, and long-played sparks to numerous, small and short sparks. As a consequence, the titania films formed in the Ti^{+3}-containing solutions are relatively thick, more uniform, composed of almost pure crystalline anatase and rutile phases of TiO_2, and contain a network of evenly distributed small pores. It has also been shown that these films are promising for applications in catalysis, sensors, and optoelectronics. The Raman spectra indicate that an increase in the electrolysis time of titanium in the Ti^{+3}-containing solution leads to the increase in the rutile content, as expected [123].

A new technique combining MAO and electrophoresis was introduced to develop a biocompatible oxide layer on the CpTi implant surface. Originally developed alkaline electrolyte containing nanoscale HA powder suspension was used in the new technique. In the electric field, nanoscale HA powder was electrophoretically moved and sintered into the gradually-formed oxide layer on titanium anode. Physio-chemical properties and *in vitro* biological performance of the newly formed surface were examined and evaluated. An 8.5-μm thick oxide layer with high surface energy and roughness, which was composed of TiO_2 and calcium phosphates as well as HA, was formed on the titanium surface by the modified MAO technique. Osteoblasts cultured on the modified MAO titanium surface showed significantly increased alkaline phosphatase activity comparing to machined titanium and MAO titanium surface. The natural oxide surface of titanium could be transformed into a hybrid oxide layer by modified MAO treatment. The modified titanium surface, which is rough and porous, contains calcium phosphates and proved to be more biocompatible *in vitro* [124].

Plasma treatment [3] is an interesting method to modify the implant surface. Not only can this treatment alter the surface charge, but this treatment can also alter the chemistry and the topography [17,125]. Thermal plasma treatment has been traditionally used as a method to utilize HA coatings on implant surfaces (plasma spraying) [126–128]. Another form of plasma treatment, the atmospheric pressure (cold) plasmas, has shown to alter the surface energy and the chemistry due to the generation of high concentration of reactive species that are generated [17]. This has been reported to be beneficial for the enhancement of osteogenic responses, since surfaces treated with atmospheric plasma significantly enhanced the wettability and improved the initial cellular interaction. Plasma surface modification has become a popular method to modify the surface structure and biological properties of biomaterials. By modifying selective surface mechanical and biological properties, conventional materials can be redesigned with their favorable bulk attributes retained. Plasma surface modification can enhance the multifunctionality, mechanical properties, as well as biocompatibility of artificial biomaterials and medical implants [129]. Titanium and its alloys are preferred materials for hard tissue replacements because of their excellent mechanical properties, corrosion resistance, and biocompatibility.

In order to improve the properties of titanium and expand its clinical application, many methods have been applied to modify the surface of titanium, which should include the application of plasma surface modification technologies (such as plasma spraying and PIII and deposition), to improve the bioactivity of titanium [130]. Plasma technology can be applied not only to metallic materials, but also to polymeric materials. For biomedical polymers, the surface properties need to be altered to promote a good cell adhesion, growth, and proliferation and to make them suitable for implants and tissue engineering scaffolds. For polymers, it is also important to know plasma polymerization and plasma grafting techniques [131].

Initial adhesion of cells to implant surfaces and subsequent behavior of the cells are important determinants for biocompatibility of the implants. It was previously reported that both adhesion of MC3T3-E1 osteoblast-like cells to titanium plates and their differentiation into more mature cells on the plates were stimulated by treatment of the plates with glow discharge plasma (GDP). However, the mechanisms of these processes have not yet been identified. Shibata et al. [132] investigated the adhesion and differentiation mechanism of osteoblast-like cells to Ti with and without GDP. The adhesion and differentiation mechanism of MC3T3-E1 osteoblast-like cells to Ti, with and without GDP, were investigated by cultivation in serum-free medium and use of a competitive inhibition test to examine the influence of extracellular matrix proteins contained in the serum and to identify cell binding proteins [132]. In addition, the amount of fibronectin adsorption on each Ti plate was investigated by enzyme-linked immunosorbent assay and fluorescein isothiocyanate labeling. It was reported that (i) adherent cells on Ti plates, with and without GDP, were significantly reduced in serum-free conditions and the presence of RGDS (Arg-Gly-Asp-Ser) peptides, (ii) fibronectin adsorption on titanium plates was increased by GDP, and (iii) stress fiber formation of cells was extremely progressive on the Ti plates treated with GDP and was not observed on the cells inhibited by the RGDS peptide. These results suggest that RGDS containing serum proteins have a major role in regulating specific adhesion of cells to Ti, and GDP promoted cell adhesion and differentiation on Ti by increasing the adsorption of proteins, concluding that the adhesion and differentiation mechanism of osteoblast-like cells to Ti, with and without GDP, can be obtained [132].

Since metallic biomaterials used for orthopedic and dental implants possess a paucity of reactive functional groups, bioactivity modification of these materials is challenging. Hu et al. [133] treated the titanium disks and rods with carbon dioxide plasma and then incubated in a modified SBF to obtain an HA layer. Surface hydrophilicity of samples, changes of surface chemistry, surface morphologies of samples, and structural analysis of formed HA were investigated by contact angle to water, XPS, SEM), Fourier transform infrared (FTIR) and XRD. The results demonstrated that hydrophilicity of titanium surface was improved and hydroxyl groups increased after modification with carbon dioxide plasma treatment. The hydroxyl groups on the surface of titanium were the richest after carbon dioxide plasma treatment under the condition of 20W for less than 30 seconds. The HA formability of titanium surface was enhanced by carbon dioxide plasma pretreatment, which was attributed to the surface chemistry. MC3T3-E1 cell as a model cell was cultured on the Ti, CPT-Ti, and CPT/SBF-Ti discs *in vitro*, and the results of the morphology and differentiation of the cell showed that CPT/SBF-Ti was the highest bioactive. The relative parameters of the new bone around the Ti and CPT/SBF-Ti rods including bone mineral density (BMD), a ratio of bone volume to total volume (BV/TV), trabecular thickness (Tb.Th.), and trabecular number (Tb.N.) were analyzed by a microcomputed tomography (micro-CT) after 4-, 8- and 12-week implantation periods *in vivo*. It was mentioned that the CPT/SBF-Ti was more advantageous for new bone formation [133].

Plasma-based ion implantation and deposition techniques are widely used in many applications, including microelectronics, biomedical engineering, and nanotechnology [134–136]. For improving biocompatibility, Chen et al. [137] conducted surface modification of different discharge gases (Ar, O_2, and Ar + O_2) plasma-treated polystyrene (PS) film by Ar plasma-induced graft polymerization, with biocompatible monomer *N*-vinyl-2-pyrrolidone (NVP). The films are characterized by attenuated total reflectance Fourier transfer infrared (ATR-FTIR) spectroscopy, XPS, and SEM. Water contact angle measurement demonstrates the modified films possess a relatively hydrophilic surface. Furthermore, the films are also examined for cell attachment and proliferation *in vitro* using mouse fibroblasts (L929 cells). The modified film surface shows a better cell distribution and growth than that of the pristine PS surface. From cell culture experiments, it is also observed that Ar + O_2 plasma is more capable of increasing cell adhesion and proliferation. This method will provide a potential and effective solution for grafting useful component in future tissue-engineering applications [137].

Titanium oxide with a rutile structure has superior optical properties and blood compatibility and is thermodynamically more stable than other oxide forms of titanium. Titanium oxide thin films are deposited on (1 0 0) silicon and SiO_2 wafers by metal plasma ion implantation and deposition. The substrates are DC biased during the film deposition and the influence of the oxygen pressure on the characteristics of the coatings is investigated. XRD indicates the existence of Ti_4O_7 in the film when the oxygen pressure is lower than 2.0×10^{-2} Pa. By increasing the oxygen pressure, the preferred orientation of the as-deposited titanium oxide film changes from the (1 0 0) low-index plane to the (2 0 0) high-index plane. The as-deposited titanium oxide films are subsequently annealed at 750 °C for 60 minutes in vacuum. The microstructure, resistance, composition, and blood compatibility of the films are assessed. Before annealing, the sheet resistance of the titanium oxide increases with higher oxygen pressure, and after vacuum annealing, the sheet resistance of some of the titanium oxide films increases by approximately 60 times. The results of the platelet adhesion experiments acquired from the annealed samples are similar to those from low-temperature isotropic pyrolytic carbon [138].

Surface modification of biomaterials modification by ion-beam processing is becoming popular for improving medical device function, biocompatibility and as a new mutation breeding method. Ion-beam-based processes, such as ion implantation and ion-beam assisted deposition can provide beneficial surface layers with desirable properties without detrimentally affecting the bulk properties [139]. Ion implantation has been successful in biomaterials modification, such as in improving the wear resistance of artificial joint components, in improving wettability, anticoagulability, anticalcific behavior of biomedical polymers, in minimizing biofouling of medical devices, and depositing HA or Ca-P compounds [140–144]. Application of the PIII technique to oxidation can be found in various references. Liu et al. [145] reported a new method of titanium surface modification through ammonia (NH_3) PIII technique and its effect on the cellular behaviors of MC3T3-E1 osteoblastic cells. The NH_3PIII-treated titanium substrates (NH_3-Ti) were characterized by XPS, which showed that NH_3-Ti had a nitrogen-rich surface. However, there was no significant difference between the surface morphology of NH_3-Ti and unmodified Ti. When MC3T3-E1 cells were cultured on NH_3-Ti substrates, it was found that cell proliferation was accelerated at 4 and 7 days of culture. Meanwhile, cell differentiation was evaluated using type I collagen (COL I), osteocalcin (OC), and bone sialoprotein (BSP) as differentiation markers. It was found that the expression of COL I and OC genes was up-regulated on NH_3-Ti substrates. However, no significant difference was found in the BSP gene expression between NH_3-Ti and unmodified Ti substrates. Therefore, findings from this study indicate that surface modification of titanium through NH_3PIII favors osteoblastic proliferation and differentiation and as a result, it may be used to improve the biocompatibility of Ti implants *in vivo* [145]. Mändl et al. [146] treated NiTi and CpTi (grade 2) in the oxygen-PIII method and found that a hard, dense and thick rutile type TiO_2 layer formed with excellent biocompatibility [146]. Surface passivation can be achieved by PIII processing in oxygen atmosphere on Ti [147,148] and NiTi [148,149]. PIII nitridization were conducted on Ti or NiTi, or both [148–150]. Byeliet al. [66] conducted PIII treated pure Ti and Zr and reported that equal channel angular pressing and nitrogen ion implantation can be efficiently used to improve bulk and surface properties of Ti- and Zr-based implants. Ti-based alloys (Ti–6Al–4V [151–153] and Ti–5Al–2.5Fe [154]) were also subjected to PIII treatment, reporting that the treated surface was covered with Ti_2N. Furthermore, when such PIII nitride Ti-based alloys were immersed into Hank's balanced salt solution, it was reported that a Ca- and P-rich surface layer was detected by X-ray photo-electron spectroscopy [153,154]. Pye had processed steel to nitride to form FeN [155]. Xie et al. [156] investigated the effects of (H_2O + H_2) implanted titanium by the PIII technique on human osteoblast cells culture and concluded that (H_2O + H_2) implanted titanium exhibited good adhesion and growth, suggesting that a practical means to improve the surface bioactivity and cytocompatibility of medical implants made of titanium [156].

The current review casts new light on surface modification of titanium and titanium alloys by ion beam implantation [157]. A similar work was reported on NiTi [158]. Both negative-ion and positive-ion are implanted for surface modification of materials. In the negative-ion implantation, we have the advantage of a nearly "charge-up-free" property for the implanted surface of insulators or insulated materials. The charging voltage on the implanted surface is no greater than plus or minus a few volts. Because of this, negative-ion implantation can include more excellent applications than those accessible only by positive-ion implantation. Negative-ion implantation can be used not only for formation of metal nanoparticles, but this technique also makes possible the manipulation of nerve cell growth by precise control of the biocompatibility of a polymer surface [159]. Ca-ion was implanted in the titanium surface [160,161], claiming that the Ca-implanted Ti specimen showed more active electrochemical behavior than nonimplanted specimen, and easier formation of apatite with a good Ca/P ratio in the range of 1.38 and 1.60, revealing its potential as a bioactive material [160]. Gallardo-Moreno et al. [162] investigated the effects of surface modification by Si-ion implantation on 316L stainless steel on the biocompatibility and bacterial adhesion and reported that Si-ion implantation was an effective way of reducing bacterial adhesion on 316L stainless steel surfaces without compromising its good biocompatibility.

Among plasma technology, the most popular application is a plasma-spraying HA on the titanium surface [163–165]. Recently, Latka et al. [166] developed suspension plasma spraying that enables the production of finely grained nanometric or submicrometric coatings. The suspension (which is formulated with the use of fine powder particles in water or alcohol) is injected into plasma jet and the liquid additives evaporate. The remaining fine solids are molten and subsequently agglomerate or remain solid. Suspension plasma coating of titanium oxide and HA were demonstrated successfully [166]. Plasma oxidation was conducted in various ways [167–169]. Montazeri et al. [167], using the plasma electrolytic oxidation which is one of the effective techniques, coated titania, and HA onto Ti–6Al–4V. It was reported that, by increasing the operation time, the amount of the formed HA increased, and the sample coated at 500 V and

15 minutes showed the best corrosion resistance in Ringer's solution. Ti was subjected to plasma oxidation and showed that improved wetting was obtained, which is potentially associated with shorter osseointegration periods [167]. Huan et al. [169] modified the surface of the NiTi shape memory alloy (SMA) by plasma electrolytic oxidation in Na_3PO_4 with an aim to produce porous NiTi surfaces for biomedical applications. It was concluded that the wettability and surface free energy of NiTi increased significantly, indicating that the plasma oxidation process shows potential for expanding the biofunctionality of NiTi [169].

Similarly, plasma nitrization can be achieved. Ti–6Al–4V and Ti–4Al–2.5 Fe [170] and Ti–24Al–10Nb intermetallic alloy [171] were plasma nitrided and TiN film was detected formed on these alloy surfaces. Fouquet et al. plasma treated Ti–6Al–4V using a N_2–H_2 gas mixture under 10 Pa [172]. It was reported that (i) the plasma treatment enables the formation of a δ-TiN layer which can act as a diffusion barrier for nitrogen, and (ii) the underneath previously formed ε-Ti_2N grains undergo a nitrogen rearrangement with the remaining α-Ti grains leading to the formation of a nitrogen poor phase that was identified as the α-$TiN_{0.26}$ phase [172].

Chrzanowski et al. [173] plasma treated NiTi since high nickel content such as in NiTi is believed to reduce the number of biomedical applications due to the reported toxicity of nickel. The reduction in nickel release and minimized exposure of the cell to nickel can optimize the biocompatibility of the alloy. Among many idea proposed to prevent Ni element release from NiTi, it was hypothesized that the native surface of NiTi supports cell differentiation and insures good biocompatibility [173]. Three types of surface modifications were investigated: thermal oxidation, alkali treatment, and plasma sputtering, and compared with smooth, ground surface. It was concluded that the most favorable cell responses were observed for ground and plasma-sputtered surfaces, suggesting that smooth, plasma-modified surfaces provide sufficient properties for cells to grow [173].

Diamond (or carbon) is highly biocompatible and has emerged as a potential biomaterial and was plasma CVD treated onto pure titanium surface under various gas ratio of CH_4 and H_2 [174]. It was reported that (i) the growth of diamond crystals and coatings on the TiC layer were observed, (ii) pre-etching of the Ti substrate with hydrogen plasma for a short time significantly increased nuclei density of diamond crystals, and (iii) plasma power had a significant effect on the surface morphology and the mechanical properties of the deposited diamond coatings [174]. Bazaka et al. treated biopolymer plasma modification to control bacterial cell attachment and biofilm formation [175].

Plasma energy can also be used for graft-polymerization. Chen et al. [176] employed the plasma-induced graft-polymerization of bioactive molecule polyacrylamide to improve corrosion behavior and biocompatibility of the titanium surface. It was reported that potentiodynamic polarization and cellular proliferation tests were implemented to validate the enhanced corrosion resistance and biocompatibility of modified Ti surface, respectively [176].

The application of atmospheric plasma is increasing in numerous situations especially in the biomedical field due to their practical capability to low temperature providing plasma that are not spatially bound or confined by electrodes [177,178]. Stachowski et al. has reported that there is a possibility to maintain the high surface energy state of the titanium implant for at least 30 days, depending on various factors such as storage conditions [178]. The reason for 30 days storage of plasma-treated implants is to simulate a scenario of large-scale production by dental implants manufacturers, where the storage after surface modification may occur for several days prior to reaching the dental practitioner [178].

Light amplification by stimulated emission of radiation (laser) is a coherent and monochromatic source of electromagnetic radiation that can propagate in a straight line with negligible divergence. As a result, laser finds diverse applications ranging from mere mundane to most sophisticated uses either for totally commercial or purely scientific purposes, and from life-saving to life-threatening causes. High power lasers can produce intense heating and perform various manufacturing operations or material processing. The manufacturing processes covered have been broadly divided into four major categories, namely, laser assisted forming, joining, machining, and surface engineering. Surface engineering means the design and modification of a surface to enhance hardness, wear resistance, heat resistance, or some other property. Although most laser surface engineering processes appear expensive compared to other technologies, in many cases they are actually more cost-effective because of their precision and speed. Due to the intrinsic properties of high coherence and directionality, laser beam can be focused onto metallic surface to perform a broad range of treatments such as remelting, alloying, and cladding, which are used to improve the wear and corrosion resistance of titanium alloys [179–183]. Romanos et al. [183] evaluated the use of different laser systems in implant dentistry. Although many case studies indicate extensive use of lasers and promising results in dental implantology, lasers may be used for uncovering submerged implants atraumatically to prevent crestal bone loss, recontouring peri-implant soft tissues, and sculpting emergence profile for prosthetic components, raising surgical flaps, osseous recontouring, and creating parabolic tissue architecture. Additionally, bone harvesting of block grafts, window preparation in sinus lift procedures, ridge splitting, and debridement of extraction sockets for immediate implant placement can be included. It was concluded that aside from the many benefits associated with the use of lasers in implant-related procedures, there are also risks to consider from the laser irradiation on the implant surface and the peri-implant tissues. Therefore, an appropriate training on laser use is mandatory to increase the clinical outcome and to control the potential of complications [183].

Laser surface modification has been extensively employed. Bandyopadhyay et al. [184] employed laser surface modification method to improve mechanical and tribological properties of Ti biomaterials (CpTi and Ti–6Al–4V). To improve tribological properties of Ti–48Al–2Cr–2Nb intermetallic alloy, laser surface modification with NiCr–Cr_3C_2 precurds or powders was conducted [185]. The appropriate level of surface roughness of titanium implant was created by laser modification to improve the bio-integration [186]. Using localized melting and rapid solidification by laser energy, the surface of machined and Al_2O_3 blasted screw-shaped Ti dental implants were treated by Nd:glass laser and reported that surface treatment seems to be promising for the improvement of the osseointegration of dental implants [187]. Laser surface treatment was used on electrophoretically deposited HA coatings on titanium to improve interfacial bonding. First, EPD was used to produce thick HA coatings on the Ti substrate. Both heat treatment and laser surface treatment were used to create a strong metal–ceramic interface. XRD results for the laser-treated surface indicated the presence of HA and Ti phases along with $CaTiO_3$. A second layer of HA was electrophoretically deposited on laser-treated coatings to improve biological properties further. It was shown that laser surface treatment can eliminate delamination of weak interface of HA coatings by forming a strong Ti-HA composite layer at the interface. The coating hardness increased to 582 ± 98 Hv compared with the base metal hardness of 306 ± 20 Hv. It was further reported that bone cell–material interactions for both laser-treated and untreated samples with human osteoprecursor cells showed no sign of toxicity due to laser processing, and increased bioactivity due to HA coatings [188].

The interaction of a transversely excited atmospheric pressure (TEA) CO_2 laser, operating at 10.6 μm wavelength and pulse duration of 100 ns (FWHM), with a titanium implant in various gas atmospheres was studied [189]. The Ti implant surface modification was typically studied at the moderate laser beam energy density/fluence of 28 J/cm^2 in the surrounding of air, N_2, O_2, or He. The energy absorbed from the TEA CO_2 laser beam is partially converted to thermal energy, which generates a series of effects, such as melting, vaporization of the molten material, shock waves, and so forth. The following titanium implant surface changes and phenomena were observed, depending on the gas used: (i) creation of cone-like surface structures in the atmospheres of air, N_2 and O_2, and dominant microholes/pores in He ambient; (ii) hydrodynamic features, most prominent in air; (iii) formation of titanium nitride and titanium oxide layers, and (iv) occurrence of plasma in front of the implant. It was concluded that the reported laser fluence and gas ambiences can effectively be applied for enhancing the titanium implant roughness and creation of titanium oxides and nitrides on the strictly localized surface area. The appearance of plasma in front of the implants indicates relatively high temperatures created above the surface. This offers a sterilizing effect, which can facilitate contaminant-free conditions [189]. Stübinger et al. [190] compared and analyzed the influence of different lasers (CO_2, Er:YAG, and diode laser) on titanium surfaces that were either polished or sandblasted with large-grit, followed by acid-etched (SLA). It was found that (i) the CO_2 and diode laser did not cause any visible surface alterations on either the polished or SLA disks, and (ii) both polished and SLA disks showed surface alterations when irradiated with the pulsed Er:YAG laser. It was concluded that it is only safe to use the Er:YAG laser for implant surface irradiation with settings no higher than 300 or 500 mJ/10 Hz [190].

In a field of the laser fabrication, a variety of applications can be found. Vorobyev et al. [191] used the femtosecond laser to surface structure of titanium implants. It was found that the femtosecond laser produces a large variety of nanostructures (nanopores, nanoprotrusions) with a size down to 20 nm, multiple parallel grooved surface patterns with a period on the sub-micron level, microroughness in the range of 1–15 μm with various configurations, smooth surface with smooth micro-inhomogeneities, and smooth surface with sphere-like nanostructures down to 10 nm. It was concluded that the femtosecond laser treatment can produce a richer variety of surface structures on titanium for implants and other biomedical applications than long-pulse laser treatments [191]. The femtosecond laser irradiation of titanium metal in an oxidizing environment was used to form a highly stable surface layer of nanostructured amorphous TiO_2. The influence of atmospheric composition on these surface structures was studied and it was found that the gas composition and pressure affect the chemical composition of the surface layer but not the surface morphology. Incorporation of nitrogen is only possible when no oxygen is present in the surrounding atmosphere [192].

Alloying can be achieved by not only conventional melting/casting method, but it can be also done by solid-state powder metallurgy, mechanical alloying, and laser alloying [193] and laser additive manufacturing [194]. Another application of laser-assisted fabrication can be found in laser processing nylon 6, 6 to enhance the wettability and bioactivity—osteoblast cell response [195]. Laser metal sintering has shown promising results, but no comparison with other commercially available surface has been performed. Witek et al. [196] evaluated the biomechanical and histological early bone response to laser sintered implants relative to alumina-blasted/acid-etched (AB/AE). Surface topography was characterized by SEM and optical interferometry. Surface chemistry was assessed by XPS. Beagle dogs received four Ti–6Al–4V implants in each radius, remaining for 1, 3, and 6 weeks *in vivo*. BIC and bone area fraction occupancy (BAFO) were evaluated. Biomechanical evaluation was done by the torque-to-interface failure analysis. The laser sintered surface presented higher S_a and S_q than AB/AE. Significantly higher torque was observed at 1 and 6 week for the laser sintered, whereas at 3 weeks no significant differences were observed. Significantly higher BIC and BAFO values were observed for the laser sintered only at 1 week, whereas no significant differences were observed at 3 and 6 weeks. It was also found that the laser sintered implants presented biocompatible and osseoconductive properties and improved biomechanical response compared with the AB/AE surface only at 1 and 6 weeks *in vivo* [196].

Laser deposition was performed to produce nanostructured TiO_2 film [197,198] and TiO_x nanoparticles [199,200]. Ca-P as well as HA can be deposited by laser treatment [201–203]. Thin films of calcium hydroxylapatite ($Ca_{10}(PO_4)_6(OH)_2$) was deposited on polished substrates of Ti–6Al–4V [202], and calcium phosphate compounds were deposited on acid- and alkali-treated Ti substrate [203], indicating that such laser treated surfaces enhance the biocompatibility of titanium and its alloys.

Laser oxidation and nitrization are another remarkable applications of laser technology. CpTi was treated using Q-switched Nd:YAG laser radiation to control early stage of oxidation, so that the oxygen content did not exceed 50 at.% (TiO) [204]. CpTi surfaces were subjected to laser nitrization [205–207]. It was reported that laser-treated CpTi was covered with δ-TiN phase [207] or tetragonal δ′-Ti_2N phase [208] and it was mentioned that films containing tetragonal Ti_2N phases possess better mechanical properties, corrosion, and wear resistance in comparison with cubic TiN [207]. Similarly, the Ti–6Al–4V alloy surface was laser-treated under various aims [208–210]. Excimer laser was employed to improve the pitting corrosion resistance of the alloy and found that pitting corrosion resistance was improved due to TiN precipitates acting as galvanic cathodes at high corrosion potentials [208]. For improving tribological properties, laser diffusion nitriding was conducted [209,210].

Queiroz et al. [211] evaluated the surfaces of CpTi implants modified by laser beam, without and with HA deposition by the biomimetic method, without and with thermal treatment, and compare them with implants with surfaces modified by acid treatment and with machined surfaces, employing topographical and biomechanics analysis. It was concluded that the laser-beam-modified implants, biomimetic-deposited implants, and heat-treated biomimetic-deposited implants presented physicochemical and topographical properties superior to those of acid-treated implants and machined implants and favored the osseointegration process in the shorter periods. In addition, the biomimetic-deposited implants showed the best results when compared with other surfaces [211].

Laser chemical vapor deposition (LCVD) is a new manufacturing process that holds great potential for the production of small and complex metal and ceramic parts [212]. A complex compound of silver nanoparticles (size 40 nm) combined with polymer blends (polyethylene glycol/poly(lactide-*co*-glycolide) was deposited through laser assisted pulsed evaporation method to cover the substrate surface with antibacterial feature [213]. Besides major surface coating and modification technology involved in the physical reaction as described above, there are still various methods available. Mishra et al. [214] investigated synthesizing HA nanorods by the microwave irradiation technique, taking ethylene diamine tetra-acetic acid as a complexing reagent. After examining calcinizing in the temperature range from 450 °C to 900 °C, it was found that the precursor was needed above 700 °C to produce nanorods with ~200 nm [214]. Nanocomposite Ti–Si–N coating was performed by reactive DC magnetron sputtering in a mixture of Ar and N_2 gases onto bio implantable 316L stainless steel substrates [215]. It was found, by XRD, that the thus processed Ti–Si–nanocomposite coatings are mainly composed of amorphous Si_3N_4 and TiN crystals as major constituents along with TiN, TiO_2, and Si_3N_4 [215]. For modifying titanium dental implants, Yoshinari et al. [216] employed a dry-process on the titanium surface, including the ion beam dynamic mixing (thin calcium phosphates), ion implantation (Ca^+, N^+, F^+), titania spraying, ion plating (TiN, alumina), and ion beam mixing (Ag, Sn, Zn, Pt) with Ar^+ to enhance surface compatibility with the host bone tissue, subepithelial connective tissue, and epithelial tissue, so that the tissue-compatible surface can be obtained. It was concluded that dry-process surface modification was useful in controlling the physicochemical nature of surfaces, including the surface energy and the surface electrical charge, and in developing tissue-compatible implants [216]. HA was cold-sprayed to the biodegradable Mg alloy and it was reported that biocompatible coatings of the order of 20–30 μm thickness was obtained by pre-heating at 400 °C prior to the cold spraying [217]. Cai et al. [218], for improving the surface biocompatibility of titanium films, used the layer-by-layer self-assembly technique, based on the polyelectrolyte-mediated electrostatic adsorption of chitosan and gelatin. It was suggested that titanium films could be modified with chitosan and gelatin [218]. The electrostatic layer-by-layer self-assembly technique was also employed for producing polymers and enzymes [219]. Since the presence of appropriate porosity is required for tissue ingrowth and for the concurrent degradation of implanted structure, the formation of sufficiently large three-dimensional nano/macroporosity in bone scaffolds is important. Zhang et al. [220] introduced a new technique of combining the slip casting and polymer sponge methods using the slips with different powders to prepare HA scaffolds with bimodal pore sizes. It was reported that (i) the scaffolds were prepared with an open, uniform, and interconnected porous structure with a bimodal pore size of 100–300 μm and (ii) the bimodal porous HA scaffold sintered at 1200 °C had a large flexural strength of 73.3 MPa and a porosity of 52.5 vol% [220].

Turner et al. [221] compared laser cleaning trials performed using a Q-switched Nd:YAG laser, $\lambda = 1.064$ μm, and a continuous wave CO_2 laser, $\lambda = 10.6$ μm, applied to aerospace-grade, contaminated titanium alloys. The mechanisms for cleaning using each laser system are modelled to determine the mode and extent of contaminant removal. The model results are then compared with the surface chemistry and microstructural results from the cleaning trials performed. The results show the dominant cleaning process for Nd:YAG cleaning to be by evaporation of the contaminant via conduction through surface heating, while for CO_2 laser cleaning the small fraction of the beam coupling directly with the contaminant is sufficient for direct heating and selective evaporation. The results for experimental cleaning, electron beam (EB) welding, and diffusion bonding align well with the model, particularly when secondary reactions are taken into account [221,222].

Polymeric biomaterial surfaces were modified by albumin grafting to improve their blood compatibility. Albumin molecules were functionalized by introducing double bonds using glycidyl acrylate [223]. The functionalized albumin was covalently attached to various biomaterial surfaces such as polypropylene, polycarbonate, and poly(vinyl chloride) by γ-irradiation. Surface-induced platelet adhesion and thrombus formation on the albumin-grafted surfaces were examined using computer-enhanced video microscopy and SEM. It was reported that (i) the amount of the grafted albumin was dependent on the γ-irradiation dose and the concentration of albumin used for adsorption, (ii) the grafted albumin molecules remained on the surface even after exposure to blood for prolonged time periods. This approach was used to graft albumin to polymeric materials of an oxygenator, (iii) the albumin grafting resulted in a substantial improvement in blood compatibility as compared to control oxygenators, and (iv) the covalent grafting of functionalized albumin by γ-irradiation obviates the need for premodification of chemically inert polymer surfaces [223].

Sandblasting with large grit and acid-etching (SLA) treatment is considered to be a reliable modification to achieve the excellent titanium surface. However, contamination of hydrocarbons would make the SLA surface hydrophobic and influence its bioactivity. Thus, appropriate methods of preservation or further treatments could be used for improvement. Li et al. [224] conducted preservation in deionized water and ultraviolet (UV) irradiation were, respectively, applied to achieve SLAed and UV-SLAed surfaces. Surface characteristics were assessed by SEM, optical profilometer and XPS as well as wettability by an optical contact angle analyzer. Additionally, biocompatibility was evaluated by the response to osteoblast-like MG63 cells. It was mentioned that (i) prevented from further contamination, the SLAed surface with fewer hydrocarbons (25.31%) remained hydrophilic and showed better affinity to mineralization of MG63 cells than the hydrophobic polluted SLA surface, and (ii) furthermore, with the lowest content of hydrocarbons (14.26%) and super-hydrophilicity, the UV-SLA surface, which had the hydrocarbons effectively decomposed by photocatalysis and meanwhile acquired abundant hydroxyl groups, had most greatly promoted the attachment, proliferation, differentiation, and mineralization of MG63 cells. Therefore, hydrocarbons were found to be an important influencing factor to compatibility of biomaterials. It was also reported that UV irradiation was recognized as a trustworthy method for surface cleaning without change of topography and roughness and could ever lead to greater biocompatibility of sandblasted and acid-etched titanium surface [224].

5.3.4. Thermal Modification

The titanium surface was hydrothermally treated at a high pressure of 6.3 MPa (at 280 °C) in the CaO solution or water to improve bioactivity and biocompatibility [225] to form calcium titanate on the titanium surface. It was reported that beside the calcium titanate, titanium oxide, and titanium hydroxide layers were also formed as processing temperature and pressure increased. After immersing the thus surface-modified titanium in an SBF, needle-like apatite precipitation was observed, suggesting that surface modification of titanium with high-pressure hydrothermal treatment seemed to improve bioactivity and biocompatibility [225]. A complex compound of a crystalline $CaTiO_3$ layer was formed on the Ti–13Nb–13Zr alloy by the hydrothermal treatment [226]. An anatase type TiO_2 along with $Ti(OH)_4$ was deposited on Ti [227], and Zn-PO_4 was coated on Ti implants, forming zinc titanium phosphate [228].

Thermal spray is an established industrial method for the surfacing and resurfacing of metal parts and one of the most successful and versatile because of the very wide range of coating materials and substrates that can be processed, for example, from tape recording heads to print rollers and bridge structures. The benefits are typically lower cost, improved engineering performance, or increased component life, or both. In addition to original equipment applications, thermal spray coatings repair worn parts and those damaged ion service, and restore dimensions to mis-machined parts [229–233]. Bioceramics such as HA mixed with TiO_2 on the Ti–6Al–4V substrate [234] and rutile type TiO_2 on the surgical stainless steel substrate [235] were thermal sprayed. Polymeric materials can also be thermal sprayed, although thermally sprayed polymer coatings are gaining significant attention from many industries, including the potential applications are limited in petrochemical, automotive, and aircraft industries [236].

HA ceramics have been prepared from α-tricalcium phosphate (α-TCP) with the addition of water or ammonia water by the hydrothermal hot-pressing (HHP) method at 300 °C under a pressure of 40 MPa for 2 hours. When the additive is water, it appears that the HA grains produced show whisker-like and plate-like features. The bending strength of the HA ceramic obtained is measured to be 24.5 MPa. When the additive is ammonia water, the obtained HA ceramic consists of HA-whiskers only. The bending strength and fracture toughness reach 56 MPa and 1.52 MPa $m^{1/2}$, respectively. It was concluded that treating α-TCP with the addition of ammonia water by the HHP method is thus a useful method for *in situ* fabrication of HA-whisker ceramics [237]. Tang et al. [238] reported a new method of preparation of uniform porous HA biomaterials. In order to obtain uniform porous biomaterials, disk samples were formed by the mixture of HA powders and monodispersed polystyrene microspheres, and then HA uniform porous materials with different diameter and different porosity (diameter: 436 ± 25 nm, 892 ± 20 nm and 1890 ± 20 nm, porosity: 46.5%, 41.3%, and 34.7%, respectively) were prepared by sintering these disk samples at 1250 °C for 5 hours. A single electro-discharge-sintering (EDS) pulse (1.0 kJ/0.7 g), from a 150 °C capacitor, was applied to atomized spherical Ti–6Al–4V powder in air to produce microporous compact. A solid core surrounded by a porous layer was self-assembled by a discharge in the middle of the compact. XPS was used to study the surface characteristics of the compact material. C, N, O, and Ti were the main constituents, with smaller amounts of Al and V. The surface was lightly oxidized and was primarily in the form of TiO_2. A lightly etched

EDS sample showed the surface form of metallic Ti, indicating that EDS breaks down the oxide film of the as-received Ti–6Al–4V powder during the discharge process. The EDS Ti–6Al–4V compact surface also contained small amounts of TiN in addition to TiO_2, resulting in the reaction between nitrogen in air and the Ti substrate in times as short as 125 μs [239].

Corrosion tests were performed on sintered and unsintered titanium porous compacts of various porosities, as well as on solid titanium which acted as a control material. The tests were conducted in the 0.9% aqueous NaCl solution maintained at 37 °C to simulate the physiological environment encountered by surgical implants in the human body. The results confirm that solid titanium and sintered porous titanium both possess a distinct passivation range. Unsintered porous titanium does not seem to passivate at all and suffers greater corrosion than solid titanium. Unsintered specimens compacted at higher pressures experienced more corrosion than those compacted at lower pressures, although sintered specimens behaved in the exact opposite fashion [240]. Dewidar et al. [241] fabricated porous-surfaced with solid core Ti–6Al–4V implant compacts by traditional powder metallurgy. The powder metallurgy technique was used to produce three different porous surfaced implant compacts 30, 50, and 70% in vacuum atmosphere. The solid core formed in the center of the compact shows a similar microstructure of near full density of Ti–6Al–4V. The compressive yield strength was up to 270 MPa and significantly depended on the surface porosity, core size, and temperature of sintering. Porous-surfaced Ti–6Al–4V implant compacts with a solid core have much higher compressive strengths compared to the human bone. The ingrowth of bone tissue into the outer porous surface layer results in part fixation, while the solid inner core region provides the necessary mechanical strength for a device used for the replacement of heavy load bearing joint regions such as the hip and knee [241]. Two-step thermal oxidation of CpTi was investigated with a focus on the formation of anatase-type TiO_2. A first-step treatment was conducted in Ar-(0.1–20)%CO atmosphere at a temperature of 500 °C to 900 °C for a holding time of 0 or 1 hour, and a subsequent second-step treatment was conducted in air at 200 °C to 600 °C for 1 hour. It was reported that (i) titanium oxides and titanium oxycarbide were obtained in the firststep, with relative amounts depending on heating temperature, holding time, and CO partial pressure, (ii) an anatase-rich layer on Ti was obtained after second-step treatment in air at 300 °C to 350 °C in cases where single-phase titanium oxycarbide formed in the first step, and (iii) the bonding strength of an anatase-rich layer with a thickness of 0.5 μm was calculated to be around 90 MPa [242].

Besides the above popular coating thermal methods, there are still several important ways for coatings. Rodionov et al. [243] employed the steam-thermal oxidation of medical titanium implants. A porous-coated Ti–6Al–4V implant was fabricated by electrical resistance sintering [244]. Shenhar et al. [245] developed power immersed reaction-assisted coating nitriding method, which is suitable for the surface modification of large complex shape orthopedic implants. The Ti–6Al–4V alloy samples were annealed at 850 °C to 1100 °C in sealed stainless steel containers that allow selective diffusion of nitrogen atoms from the atmosphere and it was reported that (i) the Ti_3Al intermetallic phase was detected at the Ti_2N/α–Ti interface acting as a barrier for nitrogen diffusion and (ii) importantly for biomedical applications, no toxic Al or V were detected in the surface layer nitrided Ti–6Al–4V alloy [246].

5.3.5. Combined Technology

There are researches which combined several methods mentioned above; some of them are conducted simultaneously while the others are done consecutively. To improve the bioactivity of TiO_2 coatings, Zhang et al. conducted MAO in an electrolyte containing Ca and P ions, and MAO in a 1M NaOH electrolyte, and reported that alkaline-treated TiO_2 surface was found to be responsible for the rapid formation of HA during a SBF soaking, and the previous introduction of Ca and P can increase the opportunity to form HA [246]. To increase osteoinductivity and corrosive-wear resistance, a hybrid treatment of microarc discharge oxidation and EPD was conducted by forming a double layer HA–TiO_2 coating on titanium alloys with HA as the top layer and a dense TiO_2 film (which is believed to be effective as chemical barriers against the *in vivo* release of metal ions from the implants) as the inner layer, so that good combination of bioactivity, chemical stability, and mechanical integrity can be expected [247]. It was reported that a hybrid combination of MAO and EPD provided a phase-pure HA top layer and anti-corrosive TiO_2 interlayer, which should show good mechanical and biochemical stability in the corrosive environment of the human body [247]. MAO was combined with hydrothermal treatment in electrolytes containing calcium glycerphosphate and calcium acetate on Ti–6Al–4V, and it was found that (i) the film with a Ca/P ratio equivalent to HA was obtained when final voltage and current density were 350 V and 200 A/m^2 in the electrolyte containing 0.06 M calcium glycerphosphate and 0.25 M calcium acetate, and (ii) after hydrothermal treatment, the HA was precipitated on the surface of the film obtained by MAO with a thickness of about 4 μm [248].

Martines et al. [249] employed a sandblasted/acid-etched (SLAed) implant versus a smooth-surface implant to compare implant mobility (MO) and clinical reactions of peri-implant tissues to experimentally induced peri-implantitis in Beagle dogs. The right and left mandibular premolars were extracted from five Beagle dogs, and two smooth-surface implants and two SLAed implants were placed in each animal. The followings were findings. After 120 days, healing abutments were connected. Fifteen days later, the prosthetic abutments were connected, the hygiene regimen was suspended, and peri-implantitis was induced by the insertion of cotton ligatures into the soft tissue around the implants. At baseline and 30, 60, and 90 days later, clinical attachment level (CAL), probing depth (PD), and MO were measured. PD increased significantly in the SLA group alone when baseline PD was compared with 30-, 60-, and 90-day evaluations. The loss in CAL was significant in both groups when the baseline value was compared with 30-, 60-, and 90-day evaluations. Comparison between the two implant groups revealed a greater loss in CAL in the SLA group at the 90-day evaluation period. A significant increase in MO was seen in both groups when baseline values and 90-day evaluations were compared. Experimentally induced peri-implantitis results in a greater loss of CAL in SLA implants than in smooth-surface implants in dogs; however, no differences in MO or in PD have been noted between the two implant groups [249].Wei et al. [250] heat-treated NiTi alloy in air at 600 °C to form a TiO_2 film and alkali-treated in NaOH solutions (1M, 2M, 3M, 5M) to improve their bioactivity, followed by soaking SBF to evaluate their *in vitro* performance, and was reported that (i) the 3 M NaOH treatment is the most appropriate method, (ii) a large amount of apatite formed within 1 day's soaking in SBF, and (iii) after 7 day's soaking TiO_2/HA composite layer formed on the NiTi surface [250].

Nishiguchi et al. [251] investigated the effects of the alkali and heat treatments on the bone-bonding behavior of porous titanium implants. Porous titanium implants had a 4.6 mm solid core and a 0.7 mm thick porous outer layer using a pure titanium plasma-spray technique. Three types of porous implants were prepared from these pieces: (i) control implant (CL implant) as manufactured, (ii) AW-glass ceramic bottom-coated implant (AW implant) in which AW-glass ceramic was coated on only the bottom of the pore of the implant, (iii) alkali- and heat-treated implant (AH implant), where implants were immersed in 5 mol/L NaOH solution at 60 °C for 24 hours and subsequently heated at 600 °C for 1 hour. The implants were inserted into bilateral femora of six dogs hemi-transcortically in a randomized manner. At 4 weeks, push-out tests revealed that the mean shear strengths of the CL, AW, and AH implants were about 10.8, 12.7, and 15.0 MPa, respectively. At 12 weeks there was no significant difference between the bonding strengths of the three types of the porous implants (16.0–16.7 MPa). It was also reported that, histologically and histomorphologically, direct bone contact with the implant surface was significantly higher in the AH implants than the CL and AW implants both at 4 and 12 weeks. Thus, the higher bonding strength between bone and alkali- and heat-treated titanium implants was attributed to the direct bonding between the bone and the titanium surface. It was concluded that alkali and heat treatments can provide porous titanium implants with earlier stable fixation [251].

Juodzbalys et al. [252] investigated to create an acid-etched implant surface that is similar to that created by sandblasting combined with acid etching and to compare it with the surfaces of various commercially available screw-type implants. CpTi (grade V) disks were machined in preparation for acid etching. Tests were carried out using different acids and combinations of them with varying time exposures. It was found that the surface most like the sandblasted/acid-etched surface was best obtained with a combination of sulfuric and hydrochloric acids. It was concluded that the new experimental acid-etched titanium surface had the features of a roughened titanium surface, with glossily microroughness and large waviness. In general, the experimental surface was significantly rougher than the selected commercially available implants and similar to a sandblasted/acid-etched surface (top Sa: 2.08 ± 0.36 μm, Sdr: 1.34 ± 0.3 μm, valleys: 1.16 ± 0.1 μm and 0.68 ± 0.1 μm, flanks: 2.24 ± 0.8 μm and 1.27 ± 0.1 μm, respectively) [252].

Increased surface roughness of dental implants has demonstrated greater bone apposition; however, the effect of modifying surface chemistry remains unknown. Buser et al. [17] evaluated bone apposition to a modified sandblasted/acid-etched (SLA) titanium surface, as compared with a standard SLA surface, during early stages of bone regeneration. Experimental implants were placed in miniature pigs, creating two circular bone defects. Test and control implants had the same topography, but differed in surface chemistry. The test surface was prepared by submerging the implant in an isotonic NaCl solution following acid-etching to avoid contamination with molecules from the atmosphere. It was shown that (i) test implants demonstrated a significantly greater mean percentage of bone–implant contact as compared with controls at 2 (49.30 vs. 29.42%) and 4 weeks (81.91*vs.*66.57%) of healing, and (ii) at 8 weeks, similar results were observed. It was, hence, concluded that a modified sandblasted/acid-etched titanium surface promoted enhanced bone apposition during early stages of bone regeneration [17].

Plasma-coated HA possesses a few crucial problems including easy dissolution or resorption in living tissue, and a potentially weak interfacial bond between the coating and a metal substrate, so that the low stability of the HA coating may lead to the failure of the implant. Besides, HA can't be deposited uniformly due to geometrical limitations such as on inner or undercut surfaces of a porous structure. Ishizawa et al. [253] employed combined methods of electrochemical and hydrothermal reactions to precipitate HA crystals on porous Ti. HA ceramic has been applied on Ti implants (which was previously modified by laser beam irradiation) to increase the corrosion resistance, gain better biocompatibility, and implant–bone tissue biological adhesion, by coating polyvinyldense fluoride/HA composite which was obtained by a casting method, and it was reported that uniform coating with a small thickness variation along the coated surface was successfully obtained [254]. Moreover, to control surface topography (roughness and blind porosity), surface chemistry, and wettability, affecting the osseointegration, Shtansky et al. [255] employed a combination of various techniques such as cold spray, selective laser sintering, pulsed electro-erosion treatment, and magnetron sputtering on Ti materials. In particular, for modifying surface chemistry, multifunctional bioactive nanostructured TiCaPCON films were deposited on cold sprayed, laser sintered, and electro-erosion treated using a composite $TiC_{0.5} + Ca_3(PO_4)_2$ target [255]. It was reported that (i) the wettability measurements showed that the cold sprayed and electro-erosion treated surfaces exhibit high values of water contact angle, and (ii) ion etching in vacuum and TiCaPCON film deposition made the samples highly hydrophilic, concluding that the combination of high surface roughness and blind porosity with hydrophilicity and biocompatibility makes the fabricated metal-ceramic materials promising candidates for applications involving tissue regeneration [255]. In order to improve the tribological properties of aluminum alloys, Sun [256] applied a process including the fabrication of a rutile-type TiO_2 coating on an aluminum alloy by the combination of sputter-deposition of a pure titanium coating on the substrate and subsequent thermal oxidation. It was found that (i) the coating has a layered structure, comprising a rutile-TiO_2 layer at the top, an oxygen and nitrogen dissolved α-Ti layer in the middle and a titanium-aluminide layer in the interfacial region, and (ii) such a hybrid coating system has good adhesion with the substrate, can significantly enhance the surface hardness and tribological properties of the aluminum alloy in terms of much reduced friction coefficient and increased wear resistance [256].

To make metals bioactive for orthopedic applications, apatite/TiO_2 composite coatings were formed on Ti and NiTi SMA using an H_2O_2-oxidation and hot water aging technique and the subsequent accelerated biomimetic process. Nanoindentation testing conducted on cross-sections of composite coatings indicated that there was no significant difference in nanohardness and elastic modulus between apatite/TiO_2 composite coatings formed on Ti and NiTi SMA samples. It was reported that (i) the enhancement of the adhesion between the apatite laye r and the metal substrates arose from the TiO_2 intermediate layer in the composite coating, (ii) the highest values of coating adhesion strength for Ti and NiTi SMA samples, as measured by scratch tests, were 22.58 N and 19.07 N, respectively, and (iii) however, compared to corresponding Ti samples, NiTi SMA samples had better tribological properties [257].

To enhance the biological performance of titanium coating, hierarchial structuring was investigated to produce a hybrid structure of nano-, micro-, and macro-scale layers in which each substructure possesses different biological functions. Such multi-function and multiscale structure was generated by sandblasting, acid etching, and alkali treating the vacuum plasma sprayed titanium coating following hot water immersing [258,259].

The effects of different thickness of HA coatings on bone stress distribution near the dental implant–bone interface are very important factors for the HA-coated dental implant design and clinical application. By means of finite element analysis, the bone stress distributions near the dental implant coated with different thicknesses from 0 to 200 μm were calculated and analyzed under the 200 N chewing load. In all cases, the maximal von Mises stresses in the bone are at the positions near the neck of dental implant on the lingual side, and decrease with the increase of the HA coatings thickness. The HA coatings weaken the stress concentration and improve the biomechanical property in the bone, however, in HA coatings thickness range of 60–120 μm, the distinctions of that benefit are not obvious. In addition, considering the technical reason of HA coatings, it was concluded that the thickness of HA coatings ranging from 60 to 120 μm would be the better choice for clinical application [260].

5.4. Coating Materials and Materials Preparation

The coating surface layer is another powerful way to achieve the surface transformation, including carburizing, oxidizing, or nitrizing. In this section, we will discuss coating materials and their preparation.

5.4.1. Metallic Materials

As we will see in this section, metal elements as well as alloys are chosen and used extensively as coating materials. A nanotopographic noble metal (Ag, Au, Pd) coating has been applied on commercial urinary catheters and used in more than 80,000 patients and was indicated that, by varying the noble metal ratio at implant surfaces, it is possible to modulate inflammation and fibrosis in soft tissue [261]. The use of silver element was due to the excellent anti-bacterial property [262]. Bioactive coatings are in high demand to increase the functions of cells for numerous medical devices. Metal element (Au,Ti) was coated on several potential orthopedic polymeric materials (specifically, ultrahigh molecular weight polyethylene, PEEK: polyetheretherketone and PTFE: polytetrafluoroethylene) by ionic plasma deposition process which creates a surface-engineered nanostructure (with features below 100 nm) and their osteoblast (bone-forming cell) adhesion was improved [263].

Solid Ti metal was widely selected as coating elements. Ti was coated on surgical 316 stainless steel substrate and it was reported that cell proliferation, alkaline phosphatase activity, migration, and adhesion were increased, and osteoblast-like cells on the grit-blasted, titanium-coated, microarc-oxidated surface were strongly adhered, and proliferated well [264]. Nanoscale titanium was coated on silicon surfaces and increased cell spreading and proliferation rates were reported on surfaces with 50 nm thick Ti coatings [265]. Nanostructures entail a high potential for improving implant surfaces, for instance, in stent applications. Ti nanoparticles were coated on an electropolished NiTi stent surface [266]. The solid solution phase of β-(Ti, Nb) [267] and Ti–6Al–4V film [268] were also selected as coating materials. Although carbon fiber-reinforced polyetheretherketone (CF/PEEK) exhibits properties suitable for load-bearing orthopedic implants, its hydrophobicity induces the deposition of a peri-implant fibrous tissue capsule preventing bone apposition. Devine et al. coated CF/PEEK screws coated with titanium by vacuum plasma spraying and PVD and found that Ti coating of CF/PEEK screws significantly improve bone apposition and removal torque compared with uncoated CF/PEEK screws [269].

Tantalum (Ta) metal has successfully been used for implants due to excellent biocompatibility [270–274]. It has been found that tantalum coatings show great potential within both industrial and medical applications [275]. Tantalum coating with a very ductile nature is suitable where a product can be improved by combining material characteristics of the substrate with an exceptional corrosion-resistant surface [276,277]. As a result, tantalum is an excellent candidate for usage as coatings for NiTi alloys to improve its anti-corrosion property and radiopacity [278]. Ta was coated on the Co–Cr alloy with excellent outcomes of good mechanical properties (high elastic modulus, high hardness value, low friction coefficient, high wear resistance) and chemical properties (high wettability, good corrosion resistance), so that it is of interest for joints presenting good biocompatibility and great longevity [279,280]. Porous tantalum, a low modulus metal with a characteristic appearance similar to cancellous bone, is currently available for use in several orthopedic applications (hip and knee arthroplasty, spine surgery, and bone graft substitute). It was reported that this transition metal maintains several interesting biomaterial properties, including: a high volumetric porosity (70%–80%), low modulus of elasticity (3MPa), and high frictional characteristics along with an excellent biocompatibility and tantalum chondrocyte composites have yielded successful early results *in vitro* and may afford an option for joint resurfacing in the future, suggesting a promising applications in orthopedic surgery [281–283]. Ta along with TaO was coated on surgical 316L stainless steel and it was mentioned that (i) the mechanical stability and repassivation properties of the material are guaranteed up to the onset of substrate plastic deformation, (ii) biocompatibility is obtained by tantalum oxide, and (iii) the ductility is achieved by the tantalum interface that, at the same time, ensures continued film adhesion, even after plastic deformation of the steel substrate [277].

Olivares-Navarrete et al. [284] deposited niobium (Nb) by magnetron sputtering as a possible surface modification for stainless steel substrates in biomedical implants and the biocompatibility of the coatings was evaluated using human alveolar bone derived cells, in terms of cellular adhesion, proliferation, and viability. It was observed that (i) no toxic response was observed for any of the surfaces, indicating that the Nb coatings act as a biocompatible, bioinert material, (ii) cell morphology test confirmed the healthy state of the cells on the Nb surface, and (iii) water contact angle measurements showed that the Nb surface is more hydrophobic than the stainless steel substrate [284]. Nb thin film and NbN were deposited on stainless steel to evaluate the biocompatibility of the surfaces by testing the cellular adhesion and viability/proliferation of human cementoblasts during different culture times, up to 7 days [285]. It was reported that (i) the niobium oxide films were amorphous and of stoichiometric Nb_2O_5, while the niobium nitride films were crystalline in the FCC phase (*c*-NbN) and were also stoichiometric with a Nb to N ratio of one, (ii) the biocompatibility of the stainless steel could be improved by any of the two films, but neither was better than the Ti–6Al–4V alloy, and (iii) on the other hand, comparing the two films, the *c*-NbN seemed to be a better surface than the oxide in terms of the adhesion and proliferation of human cemetoblasts [285].

NiTi films [286] or porous NiTi [287] and NiTi foam [288] were prepared. Liu et al. [287] evaluated bone ingrowth under actual load-bearing conditions and interfacial bonding strength by histological analysis and push-out test. It was reported that the porous NiTi materials bond very well to newly formed bone tissues and the highest average strength of 357N and best ductility are achieved from the porous NiTi materials [287].

High-purity biodegradable magnesium (Mg) is believed to exhibit excellent biocompatibility and coating of Mg element is expected to show appropriate for implant applications and to improve the interaction between the implant and the biological environment [288]. In recent years, research on magnesium alloys had increased significantly for hard tissue replacement and stent application due to their outstanding advantages, because (i) Mg alloys have mechanical properties similar to bone which avoid stress shielding, (ii) they are biocompatible essential to the human metabolism as a factor for many enzymes, (iii) main degradation product Mg is an essential trace element for human enzymes, and (iv) the most important reason is they are perfectly biodegradable in the body fluid [289–292]. Mg–Y–Nd was evaluated its feasibility as bone implant applications mainly focused on biocompatibility and corrosion resistance [293]. It was concluded that the biodegradable Mg–Y–Nd implant is superior to the control Ti–6Al–4V with respect to both bone/implant interface strength and osseointegration [293]. Mg–Zr–Sr alloys have recently been developed as biodegradable implant materials [294]. It was reported that (i) both Zr and Sr are evaluated excellent alloying elements in manufacturing biodegradable Mg alloy implants, (ii) Zr addition refined the grain size, improved the ductility, smoothed the grain boundaries, and enhanced the corrosion resistance of Mg alloys, (iii) Sr addition led to an increase in compressive strength, better *in vitro* biocompatibility, and significantly higher bone formation *in vivo*, and (iv) Mg–xZr–ySr alloys with x and $y \leq 5$wt.% would make excellent biodegradable implant materials for load-bearing applications [294]. Biodegradable Mg–Zn–Zr was also developed as an orthopedic implant material due to its biodegradable feature and suitable mechanical properties [295]. The amorphous Si film (which was prepared by plasma-enhanced CVD of SiH_4) was coated on the Mg–Y–Nd alloy for biomedical application [296]. The hemolysis test and blood platelets adhesion test were conducted, and it was reported that the hemolysis of the Mg–Y–Nd alloy decreased after being coated by Si and the platelets attached on the Si film were at the inactivated stage with a round shape [296].

The functionally graded, hard, and wear-resistant Co–Cr–Mo alloy was coated on the Ti–6Al–4V alloy and it was shown that the addition of the Co–Cr–Mo alloy significantly increased the surface hardness without any intermetallic phases in the transition region [297].

Selenium (in the form of sodium selenite) coating onto Ti material was evaluated and it was found that there was no inhibitory effect of the selenium coating on the osteoblastic cell growth, and Se coating is a promising method to reduce bacterial attachment on prosthetic material [298].

5.4.2. Polymeric Materials

Biodegradable polymers (which perform a structural application and are designed to be completely resorbed and to become weaker over time) form a unique class of materials that created an entirely new concept when originally proposed as biomaterials. Recently, in tissue engineering, a biodegradable scaffold seeded with an appropriate cell type provides a substitute for damaged human tissue while the natural process of regeneration is completed [299,300]. An adhesive biodegradable polymer, PVA, was coated on Mg-based alloys by the dip-coating technique in order to control the degradation rate and enhance the biocompatibility of magnesium alloys. Since the cytocompatibility of osteoblast cells (MC3T3) revealed high adherence, proliferation, and survival on the porous structure of PVA-coated Mg alloy, which was not observed for the uncoated samples, it was concluded that the PVA coating is a promising candidate for biodegradable implant materials, which might widen the use of Mg-based implants [110]. A biodegradable polymeric membrane fabricated by polycaprolactone and dichloromethane was coated on the Mg-based alloy to control a high corrosion rate and accumulation of hydrogen gas upon degradation hinders its clinical application [301]. Polyethylene (PE) [302] and polyhedral oligomeric silsesquioxanes (POSS) and poly(carbonate-urea)urethane (PCU) [303] were coated onto NiTi stent to control the thrombogenicity. When the Ti–6Al–4V alloy is used in several ventricular assist devices, the thrombogenecity resistance is highly required. A plasma-induced graft polymerization of 2-methacryloyloxyethyl phosphorylcholine (MPC) was carried out and poly(MPC) (PMPC) chains were covalently attached onto the Ti–6Al–4V surface [304]. It was reported that platelet deposition was markedly reduced on the PMPC grafted surfaces and platelet activation in blood that contacted the PMPC-grafted samples was significantly reduced relative to the unmodified Ti–6Al–4V and polystyrene control surfaces [304]. For bone and teeth repairs, biomaterials are demanded of both good biocompatibility and reliable mechanical properties for long periods. Since due to the nature of the HA of low fracture toughness and fracture energy, there are several ways to overcome these disadvantages of HA materials, including incorporating with ZrO_2 or Al_2O_3. Nakahara et al. infiltrated porous HA with nylon to improve fracture toughness of HA with 1.65 MPa$\sqrt{m}$ [305].

5.4.3. Ceramics—Metallic Oxides, Nitrides, and Carbides

Titanium oxides (TiO_2) have been used in different forms such as thick layer, thin film, porous and foam and nanotube, titanium nitrides and carbides along with other metals' oxides. Titanium dioxide (TiO_2, titania) is a widely abundant and inexpensive material. In bulk form it is produced as a white powder and it is the most widely used white pigment because of its brightness and very high refractive index. Applications include filler pigment in paints, cosmetics, pharmaceuticals, food products, tooth whitening gel, and toothpaste [306,307]. Bioactive TiO_2 was deposited on surface-modified polyethylene terephthalate (PET) plates by using a sol–gel method and was indicated that this modification possesses a mechanically stable surface-modified layer, excellent bone-bonding ability, osteoconductive ability, and biocompatibility in bone [308]. The Ti-O film was deposited on surgical 316L stainless steel by PIII and deposit method [309].

NiTi was surface-modified by plasma electrolytic oxidation in aqueous solutions of sodium sulfate and sodium hydroxide (Na_2SO_4–NaOH) using an AC power supply. It was found that a thick and porous oxide layer with micron-sized pores was formed on the NiTi substrate, with the thickness of the oxide layer ranging from a few μm to over 10 μm, depending on the processing time [310]. Similarly, TiO_2 thin films were deposited on the NiTi surgical alloy by the sol–gel method. It was found that, according to the *in vitro* evaluation on blood compatibility of the film and the NiTi alloy by dynamic clotting time and blood platelets adhesion tests, the NiTi alloy coated with TiO_2 film possessed an improved blood biocompatibility [311]. Titanium oxide coatings were conducted by MAO in galvanostatic regime on the biomedical NiTi alloy in H_3PO_4 electrolyte using DC power supply [312]. Sugita et al. using a slow-rate sputter deposition of molten TiO_2 nanoparticles, coated acid-etched microroughened titanium surfaces with a TiO_2 layer of 300 pm to 6.3 nm thickness that increased the surface oxygen levels without altering the existing microtopography [313]. It was reported that (i) a super-thin TiO_2 coating of pico-to-nanometer thickness enhances the biological properties of the proven microroughened titanium surfaces by controllably and exclusively modulating their surface chemistry while preserving the existing surface morphology, and (ii) the improvements in proliferation and differentiation of osteoblasts attained by this chemical modification is of great significance, providing a new insight into how to develop new implant surfaces for better osseointegration, based on the established microtopographic surfaces [313]. Titanium oxide (TiO_2) films were deposited onto the polymer substrates of PTFE, polyethylene (PE), and PET, which were pre-modified with polydopamine coating, by a simple liquid phase deposition process. It was indicated that the fabricated TiO_2 films could markedly improve the *in vitro* cytocompatibility [314]. TiO_2 was coated on the Ti–6Al–4V substrate by the air plasma spraying method. It was reported that, according to the osteoblast adhesion morphology and proliferation tests, osteoblast-like cell morphology was not influenced by process parameters, but cell proliferation was affected to some extent by surface roughness and porosity among TiO_2 [314].

Titania (which is the highest order of oxidation of Ti) has three distinct types of crystalline structures: brookite, anatase and rutile. Although most of works on TiO_2 coating did not identify the crystalline structure of the coating titania, there are several works which identified crystalline structures [315]. The anatase phase TiO_2 thin films were grown by pulsed laser deposition on SiO_2 substrates [316] and anatase-type TiO_2 coatings were grown on Ti and Si by atomic layer deposition [317]. On the other hand, a rutile-type titania film was deposited on a silicon substrate by RF-magnetron sputtering using a sintered oxide target in an argon-gas atmosphere [318] and an amorphous titania was formed by treating titanium plates by Ar and oxygen plasma treatment, and furthermore, nano-(α+rutile-TiO_2) were formed on the amorphous-like oxide layer following glow discharging. It was also mentioned that surface cleaning and oxidation modification by plasma treatments are believed to improve the biocompatibility and tissue healing [319].

Silicon substrate was also coated with titania films by different methods: by the spray pyrolysis method [320], ion irradiation [321], and sol–gel method [322]. Ultrathin film of titanium oxide (TiO_x) was coated on silicon wafers. It was found that (i) the surface sol–gel process predominantly formed homogeneous, but rough and porous titanium oxide layers and (ii) the protein adsorption was dependent primarily on the silane chemistry, packing of the alkyl chains (extent of van der Waals interaction), morphology (porosity and roughness), and wettability of the sol–gel oxide [322].

Thin porous titania film was also coated differently. Porous titania film is prepared by alkali (in NaOH) treatment of the NiTi alloy followed by soaking treatment in the HCl solution. The benefit of this porous titania film as an interlayer to improve adhesion and integrity of the sol–gel titania coating on the NiTi alloy substrate is evidenced by surface morphological observations [323]. Effective immobilization of bioactive substances such as adhesive proteins, synthetic peptides, and growth factors on metallic substrates is required for a number of medical applications. It was reported that (i) an alkoxy-derived nano-porous titanium oxide coating (which was synthesized electrochemically on titanium in methanolic electrolytes) may act as an effective interface for functionalizing a titanium surface, and (ii) nanoporous oxide coatings could facilitate fast diffusion of small organic molecules within the oxide network and form strong chemical bonds with the functional groups of these molecules at room temperature [324]. Porous TiO_2 coating was achieved on the Ti surface by MAO, and it was mentioned that the cortex-like coating was conducive to cell retention and implant stabilization [325].

Nanotubes of titania were coated. Oriented aligned TiO_2 nanotube arrays were fabricated by anodizing titanium foil in a 0.5% HF electrolyte solution [326]. A net-like structured TiO_2 film was produced with a low-temperature hydrothermal process, followed by acid washing and calcination in air, and was deposited on surgical 316L stainless steel substrate [327]. For improving cell adhesion and differentiation and as a result of these improvements, nanofibrous modification of dental and bone implants might enhance osseointegration [328]. TiO_2 nanofibers were fabricated by the electrospinning method using a mixture of Ti isopropoxide and poly(vinyl pyrrolidone) (PVP) in the acidic alcohol solution. It was reported that the diameter of the TiO_2 nanofibers was controlled within the range of 20–350 nm [328].

Titania composites were also chosen as coating materials. To improve the bioactivity of titanium, CpTi was hydrothermally treated in 0.1mol/l $MgCl_2$ solutions with different pH values (5.5, 7.5, and 9.5) at 200 °C for 24 hours. It was reported that (i) nano-sized anatase precipitations (including $MgTiO_3$ at low pH and $Mg(OH)_2$ at high pH) were obtained and (ii) hydrothermal treatment in the $MgCl_2$ solution can improve the bioactivity of titanium by immobilizing Mg into an oxide layer; however, the chemical state and amount of Mg should be well controlled [329]. Mg-incorporated titania was produced by hydrothermally treating Ti in an alkaline Mg-containing solution. It was concluded that the Mg-incorporated submicro-porous Ti oxide surface produced by hydrothermal treatment may improve implant osseointegration by enhancing the attachment, spreading and differentiation of osteoblastic cells [330]. A mixture of TiO_2 and TiN was deposited on the titanium alloy by plasma nitriding and oxidizing under glow discharge conditions. It was reported that nitriding and oxidizing under glow discharge conditions have provided new possibilities of producing nontoxic, human fibroblast-compatible surface layers on parts made of titanium alloys [331]. Ni_2O_3-doped TiO_2 nanotubes were deposited on the NiTi alloy using the electrochemical anodization method. It was reported that (i) forming of the Ni_2O_3-doped TiO_2 film on the surface of the NiTi alloy increased its wettability, especially for a 600 °C annealed sample, so the biological response is expected to be improved, and (ii) annealing the Ni_2O_3-doped TiO_2 film coated NiTi alloy at 450 °C is desirable for cardiovascular applications [332].

There are still several different types of oxides which are ready for coating processing. A mixture of TiO_2 and ZnO was sputter-coated on glass substrates [333]. To improve corrosion resistance and biocompatibility, the Fe-O film was coated on iron stents [334]. It was reported that the results of human umbilical vein endothelial cells (HUVECs) culture showed HUVECs had good adhesion and proliferation behavior on the Fe-O film, and, after depositing the Fe–O thin film by PIII and deposition technique under the low oxygen flux, the corrosion resistance and biocompatibility of pure iron were effectively improved [334].

Due to excellent mechanical stability and repassivation properties of the tantalum (Ta) are guaranteed up to the onset of substrate plastic deformation. Macionczyk et al. [277] coated TaO onto stainless steel implants and obtained results indicating that, while biocompatibility is obtained by tantalum oxide, the ductility is achieved by the tantalum interface which at the same time ensures continued film adhesion, even after plastic deformation of the steel substrate [277]. The thin TaO film was also coated on Ti material by a layer-by-layer sol-gel deposition technique [335]. A composite of TaO and carbon was coated on the Ti surface to improve its propensity to a long-term degradation in physiological conditions and its weak osseointegrative capacities [336].

Zirconia (ZrO_2) coating was evaluated by the histologic analysis, indicating that (i) bone growth is more evident around coating fixtures than in controls and (ii) a more mature bone is present in the peri-implant coated surface than in controls; hence zirconium oxide coating can enhance implant osseointegration [337]. Yan et al. [338] prepared a macroporous and nanocrystalline zirconia coating film by MAO, followed by chemical treatment in H_2SO_4 or NaOH aqueous solution to evaluate the apatite-forming ability. Monolithic zirconia and zirconia-HA composites were prepared by joining by cold isostatic pressing (at 300 MPa) and subsequently by glass-encapsulated hot isostatic pressing (at 1225 °C, for 1 hour and under 200 MPa) [339]. A zirconia (ZrO_2) was coated on Ti and Zr to exhibit lower friction and superior wear properties, suggesting that they could be used in hip and knee implants [340].

Nano Mg_2SiO_4 (Forsterite) was coated onto porous HA to enhance the compressive strength of porous HA scaffold (porosity: ~83%, mean pore size: ~740 μm) and found that (i) the coating microstructure consisted of the grains with the range between 35 and 80 nm, (ii) the compressive strength of highly porous HA was improved from 0.12 to 1.61 MPa, indicating that the scaffolds obtained provided a good mechanical support while maintaining bioactivity, and hence they could be used as tissue engineering scaffolds for low-load-bearing applications [341]. For controlling the porosity of bioglasses at the nanometric scale, a composite of silica-based glasses with organic components (in a form of new organic-inorganic hybrid material) was prepared by the sol–gel process [342]. Alumina (Al_2O_3) was deposited on the Fe–Cr–Al–Y alloy by the thermal oxidation technique [343].

Now moving to metal nitrides, the TiN film was coated on mild steel by a new combined laser/sol–gel processing technique, indicating that nano-hardness measurements revealed a hardness value of the order of 22 to 27 GPa [344]. Titanium and Ti–6Al–4V alloy samples were coated using a powder immersion reaction assisted coating nitriding method in order to modify their surface properties, and it was reported that strongly adherent single (TiN)- or double(Ti_2N/TiN)-layer coatings were obtained on both substrates, suggesting that titanium nitride coatings can provide surgical titanium alloys with the enhanced fretting wear and corrosion resistant surface thereby minimizing the ion- and particulate-generating potential of modular orthopedic implants [345]. TiN was coated on the surgical Ti–6Al–4V ELI alloy to improve tribological and corrosion properties by means of plasma etching in an argon/nitrogen atmosphere protection of surfaces [346]. The nanostructured TiN film was prepared by reactive plasma spraying in the air. The coated film was identified as mainly composed of TiN (max. 86.3%) and a small quantity of Ti_3O [347]. Sinter-coating combines sintering and TiN coating in one step by sintering the green specimens in N_2 atmosphere was conducted on titanium foam to produce the TiN film layer [348]. It was reported that, after the alkali treatment by soaking the foams in the NaOH solution and then heating at 600 °C, treated foams were immersed into SBF to induce a bone-like apatite layer on foam surface [348]. TiN-based composite coatings with and without the addition of Cr were prepared deposited by reactive plasma spraying in air. Both sintered and mixed powder of Ti and B_4C were used for this process. It was found that the coating deposited using sintered Ti and B_4C powder is composed of two main phases (TiN and $TiN_{0.3}$), two minor phases ($Ti_2O_3$and TiB_2), and a small fraction of TiC phase, and the composition of the coating deposited using the mixed powder with Cr added is predominantly in the TiN and TiB_2 phases, a smaller phase fraction of Ti_2O_3 and TiO_2, and some unreacted Cr [349]. The TiN/Ti multilayer was deposited on 304 stainless steel by magnetron sputtering to improve pitting corrosion resistance [350]. TiN was also coated on cellulosic fiber substrates by atomic layer deposition to produce biocompatible cellulose and other implant materials [351].

In the TiN group, there are several composites prepared for coating purposes. To improve cytotoxicity, cell-adherency, and tribological performance, TiN particle reinforced Ti–6Al–4V composite coatings were prepared. It was found that (i) the composite coatings contain distinct TiN particles embedded in the $\alpha + \beta$ phase matrix, (ii) the average top surface hardness of the Ti–6Al–4V alloy increased from 394 ± 8 HV to 1138 ± 61 HV with 40 wt% TiN reinforcement, and (iii) among the composite coatings, the coatings reinforced with 40 wt% TiN exhibited the highest wear resistance of 3.74×10 to 6 mm^3/Nm, which is lower than the wear rate, 1.04×10–5 mm^3/Nm, of the laser processed Co–Cr–Mo alloy tested under identical experimental conditions [352]. Titanium nitride oxide ($TiNO_x$) coating was preformed on roughened Ti and stainless steel by the plasma/PVD deposition technique and on cellulose fiber substrates by atomic layer deposition [353]. It was reported that $TiNO_x$ coatings yield similar proliferation and differentiation rates when applied onto roughened Ti and stainless steel, suggesting that a more effective osseointegration of endosseous implants can be produced [353].

Titanium aluminum nitride (Ti,Al)N was coated on 304 stainless steel substrate. After thus coated implants were placed into the mid-shaft of the femur of Wistar rats, it was found that (i) all implants exhibited a favorable response in bone with no evidence of fibrous encapsulation, (ii) there was no significant difference in the amount of new bone formed around the different rods (osseoconduction), and (iii) however, there was a greater degree of shrinkage separation of bone from the coated rods than from the plain rods, suggesting that titanium aluminum nitride coating may result in reduced osseointegration between bone and implant [354] Mukherjee et al. [355] coated the hard Ti-based coating TiAlN on stainless steel by PIII -assisted deposition to improve wear resistance in orthopedic conditions. Furthermore, titanium aluminum nitride oxide (TiAlNO) coatings were deposited on the Corning glass by means of the co-sputtering technique. It was indicated that TiAlNO is versatile material that could be used for both mechanical and electronic applications; however, it is important to control fabrication conditions [356]. Shtansky et al. [357] studied complicate composite of TiCaPCON films which were prepared by DC magnetron sputtering of composite comprising $TiC_{0.5}$ and $Ca_3(PO_4)_2$ target produced by self-propagating high-temperature synthesis. It was reported that (i) the *in vitro* studies showed that human fibroblasts well adhered and spread on the surface of the PTFE sample coated with TiCaPCON films, and (ii) the *in vivo* studies using rat hip and rabbit calvarial defect models demonstrated a high osseointegration potential of the TiCaPCON/PTFE implants [357].

Titanium carbide (TiC) was coated on the titanium substare by a pulsed laser deposition method to improve implant hardness, biocompatibility through surface stability, and osseointegration through improved bone growth [358], and TiC and TiB (titanium boride) were coated by a laser surface alloying of Ti–6Al–4V with graphite and boron mixed powders to enhance wear resistance [359]. Levashov et al. [360] coated composite of TiCCaPCON on NiTi by rapid plastic deformation technology, thermomechanical treatment, and magnetron sputtering.

5.4.4. Ceramcis—Nonmetallic Compounds

In recent years, implants coated with bioactive layers to promote fixation through osseointegration mechanism has become increasingly common. Fabrication routes that provide control over features such as biocompatibility and bioreactivity through management of coating chemistry and structure are still being developed. Current coating fabrication technology includes plasma spraying, rf sputtering, CVD, lasers ablation and sol–gel processing, although plasma spraying is used to produce most commonly available bioceramic coatings for orthopedic and dental implants [361].

The term apatite denotes a family of crystals with the formula $M_{10}(RO_4)_6X_2$, where *M* is usually calcium, *R* is usually phosphorus, and *X* is hydroxide or a halogen such as fluorine. Bone mineral was found to be quite complex and included various types of hydrated calcium phosphates, the most common being calcium HA—$Ca_{10}(PO_4)_6(OH)_2$ [362]. Although no standard manufacturing guideline exists for depositing HA—($Ca_{10}(PO_4)_6(OH)_2$)—on implant surfaces, HA depositions have been widely applied to generate bioactive surfaces in simulated biological environments [363,364]. HA was coated on titanium plates [365–368]. HA coating on titanium was performed by a sol–gel process combined with conventional heat treatment and with UV irradiation at ambient temperature [367]. It was reported that the sol–gel coated titanium had slightly higher bone apposition than uncoated titanium as a control material [367]. In order to improve biocompatibility of Ti substrates, Hahn et al. [368] coated 1-μm thick nano-structured HA, deposited on the substrates through aerosol deposition, which sprays HA powder with an average particle size of 3.2 μm at room temperature in vacuum. Ti–6Al–4V is also a popular biomedical metallic substrate for HA coating [369–372]. Hung et al. [371] coated HA on Ti–6Al–4V ELI surfaces by a plasma spraying method. HA-coated surfaces were immersed in a SBF. It was found that (i) after 28 days, the crystallinity level of the HA coatings in the SBF increased from 54.88% to 74.39%, (ii) the released calcium ion concentration increased from 44.9 ppm up to 79.27 ppm, and (iii) the coatings contained no significant phase components such as tricalcium phosphate (α-TCP or β-TCP) or tetracalcium phosphate [371]. The NiTi SMA was coated with HA for improving biocompatibility and bioactivity, and TiO_2 for preventing Ni ion release [373]. Gopi et al. [374] passivated surgical grade stainless steel (316L) in borate through poly-*ortho*-phenylenediamine and subsequently HA was coated by a dip coating method to minimize the release of metallic ions. Non-metallic substrates are also subjected to HA coatings. In order to improve bioactivity and to enhance osseointegration of titanium implant materials, a nanotubular TiO_2 structure was subject to HA coating, and the bond strength was further improved by annealing the HA-coated nanoporous titania in an argon atmosphere [375]. Cao et al. [376] coated the fusion-cage-like carbon fiber reinforced carbon composite implants with HA by the plasma spraying technique for bone tissue reconstruction. After autogenously bone filled fusion-cage-like implants were grafted in hybrid goats' tibia for 328 days, it was reported that the coating can significantly speed up the bone defect healing process and improve the surface bioactivity of carbon fiber reinforced carbon composites [376]. Nanocomposite ZrO_2–Al_2O_3 was HA-coated for improving biocompatibility, and, from the mechanical and biological evaluations, it was concluded that a mixture of coated HA with 30 vol% and 70 vol% of ZrO_2–Al_2O_3 composite was found to be the optimal composition for load-bearing biological applications [377].

HA material as a coating species is not limited in form of a relatively thick solid layer, but it can be formed in various shapes. HA thin films for applications in the biomedical field were grown by pulsed laser deposition and radio-frequency magnetron sputtering techniques [378–383]. Nelea et al. [378] coated HA thin film on Ti–5Al–2.5Fe alloys substrates with controlled thickness from 1 μm to 350 nm. To achieve excellent biocompatibility of metal-based implants, an HA thin film was coated on nanotube-formed Ti–35Nb–10Zr alloys after femtosecond laser texturing [383]. The thus treated surface was found to be a composite with TiO_2, Nb_2O_5, and ZrO_2. It was furthermore reported that (i) the HA-coated surface on the nanotubes showed the lowest contact angle compared with the other surfaces, and (ii) from FE-SEM observations, cell attachment and spreading of MG 63cells showed significantly higher tendency for surfaces covered by HA coating and nanotubes [383]. Not only thickness but the size is also controlled for coating HA material [384–386]. Lee et al. [384] coated a nano-sized HA layer on a Ti substrate with a titanium oxide (TiO_2) buffer layer by the electron-beam deposition method and concluded that the nano-sized HA coating with the TiO_2buffer layer holds great promise as a bioactive coating system [384]. A highly crystalline nano HA was coated CpTi using inductively coupled radio frequency plasma spray [386]. It was characterized that (i), depending on the plasma processing conditions, a coating thickness between 300 and 400 μm was achieved where the adhesive bond strengths were found to be between 4.8 and 24 MPa, (ii) the coating was made of multi-grain HA particles of ~200 nm in size, which consisted of recrystallized HA grains in the size range of 15–20 nm [386].

In most cases, HA has been prepared as synthetic material, but Duta et al. [387] prepared HA as the synthesis of novel ovine and bovine derived HA thin films and coated it on titanium substrates by pulsed laser deposition. It was reported that (i) the micrographs of the films showed a uniform distribution of spheroidal particulates with a mean diameter of ~2 μm, (ii) pull-off measurements demonstrated excellent bonding strength values between the HA films and the titanium substrates, and (iii) because of their physiochemical properties and low-cost fabrication from renewable resources, these new coating materials could be considered as a prospective competitor to synthetic HA used for implantology applications [387]. Based on this variation possibility, there are several ion substitutions inside the HA structure (which is a hexagonal closed-packed crystalline structure). Among proposed variations, fluoridated HA seems to be major one [388–390]. Mohammadi Zahrani et al. [388] prepared nanocrystalline fluoridated HA powders with a chemical composition of $Ca_{10}(PO_4)_6OH_{2-x}F_x$ (where x values were selected equal to 0.0 ,0.5, 1.0, 1.5, and 2.0) through a modified simple sol–gel technique. Similarly, the sol–gel technique was applied to produce fluoridated HA [389,390]. Carbon can be incorporated in the HA structure to show bi-function of excellent mechanical property of carbon in form of nanotube [391] or carbonate [392,393] with biocompatible HA. Li et al. [394] coated Na-doped HA (which was Ca-deficient) directly prepared onto carbon/carbon composites using electrochemical deposition. It was reported that (i) the Na/P molar ratios of the coating formed on carbon/carbon substrate was 0.097, (ii) the mean thickness of the coating was approximately 10 ± 2 μm, (iii) the average shear bonding strength of Na-HA coating on carbon/carbon was 5.55 ± 0.77 MPa and (vi), after soaking the samples in a SBF for 14 days, the Na-HA coated carbon/carbon composites can rapidly induce bone-like apatite nucleation and growth on its surface in SBF, suggesting that the Na-HA coating might be an effective method to improve the surface bioactivity and biocompatibility of carbon/carbon composites [394]. Silicon-substituted HA was prepared and was coated on the Ti substrate via a magnetron co-sputtering technique and coated surfaces were subjected to an *in vitro* study using primary human osteoblast cells to evaluate their biological property [395]. It was reported that (i) although human osteoblast cells showed initial poor adhesion and spreading on the hydrophobic Ti surface, Si-incorporated HA coatings on Ti substrates renders the surface more hydrophilic, with water contact angles between 30 and 40°, (ii) human osteoblast cells attached, spread, and proliferated well on these coatings, (iii) enhanced calcification (formation of calcium phosphate nodules across the collagenous matrices) was observed on Si-HA coatings with increasing Si content, suggesting that Si-incorporation into the HA structure enhances the surface wettability and promotes cell proliferation and calcification [395]. Guo et al. [396] investigated the physicochemical properties and biocompatibilities of La-containing apatites with the formula $La_2Ca_8(PO_4)_6O_2$ as typical one. It was reported that the sintered La-incorporated apatite block achieves a maximal flexure strength of 66.69 ± 0.98 MPa at 5% La content with 320% increase when compared with the La-free apatite, suggesting that the La-incorporated apatite possesses application potential in developing a new type of bioactive coating material for metal implants and also as a promising La carrier for further exploring the beneficial functions of La in the human body [396]. Sr (strontium)-substituted HA was prepared with 10mol% Ca^{2+} replaced by Sr^{2+} and the implant fixation in ovariectomized rats was investigated after Sr-HA was coated on Ti implant by the sol–gel dip methods [397]. It was reported that (i) Sr-HA coated implants revealed improved osseointegration compared to HA, with the bone area ratio and BIC increased by 70.9% and 49.9% in histomorphometry, (ii) the bone volume ratio and percent osseointegration by 73.7% and 45.2% in micro-CT evaluation, and (iii) the maximal push-out force and ultimate shear strength by 107.2% and 132.9% in push out test, suggesting that the feasibility of using Sr-HA coatings to improve implant fixation in osteoporotic bone [397]. Similarly, Sr-HA was coated on Mg-Sr (with Sr in the range of 0.3–2.5%) [398].

HA-based composites are also prepared. Ji et al. [406] prepared hydroxyapatite-carbon nanotube/titania double layer and coated it on titanium substrates intended for biomedical applications, reporting that the composite HA coating promoted the adhesion of preosteoblasts and the unique surfaces combined with the osteoconductive properties of HA exhibited the excellent mechanical properties [406]. A double coating layer of the first thin pre-coating made with polyalkoxysilanes was prepared to promote the adhesion of HA/polyalkoxysilanes composite second layer [400]. Furthermore, HA was admixed with TCP with a Ca/P molar ratio from 1.56 to 1.77 [401], with TiO_2 with bonding strength between HA coating and substrate of 27.2 ± 1.6 MPa [402] and ZrO_2 [403].

Biocompatible calcium-phosphate (Ca-P) has been widely employed as coating materials for improving the substrate's biocompatibility. Ca-P was coated on CpTi substrates [404–410], and various Ti-based alloys including Ti–6Al–4V [411–413], Ti–7.5Mo alloy [77], and Ti–3Zr–2Sn–3Mo–25Nb [414]. Uniquely, Wang et al. [415] prepared functionally graded bioceramic coating composed of essentially calcium phosphate compounds. It was expected that the coating was graded in accordance to adhesive strength, bioactivity, and bioresorbability; that is, the bond coat on the Ti–6Al–4V substrate is deposited with a particle range of the HA that provides a high adhesive strength and bioactivity but have poor bioresorption properties, while the top coat is composed of predominantly α-TCP that is highly bioresorbable [415]. Chen et al. [416] employed electrochemically deposited dicalcium phosphate dihydrate coating of a porous substrate on the CpTi implant surface and reported that Ca_2P coatings improve the extent of cancellous bone ingrowth in the early post-operative phase following uncemented arthroplasty [416].

The titanium substrate has been also coated with another type of Ca-containing species. Load-bearing Ti implants were coated with TCP [417,418]. Ti was also coated with composite of Ag-HA composite [419] or TCP doped by Mg element in form of $Ca_{2.8}Mn_{0.2}(PO_4)_2$ [420]. The Ti–6Al–4V alloy was coated with bioactive calcium alkali phosphate [413], Ca_2SiO_4 [421], $CaTiSiO_5$ (sphene) [422], TiO_2 + CaP compound [423], corrosion-resistant zeolite (aluminosilicate) for eliminating the release of cytotoxic Al and V ions [424], or ceramics treated in K_4ZrF_6–H_3PO_4 and $NaAlO_2$–Na_3PO_4solutions [425].

Bioglass should be included in this group as biocompatible coating material. CpTi as well as Ti-based alloys were coated with bioglass; two phase ($\alpha + \beta$) Ti–6Al–7Nb titanium alloy was coated with a composite PEEK + Bioglass [426], and Ti–6Al–4V was coated with bioactive borate glass comprised of Na_2O-CaO-B_2O_3 system, modified by additions of SiO_2, Al_2O_3, and P_2O_5 with adhesive strengths of 36 ± 2 MPa [427], or alkali-free bioglass thin films with the highest mean value of pull-out adherence (60.3 ± 4.6 MPa) [428].

5.4.5. Composites, Hybrids, Functional Gradient Materials, and Biomimetic Materials

There are a huge number of papers published on HA-based biocompatible composites. HA–TiO_2 composites [167,234,257,429–433] and HA–ZrO_2 composites [434,435] are prepared. Moreover, HA–glass composites [436,437], HA-carbon composites [438,439], and HA–Wollastonite ($CaSiO_3$) composites [440–442] are produced. In order to enhance the hard tissue biocompatibility and an excellent osteoconductivity, HA was admixed with chitosan [443–445]. In order to improve bioactivity, the initial cell proliferation, and finally the osseointegration, HA has been also incorporated with collagen [446–448]. For promoting implant osseointegration or bone tissue engineering, biomimetic coating materials were introduced: for example, HA-amelogenin composite [449] and HA-fibronection [450].

Titania (TiO_2) has been admixed/incorporated with Zn element [451], Ag element [452], carbon [453], $CaTiSiO_5$ (sphene) [454], SiO_2 [455], and $CaSiO_3$ [456]. Similarly, zirconia (ZrO_2) is mixed with Ca-P [457] or with poly-pyrrole [458], for improving corrosion resistance and biocompatibility. As nitride composites, there are reports on AlN–SiO_2 [459] and TiN–carbon composites [460].

Other metallic oxide composites are also prepared. Gurappa [461] deposited a mixture of alumina, magnesia-stabilized zirconia and yttria-stabilized zirconia with different thicknesses on a 316L stainless steel substrate by the air plasma spray technique to improve corrosion resistance [461]. Dense and ultrafine alumina–zirconia composites (Al_2O_3–16wt%ZrO_2 and ZrO_2–20wt%Al_2O_3) were prepared to enhance the bioactivity [462]. Nelson et al. [463] deposited a mixture of powders of titanium alloy (Ti–6Al–4V) and bioactive glass by flame spraying to fabricate composite porous coatings for potential use in bone fixation implants. After immersing samples in SBF, it was reported that HA was found on the bioactive glass–alloy composite coatings after 7 days of immersion, while no HA was observed after 14 days on the pure titanium alloy control coating [463]. Balasubramanian et al. [215] prepared nanocomposite Ti–Si–N coatings by reactive DC magnetron sputtering in a mixture of Ar and N_2gases and deposited the composite on implantable 316L stainless steel substrates. It was reported that the Ta–Si–N nanocomposite coatings exhibited superior corrosion resistance compared with the Si_3N_4, TiN single layer, and the bare substrate in the SBF solution [215].

With an attempt at achieving faster osseointegration to hasten the overall treatment process, the use of biomimetic agents represents a growing area of research in implant dentistry. Major biomimetic agents should include (i) biocompatible ceramics, (ii) bioactive agents, (iii) ions, and (iv) polymers, and their respective importance in the early stages of osseointegration. The potential bioactive agents include bone morphogenetic proteins, growth factors, type I collagen, RGD peptide, fluoride, or chitosan, among others. The ideal characteristics that biomimetic agents should uphold and factors that may influence their effectiveness are reviewed [464]. It was pointed out that (i) some of these agents, such as bioceramics (calcium phosphate salts) or ions (fluoride), are already commercially available and have shown clinical success, (ii) others such as bone morphogenetic proteins are very promising, with an excellent therapeutic potential, and (iii) a specific implant surface coating may enhance the percentage of BIC as well as speed of osseointegration that allows clinicians to overcome many challenging clinical scenarios [464]. In implantolgy, in particular dental implants, the increased demand on implant performance and the broadened treatment indications have led to the development of new moderately rough surfaces and alterations in both the surface chemistry and topography for chemical influences on bone tissue (or bioactivity) [465–469]. Furthermore, surface alterations should include manipulations for surface energy, surface wettability, cellular maturation state, nutrition status, and microstresses alter the degree of bioactivity [466,467]. It was reported that implant roughness promotes bacterial colonization [470]. In order to enhance bone formation, implants have been coated with bone-specific biomolecules [2,471–473].

Based on the aforementioned background, there have been many ideas as well as coating materials proposed toward the promising biomimetic materials for surface engineering for biomaterials. For the particular case of artificial bone grafts, synthetic materials which are to be used in biological environments must display an adequacy of both their surface and bulk characteristics in order to fulfill the dual requirements of biocompatibility and suitable mechanical properties for the given application [474,475]. Otherwise, due to a poor biocompatibility of improper compounds, fibrous tissues always encapsulate the implants made from such materials, which prolong the healing time [474]. Since in surgical discipline in both dental and medical fields, where bones have to be repaired, augmented or improved, an interest has dramatically increased in application of synthetic bone grafts with excellent mechanical stability [474].

The surface microtopography of implant influences distinctly the rate of bone-formation and the ratio of bone–implant contact. However, it is indicated that the surface of titanium implant existed contamination after different surface treatments. Chitosan is one of the most abundant natural polymers for its adsorption property for metal ions. He et al. [476] reported on the pretreatment of the metal surface and comparison of the efficacy of three treatments for the binding ability of collagen and chitosan. The compound of collagen and chitosan was immobilized on the titanium oxide and the morphology and chemical composition were used to characterize the titanium surfaces by SEM, and X-ray photoelectron spectrometry. The results showed that the surface displayed irregularities after roughness treatments and the rough surface was beneficial to the adsorption and attachment of collagen and chitosan [476]. Collagen is a highly versatile material, extensively used in the medical, dental, and pharmacological fields. Resorbable forms of collagen have been used to dress oral wounds, for closure of graft and extraction sites, and to promote healing. Collagen-based membranes have also been used in periodontal and implant therapy as barriers to prevent epithelial migration and allow cells with regenerative capacity to repopulate the defect area [477]. In particular, collagen type-I is a major component of the extracellular matrix of most tissues and it is increasingly utilized for surface engineering of biomaterials to accelerate receptor-mediated cell adhesion [478]. Collagen was coated on Ti-based [479,480], Co-based biomaterials [478], or stainless steel [481], suggesting that collagen coating can enhance the rate of bone healing and increase new bone formation at the implant surface. Collagen was even coated on poly(DL-lactide-co-glycolide) fiber [482] and TiO_x surface oxide layer [483].

Fibronectin functions in cell adhesion, migration, survival, proliferation, and differentiation as well as tissue organization and interacts with other biomolecules, such as collagen, proteoglycan, heparin, hyaluronic acid, fibrin/fibrinogen, plasmin, gangliosides, complement components, and also integral proteins of cell plasma membrane-integrins, as well as with itself [484,485]. Fibronection was coated on the Ti surface [485–487] and the porous TiO_2/perlite composite [488,489], reporting that fibronection coating improved cellular spreading and enhance the tissue ingrowth.

Immobilization of bone morphogenetic proteins as growth factor onto material surfaces is a promising since these proteins can accelerate or enhance, or both, the quality of osseointegration [490,491]. Protein was coated on the Ti substrate [218,492,493] and on Ti–6Al–4V [492]. Fe-Pd-based ferromagnetic shape memory actuators for medical applications were also coated with protein [494].Covalently bound recombinant human tropoelastin as a major regulator of vascular cells *in vivo was prepared to enhance* endothelial cell interactions, suggesting that such coating for metal alloys with multifaceted biocompatibility can resist delamination and is nonthrombogenic, with implications for improving coronary stent efficacy [495].

The prevention of bacterial colonization and formation of a bacterial biofilm on implant surfaces has been a challenge in orthopedic surgery [496]. The antimicrobial peptide was coated on Ti biomaterials [497–500], suggesting that the integration of soft tissue on titanium dental implants was improved by significantly protecting implants from peri-implant inflammation and enhancement long-term implant stabilization. Similarly, for the prevention of the peri-implant infection in orthopedics, the Ca-P coated titanium surface was coated with the peptide [501]. To prevent the unwanted infection on and around titanium implants, antibacterial coatings were performed on titanium implants [502,503]. Reyes et al. [504] coated titanium implant surface with glycine-phenylalanine-hydroxyproline-glycine-glutamate-arginine collagen-mimetic peptideto improve osseointegration and reported that a biologically active and clinically relevant implant-coating that enhances bone repair and orthopedic implant integration was developed [504]. Chitosan is the deacetylated derivative of the natural polysaccharide, chitin. Chitosan has been shown to be biocompatible, biodegradable, osteoconductive, and to accelerate wound healing [505,506]. Ti was coated with chitosan to promote osteointegration [507].

Frosch et al. [508] coated titanium implant surfaces with stem cell to evaluate the partial surface replacement of the knee and to provide a basis for a successful treatment of large osteochondral defects, indicating that a partial joint resurfacing of the knee with stem cell-coated titanium implants occur. Similarly, a stem cell was coated to functionalized titanium films, reporting that stem-cell coated titanium films are beneficial for sustained *in situ* inducing osteoprogenitor cells to differentiate into mature osteoblasts over long time [509]. Achneck et al. [510] evaluated the viability and adherence of peripheral blood-derived porcine endothelial progenitor cells on thin Ti layers and reported that (i) peripheral blood-derived cells adhere and function normally on Ti surfaces, and (ii) the cells may be used to seed cardiovascular devices prior to implantation to ameliorate platelet activation and thrombus formation [510]. Moreover, electrochemically functionalized Ti-alloy surfaces were coated with a cell specificaptamer in order to enhance the cell adhesion and by aptamer-based capture molecules on cell adhesion [511].

5.4.6. Others

Siegel et al. [512] modified surface properties of polymer foils (PEEK and PTFE) by flash evaporation of carbon layers and it was found that maximal stimulation of the adhesion and proliferation of vascular smooth muscle cells on carbon-coated polymers depends on the surface roughness and contact angle of cell carriers used [512]. Carbon nanotubes are molecular-scale tubes of graphitic carbon possessing excellent mechanical properties such as modulus of elasticity as high as 1TPa and tensile strengths of up to 63 GPa [513], suggesting that such material can be used as reinforcing and improving brittle materials. Gopi et al. [514] coated titanium substrates with carbon nanotube-reinforced HA. Moreover, a carbon nanofiber film was coated onto bulk pure titanium via hybrid surface mechanical attrition treatment [515].

Diamond-like carbon (DLC) thin films may provide next generation medical device surfaces with unique hardness, tribological resistance (against friction and wear), corrosion, and cell interaction properties [516–518]. The Ti–6Al–4V alloy [519–521] and Ti–6Al–7Nb [521] were coated with DLC. Similarly, Batory et al. [522] coated surgical 316L stainless steel with silver (Ag) doped DLC using radio frequency plasma assisted CVD/magnetron sputtering technique, reporting a good adhesion, beneficial topography, and high applicability for medical applications [522]. Koistinen et al. [523] examined possibility of reducing the torque and failures of bone screws by coating high-quality amorphous diamond on stainless steel screws, reporting that amorphous DLC coating provides a stable, smooth surface and reduces the risk of screw failures [523]. It was reported that Ti material incorporated with amorphous carbon nitride films by direct current magnetron sputtering enhanced biocompatibility of Ti alloy [524].

Since postoperative infection associated with implants remains a serious complication in orthopedic surgery, several biomaterial surface treatments have been proposed as a means of reducing the incidence of implant-associated infections. A clinical trial tests were conducted using an iodine-supported titanium that suppresses the microbial activities. It was reported that (i) the iodine-supported titanium implants can be very effective for preventing and treating infections after orthopedic surgery, and (ii) cytotoxicity and adverse effects were not detected [525,526].

Although pure iron is evaluated to be a potential material applying for coronary artery stents based on its biocorrodible and nontoxic properties, Zhu et al. [527] doped pure iron with lanthanum ions by metal vapor vacuum arc source to improve its corrosion resistance and biocompatibility. It was reported that (i) the systematic evaluation of blood compatibility (including *in vitro* platelets adhesion, prothrombin time, and thrombin time) indicated that the number of platelets adhesion, activation, aggregation, and pseudopodium on the surface of the La-implanted samples were remarkably decreased compared with pure iron and 316L stainless steel, and (ii) lanthanum ion implantation could effectively improve the corrosion resistance and blood compatibility of pure iron [527].

Polypyrrole (with basic properties of hydrophilicity and surface roughness) is an inherently conducting polymer that has shown great promise for biomedical applications within the nervous system [528]. In order to improve the biocompatibility, the functionalized polypyrrole-coated 316L stainless steel surfaces were examined to covalent attachment to proteins [529].

Taxt-Lamolle et al.[530] treated titaniumimplant surface with HF acid to make Ti surface doped with fluorine ions and it was reported that the surface modification of titanium implants with low concentrations of HF using cathodic reduction improved osseointegration properties. The Ti–6Al–4V surface was incorporated strontium (Sr) ions by hydrothermal treatment using a Sr-containing solution, and it was reported that the Sr-containing oxide layer produced by hydrothermal treatment may be effective in improving the osseointegration of Ti–6Al–4V alloy implants by enhancing differentiation of osteoblastic cells, removal torque forces and bone apposition in both cortical and cancellous bones [531].

The GnG composite was investigated for surface modification of titanium in addition to insure biocompatibility on dental implants or biomaterials [114], with characteristics that this composite was constructed by gelatin and hydrogen tetrachloroaurate in the presence of reducing agent, sodium borohydrate ($NabH_4$). It was shown that (i) titanium surface coated with the GnG composite exhibited a good biocompatibility for osteoblast growth and attachment, (ii) it offers good communication between cell and implant surfaces by regulating cell signaling and adherent molecules, which are useful to enhance the biocompatibility of titanium surfaces [114].

References

1. Coelho, P.G., Granjeiro, J.M., Romanos, G.E., Suzuki, M., Silva, N.R, Cardaropoli, G., Thompon, V.P. and Lemons, J.E., 2009, Basic research methods and current trends of dental implant surfaces, *J Biomed Mater Res B Appl Biomater* 88:579–596. doi: http://dx.doi.org/10.1002/jbm.b.31264
2. Jimbo, T., Sawase, T., Shibata, Y., Hirata, K., Hishikawa, Y., Tanaka, Y., Bessho, K., Ikeda, T. and Atsuta, M., 2007, Enhanced osseointegration by the chemotactic activity of plasma fibronectin for cellular fibronectin positive cells, *Biomaterials* 28:3469–3477. doi: http://dx.doi.org/10.1016/j.biomaterials.2007.04.029
3. Coelho, P.G., Giro, G., Teixeira, H.S., Marin, C., Witek, L., Thompson, V.P., Tovar, N. and Silva, N.R., 2012, Argon-based atmospheric pressure plasma enhances early bone response to rough titanium surfaces, *J Biomed Mater Res A* 100:1901–1906. doi: http://dx.doi.org/10.1002/jbm.a.34127
4. von Wilmowsky, C., Moest, T., Nkenke, E., Stelzle, F., and Schlegel, K.A., 2013, Implants in bone: Part I. A current overview about tissue response, surface modifications and future perspectives, *Oral Maxillofac Surg.* doi: http://dx.doi.org/10.1007/s10006-013-398-1

5. Wennerberg, A. and Albrektsson, T., 2010, On implant surfaces: A review of current knowledge and opinions, *Int J Oral Maxillofac Implants* 25:63–74.
6. Albrektsson, T., Buser, D. and Sennerby, L., 2012, On crestal/marginal bone loss around dental implants, *Int J Oral Maxillofa Implants* 27:73–738.
7. Albrektsson, T., Buser, D. and Sennerby, L., 2012, On crestal/marginal bone loss around dental implants, *Int J Prosthodon* 25:320–322.
8. Göransson, A., Arvidsson, A., Currie, F., Franke-Stenport, V., Kjellin, P., Mustafa, K., Sul, Y.T. and Wnnerberg, A., 2009, An in vitro comparison of possibly bioactive titanium implant surface, *J Biomed Mater Res A* 88:1037–1047. doi: http://dx.doi.org/10.1002/jbm.a.31911
9. Kang, B.S., Sul, Y.T., Oh, S.J., Lee, H.J. and Albrektsson, T., 2009, XPS, AES, and SEM analysis of recent dental implants, *Acta Biomat* 5:2222–2229. doi: http://dx.doi.org/10.1016/j.actbio.2009.01.049
10. Jimbo, R., Sotres, J., Johansson, C., Breding, K., Currie, F. and Wennerberg, A., 2012, The biological response to three different nanostructures applied on smooth implant surfaces, *Clin Oral Implants Res* 23:706–712. doi: http://dx.doi.org/10.1111/j.1600-0501.2011.02182.x
11. Karlsson, J., Jimbo, R., Fathali, H.M., Schwartz-Filho, H.O., Hayashi, M., Halvarsson, M., Wennerberg, A. and Andersson, M., 2012, In vivo biomechanical stability of osseo-integrating mesoporous TiO_2 implants, *Acta Biomat* 8:4438–4446. doi: http://dx.doi.org/10.1016/j.actbio.2012.07.035
12. Foest, R., Kindel, E., Ohl, A., Stieber, M. and Weltmann, K.D., 2005, Non-thermal atmospheric pressure discharges for surface modification, *Plasma Phys Control Fusion* 47:B52–B536. doi: http://dx.doi.org/10.1088/0741-3335/47/12B/S38
13. Singh, R. and Dahotre, N.B., 2007, Corrosion degradation and prevention by surface modification of biometallic materials, *J Mater Sci Mater Med* 18:725–751. doi: http://dx.doi.org/10.1007/s10856-006-0016-y
14. Shi, J.Z., Chen, C.Z., Zhang, S. and Wu, Y., 2007, Application of surface modification in biomedical materials research, *Surf Rev Lett* 14:361–369. doi: http://dx.doi.org/10.1142/S0218625X07009669
15. Yeo, I-S., Han, J-S. and Yang, J-H., 2008, Biomechanical and histomorphometric study of dental implants with different surface characteristics, *J Biomed Mater Res Part B Appl Biomater* 87:303–311. doi: http://dx.doi.org/10.1002/jbm.b.31104
16. Carlsson, L.V., Alberktsson, T. and Berman, C., 1989, Bone response to plasma-cleaned titanium implants, *Int J Oral Maxillofac Implants* 4:199–204.
17. Buser, D., Broggini, N., Wieland, M., Schenk, R.K., Denzer, A.J., Cochran, D.L., Hoffman, B., Lussi, A. and Steinemann, S.G., 2004, Enhanced bone apposition to a chemically modified SLA titanium surface, *J Dent Res* 83:529–533. doi: http://dx.doi.org/10.1177/154405910408300704
18. Santos, O., Svendsen, I.E., Lindh, L. and Arnebrant, T., 2011, Adsorption of HSA, IgG and laminin-1 on model titania surfaces—effects of glow discharge treatment on competitively adsorbed film composition, *Biofouling* 27:1003–1015. doi: http://dx.doi.org/10.1080/08927014.2011.622440
19. Jimbo, R., Ivarsson, M., Koskela, A., Sul, Y.T. and Johansson, C.B., 2010, Protein adsorption to surface chemistry and crystal structure modification of titanium surfaces, *J Oral Maxillofac Res* l:e3p1–e3p9.
20. Guastaldi, F.P.S., Yoo, D., Marin, C., Jimbo, R., Tovar, N., Zanetta-Barbosa, D. and Coelho, P.G., 2013, Plasma treatment maintains surface energy of the implant surface and enhances osseointegration, *Int J Biomat* 2013: Article ID 354125. doi: http://dx.doi.org/10.1155/2013/354125

21. Manero, J. M., Salsench, J., Nogueras, J., Aparicio, C., Padrós, A., Balcells, M., Gil, F.J. and Planell, J.A, Growth of bioactive surfaces on dental implants, *Implant Dent* 11:170–175.
22. Le Guéhennec, L., Soueidan, A., Layrolle, P. and Amouriq, Y. 2007, Surface treatments of titanium dental implants for rapid osseointegration, *Dent Mater* 23:844–854. doi: http://dx.doi.org/10.1016/j.dental.2006.06.025
23. Munisamy, S., Vaidyanathan, T.K. and Vaidyanathan, J., 2008, A bone-like precoating strategy for implants: Collagen immobilization and its mineralization on pure titanium implant surface, *J Oral Implant* 34:67–75. doi: http://dx.doi.org/10.1563/1548-1336(2008)34[67:ABPSFI]2.0.CO;2
24. Wang, F., Shi, L., He, W-X., Han, D., Yan, Y., Niu, Z-Y. and Shi, S-G., 2013, Bioinspired micro/nano fabrication on dental implant–bone interface, *Appl Surf Sci* 265:480–488. doi: http://dx.doi.org/10.1016/j.apsusc.2012.11.032
25. Kasemo, B. and Gold, J., 1999, Implant surfaces and interface processes, *Adv Dent Res* 13:8–20. doi: http://dx.doi.org/10.1177/08959374990130011901
26. Wang, J., Tang, J., Zhang, P., Li, Y., Wang, J., Lai, Y. and Qin, L., 2012, Surface modification of magnesium alloys developed for bioabsorbable orthopedic implants: A general review, *J Biomed Mater Res Part B Appl Biomater* 100:1691–1701. doi: http://dx.doi.org/10.1002/jbm.b.32707
27. Oshida, Y., 2007, *Bioscience and Bioengineering of Titanium Materials*, 1st ed. Elsevier, London, UK.
28. Oshida, Y., 2013, *Bioscience and Bioengineering of Titanium Materials*, 2nd ed. Elsevier London, UK.
29. Tucker, R.C., 2002, Surface engineering, *JOM* 160:1–3.
30. Allen, P., 1996, Titanium alloy development, *Adv Mater Process* 154:35–37.
31. Oshida, Y., Hashem, A., Nishihara, T. and Yapchulay, M.V., 1994, Fractal dimension analysis of mandibular bones—Toward a morphological compatibility of implants, *J Bio-Med Mater Eng* 4:397–407.
32. Oshida, Y., 2007, *Bioscience and Bioengineering of TitaniumMaterials*, Elsevier, London, UK, pp. 314–315.
33. Wen, X., Wang, X. and Zhang, N., 1996, Microrough surface of metallic biomaterials: A literature review. *Biomed Mater Eng* 6:173–189.
34. Piattelli, A., Scarano, A., Corigliano, M. and Piattelli, M., 1996, Presence of multinucleated giant cells around machined, sandblasted and plasma-sprayed titanium implants: A histological and histochemical time-course study in rabbit. *Biomaterials* 17:2053–2058. doi: http://dx.doi.org/10.1016/0142-9612(96)00052-X
35. Citeau, A., Guicheux, J., Vinatier, C., Layrolle, P., Nguyen, T.P., Pilet, P. and Daculsi, G., 2005, In vitro biological effects of titanium rough surface obtained by calcium phosphate grid blasting, *Biomaterials* 26:157–165. doi: http://dx.doi.org/10.1016/j.biomaterials.2004.02.033
36. Miyakawa, O., Watababe, K., Okawa, S., Shiokawa, N., Kobayashi, M. and Tamura, H., 1990, Grinding of titanium, Part 1: Commercial and experimental wheels made of silicon carbide abrasives, *Dent Mater J* 9:30–41.
37. Miyakawa, O., Watanabe, K., Okawa, S., Nakano, S., Shiokawa, N., Kobayashi, M. and Tamura, H., 1990, Grinding of titanium, Part 2: Commercial vitrified wheels made of alumina abrasives, *Dent Mater J* 9:42–52.
38. Miyakawa, O., Watanabe, K., Okawa, S., Kanatani, M., Nakano, S. and Kobayashi, M., 1996, Surface contamination of titanium by abrading treatment, *Dent Mater J* 15:11–21. doi: http://dx.doi.org/10.4012/dmj.15.11
39. Balza, J.C., Zujur, D., Gil, L., Subero, R., Dominguez, E., Delvasto, P. and Alvarez, J., 2013, Sandblasting as a surface modification technique on titanium alloys for biomedical

applications: abrasive particle behavior, *IOP Conf Ser: Mat Sci Eng* 45. doi: http://dx.doi.org/10.1088/1757-899X/45/1/012004
40. Mandelbrot, B.B., 1983, *The Fractal Geometry of Nature,* Freeman, New York, NY, p. 34.
41. Chesters, S., Wen, H.Y., Lundin, M. and Kasper, G., 1989, Fractal-based characterization of surface texture, *Appl Surf Sci* 40:185–192. doi: http://dx.doi.org/10.1016/0169-4332(89)90001-9
42. Sayles, R.S. and Thomas, T.R., 1978, Surface topography as a non-stationary random process, *Nature* 271:431–434. doi: http://dx.doi.org/10.1038/271431a0
43. Oshida, Y., Munoz, C.A., Winkler, M.M., Hashem, A. and Ito, M., 1993, Fractal dimension analysis of aluminum oxide particle for sandblasting dental use, *J Biomed Mater Eng* 3:117–126.
44. Miyakawa, O., Okawa, S., Kobayashi, M. and Uematsu, K., 1998, Surface contamination of titanium by abrading treatment, *Dent Mater J* 34:90–96.
45. Oshida, Y. unpublished data, 2013.
46. Mustafa, K., Lopez, B.S., Hultenby, K. and Arvison, K., 1997, Attachment of HGF of titanium surfaces blasted with TiO_2 particles, *J Dent Res* 76:85.
47. Wennerberg, A., Albrektsson, T., Johnsson, C. and Andersson, B., 1996, Experimental study of turned and grit-blasted screw-shaped implants with special emphasis on effects of blasting material and surface topography, *Biomaterials* 17:15–22. doi: http://dx.doi.org/10.1016/0142-9612(96)80750-2
48. Johansson, C.B., Albrektsson, T., Thomsen, P., Snnerby, I., Lodding, A. and Odelius, H., 1992, Tissue reactions to titanium-6aluminum-4vanadium alloy, *Eur J Exp Musculoskel Res* 1:161–169.
49. Wang, C-S., 2004, *Surface Modification of Titanium for Enhancing Titabium-Pocelain Bond Strength.* Indiana University Master Degree Thesis.
50. Peutzfeld, A. and Asmussen, E., 1996, Distortion of alloy by sandblasting, *Am J Dent* 9:65–66.
51. Peutzfeld, A. and Asmussen, E., 1996, Distortion of alloys caused by sandblasting, *J Dent Res* 75:259.
52. Oshida, Y. and Daly, J., 1990, Fatigue damage evaluation of shot peened high strength aluminum alloy. In: S.A.Meguid ed., *Surface Engineering,* Elsevier Applied, New York, NY, pp. 404–416. doi: http://dx.doi.org/10.1007/978-94-009-0773-7_42
53. Metal Improvement Company, Inc. 1990, *Shot Peening Applications*, 7th ed.
54. Oshida Y. unpublished report, 2012.
55. Guo, C.Y., Matinlinna, J.P. and Tang, A.T.H., 2012, A novel effect of sandblasting on titanium surface: Static charge generation, *J Adhes Sci Tech* 26:2603–2613. doi: http://dx.doi.org/10.1080/01694243.2012.691007
56. DeWald, A.T., Rankin, J.E., Hill, M.R., Lee, M.J. and Chen, H-L., 2004, Assessment of tensile residual stress mitigation in Alloy 22 welds due to laser peening, *J Eng Mater Tech, Trans ASME* 126:81–89.
57. Fairland, B.P., Wilcox, B.A., Gallagher, W.J. and Williams, D.N., 1972, Laser shock-induced microstructural and mechanical property changes in 7075 aluminum, *J Appl Phys* 43:3893–3895. doi: http://dx.doi.org/10.1063/1.1661837
58. Fairland, B.P. and Clauer, A.H., 1979, Laser generation of high amplitude stress waves in materials, *J Appl Phys* 50:1497–1502. doi: http://dx.doi.org/10.1063/1.326137
59. Dane, C.B., Hackel, L.A., Daly, J. and Harrison, J., 2000, High power laser for peening of metals enabling production technology, *Mater Manuf Process* 15:81–96. doi: http://dx.doi.org/10.1080/10426910008912974
60. Cho, S-A. and Jung, S-K., 2003, A removal torque of the laser-treated titanium implants in rabbit tibia, *Biomaterials* 24:4859–4863. doi: http://dx.doi.org/10.1016/S0142-9612(03)00218-7

61. Gaggl, A., Schultes, G., Muller, W.D. and Karcher, H., 2000, Scanning electron microscopical analysis of laser-treated titanium implants surfaces—a comparative study, *Biomaterials* 21:1067–1073. doi: http://dx.doi.org/10.1016/S0142-9612(00)00002-8
62. Jindal, S., Bansal, R., Singh, B.P., Pandey, R., Shankar Narayanan, T.S.N., Wani, M. and Singh, V., 2012, Enhanced osteoblast proliferation and corrosion resistance of c p-Ti through surface nanostructuring by ultrasonic shot peening and stress relieving, *J Oral Implant* doi: http://dx.doi.org/10.1563/AAID-JOI-D-12-00006.1
63. Harcuba, P., Bačáková, L., Stráský, J., Bačáková, M., Novotná, K. and Janeček, M., 2012, Surface treatment by electric discharge machining of Ti–6Al–4V alloy for potential application in orthopaedics, *J Mech Behav Biomed Mater* 7:96–105. doi: http://dx.doi.org/10.1016/j.jmbbm.2011.07.001
64. Otsuka, F., Kataoka, Y. and Miyazaki, T., 2012, Enhanced osteoblast response to electrical discharge machining surface, *Dent Mater J* 31:309–315. doi: http://dx.doi.org/10.4012/dmj.2011-039
65. Valiev, R.Z. and Langdon, T.G., 2011, Achieving exceptional grain refinement through severe plastic deformation: New approaches for improving the processing technology, *Metall Mater Trans A* 42:2942–2951. doi: http://dx.doi.org/10.1007/s11661-010-0556-0
66. Byeli, A.V., Kukareko, V.A. and Kononov, A.G., 2012, Titanium and zirconium based alloys modified by intensive plastic deformation and nitrogen ion implantation for biocompatibleimplants, *J Mech Behav Biomed Mater* 6:89–94. doi: http://dx.doi.org/10.1016/j.jmbbm.2011.05.034
67. Hansson, S. and Hansson, K.N., 2005, The effect of limited lateral resolution in the measurement of implant surface roughness: A computer simulation, *J Biomed Mater Res A* 75:472–477. doi: http://dx.doi.org/10.1002/jbm.a.30455
68. Elias, C.N., Oshida, Y., Lima, J.H.C. and Muller, C.A., 2008, Relationship between surface properties (roughness, wettability and morphology) of titanium and dental implant removal torque, *J Mech Behav Biomed Mater* 1:234–242. doi: http://dx.doi.org/10.1016/j.jmbbm.2007.12.002
69. Ajami, E. and Aguey-Zinsou, K-F., 2011, Formation of OTS self-assembled monolayers at chemically treated titanium surfaces, *J Mater Sci Mater Med* 22:1813–1824. doi: http://dx.doi.org/10.1007/s10856-011-4356-x
70. Variola, F., Yi, J-H., Richert, L., Wuest, J.D., Rosei, F. and Nanci, A., 2008, Tailoring the surface properties of Ti6Al4V by controlled chemical oxidation, *Biomaterials* 29:1285–1298. doi: http://dx.doi.org/10.1016/j.biomaterials.2007.11.040
71. Pisarek, M., Roguska, A., Andrzejczuk, M., Marcon, L., Szunerits, S., Lewandowska, M. and Janik-Czachorm, M., Effect of two-step functionalization of Ti by chemical processes on protein adsorption, *Appl Surf Sci* 257:8196–8204.
72. Kawai, T., Takemoto, M., Fujibayashi, S., Akiyama, H., Yamaguchi, H., Pattanayak, D.P., Doi, K., Matsushita, T., Nakamura, T. and Kokubo, T., 2013, Osteoconduction of porous Ti metal enhanced by acid and heat treatments, *J Mater Sci Mater Med* 24:1707–1715. doi: http://dx.doi.org/10.1007/s10856-013-4919-0
73. Yoneyama, Y., Matsuno, T., Hashonoto, Y. and Satoh, T., 2013, In vitro evaluation of H_2O_2 hydrothermal treatment of aged titanium surface to enhance biofunctional activity, *Dent Mater* 32:115–121.
74. Li, Y., Zou, S., Wang, D., Feng, G., Bao, C. and Hu, J., 2010, The effect of hydrofluoric acid treatment on titanium implant osseointegration in ovariectomized rats, *Biomaterials* 31:3266–3273. doi: http://dx.doi.org/10.1016/j.biomaterials.2010.01.028
75. Viornery, C., Chevolot, Y., Léonard, D., Aronsson, B-O., Péchy, P., Mathieu, H.J., Descouts, P. and Grätzel, M., 2002, Surface modification of titanium with phosphonic acid

to improve bone bonding: Characterization by XPS and ToF-SIMS, *Langmuir 18*:2582–2589. doi: http://dx.doi.org/10.1021/la010908i
76. Park, J-W., Kim, Y-J., Jang, J-H., Kwon, T-G., Bae, Y-C. and Suh, J.Y., 2010, Effects of phosphoric acid treatment of titanium surfaces on surface properties, osteoblast response and removal of torque forces, *Acta Biomat* 6:1661–1670. doi: http://dx.doi.org/10.1016/j.actbio.2009.10.011
77. Hsu, H-C., Wu, S-C., Fu, C-E. and Ho, W-F., Formation of calcium phosphates on low-moldulus Ti-7.5 Mo alloy by acid and alkali treatments, *J Mater Sci* 45:3661–3670.
78. Szmukler-Moncler, S., Bischof, M., Nedir, R. and Ermrich, M., 2010, Titanium hydride and hydrogen concentration in acid-etched commercially pure titanium and titanium alloy implants: A comparative analysis of five implant systems, *Clin Oral Implants Res* 21:944–950.
79. de Souza, G.B., Lepienski, C.M., Foerster, D.E., Kuromoto, N.K., Soares, P. and de Araújo Ponte, H., 2011, Nanomechanical and nanotribological properties of bioactive titanium surfaces prepared by alkali treatment, *J Mech Behav Biomed Mater* 4:756–765. doi: http://dx.doi.org/10.1016/j.jmbbm.2010.07.005
80. Xie, J. and Juan B.L., 2008, Formation of hydroxyapatite coating using novel chemo-biomimetic method, *J Mater Sci Mater Med* 19:3211–3220. doi: http://dx.doi.org/10.1007/s10856-008-3451-0
81. Park, I.S., Choi, U.J., Yi, H.K., Park, B.K., Lee, M.H. and Bae, T.S., 2008, Biomimetic apatite formation and biocompatibility on chemically treated Ti–6Al–7Nb alloy, *Surf Interf Anal* 40:37–42. doi: http://dx.doi.org/10.1002/sia.2666
82. Guslitzer-Okner, R. and Mandler, D., 2011, Applications of electrochemistry and nanotechnology in biology and medicine, I: Electrochemical coating of medical implants, *Mod Aspect Electroc* 52:291–342.
83. Gao,Y., Gao, B., Wang, R., Wu, J., Zhang, L.J., and Hao, Y.L. and Tao, X.J., 2009, Improved biological performance of low modulus Ti–24Nb–4Zr–7.9Sn implants due to surface modification by anodic oxidation, *Appl Surf Sci* 255:5009–5015. doi: http://dx.doi.org/10.1016/j.apsusc.2008.12.054
84 Minagar, S., Berndt, C.C.,Wang, J., Ivanova, E. and Wen, C., 2012, A review of the application of anodization for the fabrication of nanotubes on metal implant surfaces, *Acta Biomater* 8:2875–2888. doi: http://dx.doi.org/10.1016/j.actbio.2012.04.005
85. Oshida, Y., 2013, *Bioscience and Bioengineering of Titanium Materials*, 2nd ed. Elsevier, London, UK, pp. 96–97.
86. Xiao, X., Ouyang, K., Liu, R. and Liang, J., 2009, Anatase type titania nanotube arrays direct fabricated by anodization without annealing, *Appl Surf Sci* 255:3659–3663. doi: http://dx.doi.org/10.1016/j.apsusc.2008.10.014
87. Necula, B.S., Apachitei, I., Fratila-Apachitei, L.E., van Langelaan, E.J. and Duszczyk, J., 2013, Titanium bone implants with superimposed micro/nanoscale porosity and antibacterial capability, *App Sur Sci* 273:310–314. doi: http://dx.doi.org/10.1016/j.apsusc.2013.02.036
88. Xie, J., Luan, B.L., Wang, J., Liu, X.Y., Rorabeck, C. and Bourne, R., 2008, Novel hydroxyapatite coating on new porous titanium and titanium-HDPE composite for hip implant, *Surf Coat Tech* 201:2960–2968. doi: http://dx.doi.org/10.1016/j.surfcoat.2007.10.040
89. Iwaniak, A., Nawrat, G., Maciej, A., Michalska, J., Radwański, K., Gazdowicz, J. and Simka, W., 2009, Modification of titanium oxide layer by calcium and phosphorus, *Electrochimica Acta* 54:6983–6988. doi: http://dx.doi.org/10.1016/j.electacta.2009.07.010
90. Simka, W., Krząkała, A., Korotin, D.M., Zhidkov, I.S., Kurmaev, E.Z., Cholakh, S.O., Kuna, K., Dercz, G., Michalska, J., Suchanek, K. and Gorewoda, T., 2013, Modification

of a Ti–Mo alloy surface via plasma electrolytic oxidation in a solution containing calcium and phosphorus, *Electrochimica Acta* 96:180–190. doi: http://dx.doi.org/10.1016/j.electacta.2013.02.102

91. Chávez-Valdez, A., Herrmann, H. and Boccaccini, A.R.,2012, Alternating current electrophoretic deposition (EPD) of TiO_2 nanoparticles in aqueous suspensions, *J Colloid and Interface Sci* 375:102–105. doi: http://dx.doi.org/10.1016/j.jcis.2012.02.054
92. Sharma, S., Soni, V.P. and Bellare, J.R., 2009, Chitosan reinforced apatite-wollastonite coating by electrophoretic deposition on titanium implants, *J Mater Sci* 20:1427–1436.
93. Morcos, B.M., O'Callaghan, J.M., Amira, M.F., Van Hoof, C. and de Beeck, M.O., 2013, Electrodeposition of platinum thin films as interconnects material for implantable medical applications electrochemical/electroless deposition, *J Electrochem Soc 160:*D300-D306. doi: http://dx.doi.org/10.1149/2.024308jes
94. Sebaa, M.A., Dhillon, S. and Liu, H., 2013, Electrochemical deposition and evaluation of electrically conductive polymer coating on biodegradable magnesium implants for neural applications, *J Mater Sci Mater Med* 24:307–316. doi: http://dx.doi.org/10.1007/s10856-012-4796-y
95. Chung, K.H., Liu, G.T., Duh, J.G. and Wang, J.H., 2004, Biocompatibility of a titanium–aluminum nitride film coating on a dental alloy, *Surf Coat Tech* 188/189:745–749. doi: http://dx.doi.org/10.1016/j.surfcoat.2004.07.050
96. Kim, K-H. and Ramaswamy, N., 2009, Electrochemical surface modification of titanium in dentistry, *Dent Mater J* 28:20–36. doi: http://dx.doi.org/10.4012/dmj.28.20
97. Sanchez, A.G., Schreiner, W., Duffó, G. and Ceré, S., 2013, Surface modification of titanium by anodic oxidation in phosphoric acid at low potentials. Part 1. Structure, electronic properties and thickness of the anodic films, *Surf Interf Anal* 45:1037–1046. doi: http://dx.doi.org/10.1002/sia.5210
98. Oshida, Y., 2007, Bioscience and bioengineering of titanium materials, Elsevier, London, UK, pp. 81–90.
99. Lee, I.G., Kim, Y.K., Park, I.S., Park, J.M., Lee, M.H., Bae, T.S. and Park, C.W., 2008, Influence of electrolyte temperature on pure titanium modified by electrochemical treatment for implant, *Surf Interf Anal* 40:1538–1544. doi: http://dx.doi.org/10.1002/sia.2930
100. Brinker, C.J., Hurd, A.J. Shunrk, P.R., Frye, G.C. and Asley, C.S., 1992, Review of sol-gel thin film formation, *J Non Cryst Solids* 147:424–436. doi: http://dx.doi.org/10.1016/S0022-3093(05)80653-2
101. Wright, J.D. and Sommerdijk, N.A.J., 2001, *Sol–Gel Materials Chemistry and Applications*, CRC Press, OPA Overseas Publishers Association.
102. Wang, D. and Bierwagen, G.P., 2009, Sol–gel coatings on metals for corrosion protection, *Progress Org Coat* 64:327–338. doi: http://dx.doi.org/10.1016/j.porgcoat.2008.08.010
103. Durán, A., Castro, Y., Aparicio, M., Conde, A. and de Damborenea, J. J., 2007, Protection and surface modification of metals with sol–gel coatings, *Int Mater Rev* 52:175–192. doi: http://dx.doi.org/10.1179/174328007X160263
104. Velu, G. and Gopal, B., 2009, Preparation of nanohydroxyapatite by a sol–gel method using alginic acid as a complexing agent, *J Am Ceramic Soc* 92:2207–2211. doi: http://dx.doi.org/10.1111/j.1551-2916.2009.03221.x
105. Ben-Nissan, B. and Chai, C., 1995, Sol-gel derived bioactive hydroxyapatite coatings , *NATO ASI Series* 294:265–273.
106. Ballarre, J., López, D.A., Schreiner, W.H., Durán, A. and Ceré, S.M., 2007, Protective hybrid sol–gel coatings containing bioactive particles on surgical grade stainless steel: Surface characterization, *Appl Surf Sci* 253:7260–7264. doi: http://dx.doi.org/10.1016/j.apsusc.2007.03.007

107. Montenero, A., Gnappi, G., Ferrari, F., Cesari, M., Salvioli, E., Mattogno, L. and Kaciulic, S., 2000, Sol-gel derived hydroxyapatite coatings on titanium substrate. *J Mater Sci* 35:2791–2797. doi: http://dx.doi.org/10.1023/A:1004738900778
108. Macwan, D.P. and Dave, P.N., 2011, A review on nano-TiO_2 sol–gel type syntheses and its applications, *J Mater Sci* 46:3669–3686. doi: http://dx.doi.org/10.1007/s10853-011-5378-y
109. Schulze, K, and Kirstein, S., 2005, Layer-by-layer deposition of TiO_2 nanoparticles, *Appl Surf Sci* 246:415–419. doi: http://dx.doi.org/10.1016/j.apsusc.2004.11.064
110. Abdal-hay, A., Dewidar, M., Lim, J.K., 2012, Biocorrosion behavior and cell viability of adhesive polymer coated magnesium based alloys for medical implants, *Appl Surf Sci* 261:536–546. doi: http://dx.doi.org/10.1016/j.apsusc.2012.08.051
111. Kim, H-W., Yoon, B-H., Koh, Y-H. and Hyoun-Ee Kim, H.E., 2006, Processing and performance of hydroxyapatite/fluorapatite double layer coating on zirconia by the powder slurry method, *J Am Ceramic Soc* 89:2466–2472. doi: http://dx.doi.org/10.1111/j.1551-2916.2006.01114.x
112. Kado, T., Hidaka, T., Aita, H., Endo, K. and Furuichi, Y., 2012, Enhanced compatibility of chemically modified titanium surface with periodontal ligament cells, *Appl Surf Sci* 262:240–247. doi: http://dx.doi.org/10.1016/j.apsusc.2012.07.091
113. Reis, A., Valente, M.L.C., Shimano, A.C. and Marcantonio, E. J., 2013, Relationship between the surface chemical composition of implants and contact with the substrate; *J Oral Implant*. doi: http://dx.doi.org/10.1563/AAID-JOI-D-11-00227
114. Lee, Y-H., Bhattarai, G., Aryal, S., Lee, N-H., Lee, M-H., Kim, T-G., Jhee, E-C., Kim, H-Y. and Yi, H-K., 2010, Modified titanium surface with gelatin nano gold composite increases osteoblast cell biocompatibility, *Appl Surf Sci* 256:5882–5887. doi: http://dx.doi.org/10.1016/j.apsusc.2010.03.069
115. Wu, J., Liu, Z-M., Zhao, X-H., Gao, Y., Hu, J. and Bo Gao, B., 2010, Improved biological performance of microarc-oxidized low-modulus Ti–24Nb–4Zr–7.9Sn alloy, *J Biomed Mater Res B Appl Biomater* 92:298–306.
116. Fan, X., Feng, B., Di, Y., Lu, X., Duan, K., Wang, J. and Jie Weng, J., 2012, Preparation of bioactive TiO film on porous titanium by microarc oxidation, *Appl Surf Sci* 258:7584–7588. doi: http://dx.doi.org/10.1016/j.apsusc.2012.04.093
117. Liu, Z., Wang, W., Liu, H., Wang, T. and Min Qi, M., 2013, Formation and characterization of titania coatings with cortex-like slots formed on Ti by microarc oxidation treatment, *Appl Surf Sci* 266:250–255. doi: http://dx.doi.org/10.1016/j.apsusc.2012.12.004
118. Yu, S., Yang,X., Yang, L., Liu, Y. and Yu, Y., 2007, Novel technique for preparing Ca- and P-containing ceramic coating on Ti–6Al–4V by microarc oxidation, *J Biomed Mater Res B Appl Biomater* 83:623–627. doi: http://dx.doi.org/10.1002/jbm.b.30836
119. Gan, J., Tan, L., Yang, K., Hu, Z., Zhang, Q., Fan, X., Li, Y. and Li, W., 2013, Bioactive Ca–P coating with self-sealing structure on pure magnesium , *J Mater Sci Mater Med* 24:889–901. doi: http://dx.doi.org/10.1007/s10856-013-4850-4
120. Abbasi, S., Golestani-Fard, F., Rezaie, H.R. and Mirhosseini, S.M.M., 2012, MAO-derived hydroxyapatite/ TiO_2 nanostructured multi-layer coatings on titanium substrate, *Appl Surf Sci* 261:37–42. doi: http://dx.doi.org/10.1016/j.apsusc.2012.07.044
121. Song, H-J., Kim, J-W., Kook,M-S., Moon, W-J. and Park, Y-J., 2010, Fabrication of hydroxyapatite and TiO_2 nanorods on microarc-oxidized titanium surface using hydrothermal treatment, *Appl Surf Sci* 256:7056–7061. doi: http://dx.doi.org/10.1016/j.apsusc.2010.05.024
122. Zhna, Z., Chen, X.,Chen, A., Huo, G. and Li, H., 2009, Preparation of K2Ti6O13/TiO2 bio-ceramic on titanium substrate by microarc oxidation, *J Mater Sci* 44:6310–6316. doi: http://dx.doi.org/10.1007/s10853-009-3869-x

123. Galevičius, R., Stalnionis, G., Niaura, G. and Jagminas, A., 2008, Microarc oxidation of Ti in a solution of sulfuric acid and Ti^{+3} salt, *Appl Surf Sci* 254:1608–1613. doi: http://dx.doi.org/10.1016/j.apsusc.2007.07.111
124. Ma, P.W., Wang, S-H., Wu, G-F., Liu, B-L., Wei, J-H., Xie, C. and Li, D-H., 2010, Preparation and *in vitro* biocompatibility of hybrid oxide layer on titanium surface, *Surf Coat Tech* 205: 61736–1742. doi: http://dx.doi.org/10.1016/j.surfcoat.2010.07.113
125. Foest, R., Schmidt, M. and Becker, K., 2006, Microplasmas, an emerging field of low-temperature plasma science and technology, *Int J Mass Spectrometry* 248:87–102. doi: http://dx.doi.org/10.1016/j.ijms.2005.11.010
126. Quaranta, A., Iezzi, G., Scarano, A., Soelho, P.G., Vozza, I., Marincola M. and Piattelli, A., 2010, A histomorphometric study of nanothickness and plasma-sprayed calcium-phosphorous-coated implant surfaces in rabbit bone, *J Periodont* 81:556–561. doi: http://dx.doi.org/10.1902/jop.2010.090296
127. Laroussi, M. and Akan, T., 2007, Arc-free atmospheric pressure cold plasma jets: A review, *Plasma Process Polym* 9:777–788. doi: http://dx.doi.org/10.1002/ppap.200700066
128. Eliasson, B. and Kogelschatz, U., 1991, Modeling and applications of silent discharge plasmas, *IEEE Trans Plasma Sci* 19:309–323. doi: http://dx.doi.org/10.1109/27.106829
129. Chu, P.K., 2007, Plasma surface treatment of artificial orthopedic and cardiovascular biomaterials, *Surf Coat Tech* 201:5601–5606. doi: http://dx.doi.org/10.1016/j.surfcoat.2006.07.003
130. Liu, X., Poon, R.W.Y., Kwoka, S.C.H., Chu, P.K. and Ding. C., 2004, Plasma surface modification of titanium for hard tissue replacements, *Surf Coat Tech* 186:227–233. doi: http://dx.doi.org/10.1016/j.surfcoat.2004.02.045
131. Jacobs, T., Morent, R., De Geyter, N., Dubruel, P. and Leys, C., 2012, Plasma surface modification of biomedical polymers: Influence on cell–material interaction, *Plasma Chem Plasma Process* 32:1039–1073. doi: http://dx.doi.org/10.1007/s11090-012-9394-8
132. Shibata, Y., Hosaka, M., Kawai, R. and Miyazaki, T., 2002, Glow discharge plasma treatment of titanium plates enhances adhesion of osteoblast-like cells to the plates through the integrin-mediated mechanism, *Intl J Oral Maxillofac Implants* 17:771–777.
133. Hu, X., Shen, H., Shuai, K., Zhang, E., Bai, Y., Cheng, Y., Xiong, X., Wang, S., Fang, J. and Shicheng Wei, S., 2011, Surface bioactivity modification of titanium by CO_2 plasma treatment and induction of hydroxyapatite: In vitro and in vivo studies, *Appl Surf Sci* 257:1813–1823. doi: http://dx.doi.org/10.1016/j.apsusc.2010.08.082
134. Chu, P.K., 2010, Recent applications of plasma-based ion implantation and deposition to microelectronic, nano-structured, and biomedical materials, *Surf Coat Tech* 204:2853–2863. doi: http://dx.doi.org/10.1016/j.surfcoat.2010.01.045
135. Chu, P.K., 2009, Applications of plasma-based technology to microelectronics and biomedical engineering, *Surf Coat Tech* 203:2793–2798. doi: http://dx.doi.org/10.1016/j.surfcoat.2009.02.131
136. Jagielski, J., Piatkowska, A., Aubert, P., Thomé, L., Turos, A. and Kader, A., 2006, Ion implantation for surface modification of biomaterials, *Surf Coat Tech* 200:6355–6361. doi: http://dx.doi.org/10.1016/j.surfcoat.2005.11.005
137. Chen, Y., Gao, Q., Wan, H., Yi, J., Wei, Y. and Liu, P., 2013, Surface modification and biocompatible improvement of polystyrene film by Ar, O_2 and Ar + O_2 plasma, *Appl Surf Sci* 265:452–457. doi: http://dx.doi.org/10.1016/j.apsusc.2012.11.027
138. Leng, Y.X., Huang, N., Yang, P., Chen, J.Y., Sun, H., Wang, J., Wan, G.J., Leng, Y. and Chu, P.K., 2002, Influence of oxygen pressure on the properties and biocompatibility of titanium oxide fabricated by metal plasma ion implantation and deposition, *Thin Solid Films* 420/421:408–413. doi: http://dx.doi.org/10.1016/S0040-6090(02)00814-3

139. Gupta, D., 2011, Plasma immersion ion implantation (PIII) porcess—physiscs and technology, *Intl J Adv Tech* 2:471–490.
140. Mändl, S., Krause, D., Thorwarth, G., Sader, R., Zeilhofer, F., Horch, H.H. and Rauschenbach, B., 2001, Plasma immersion ion implantation treatment of medical implants, *Surf Coat Tech* 142/144:1046–1050. doi: http://dx.doi.org/10.1016/S0257-8972(01)01066-0
141. Cui, F.Z. and Luo, Z.S., 1999, Biomaterials modification by ion-beam processing, *Surf Coat Tech* 112:278–285. doi: http://dx.doi.org/10.1016/S0257-8972(98)00763-4
142. Lee, I-S., Zhao, B., Lee,G-H., Choi, S-H. and Chung, S-M., 2007, Industrial application of ion beam assisted deposition on medical implants, *Surf Coat Tech* 201:5132–5137. doi: http://dx.doi.org/10.1016/j.surfcoat.2006.07.112
143. Sioshansi, P. and Tobin, E.J., 1996, Surface treatment of biomaterials by ion beam processes, *Surf Coat Tech* 83:175–182. doi: http://dx.doi.org/10.1016/0257-8972(95)02838-2
144. Sawase, T., Wennerberg, A., Baba, K., Tsuboi, Y., Sennerby, L., Johansson, C.B. and Albrektsson, T., 2001, Application of oxygen ion implantation to titanium surfaces: Effects on surface characteristics, corrosion resistance, and bone response, *Clin Implant Dent Related Res* 3:221–229. doi: http://dx.doi.org/10.1111/j.1708-8208.2001.tb00144.x
145. Liu, F., Li, B., Sun, J., Li, H., Wang, B. and Zhang, S., 2012, Proliferation and differentiation of osteoblastic cells on titanium modified by ammonia plasma immersion ion implantation, *Appl Surf Sci* 258:4322–4327. doi: http://dx.doi.org/10.1016/j.apsusc.2011.12.107
146. Mändl, S., 2007, PIII treatment of Ti alloys and NiTi for medical applications, *Surf Coat Tech* 201:6833–6838. doi: http://dx.doi.org/10.1016/j.surfcoat.2006.09.039
147. Yankov, R.A., Shevchenko, N., Rogozin, A., Maitz, M.F., Richter, E., Möller, W., Donchev, A. and Schütze, M., 2004, Reactive plasma immersion ion implantation for surface passivation, *Surf Coat Tech* 201:6752–6758. doi: http://dx.doi.org/10.1016/j.surfcoat.2006.09.010
148. Shevchenko, N., Pham, M-T. and Maitz, M.F., 2004, Studies of surface modified NiTi alloy, *Appl Surf Sci* 235:126–131. doi: http://dx.doi.org/10.1016/j.apsusc.2004.05.273
149. Qi, H. and Wu, H. Y., 2013, Effect of surface modification of pure Ti on tribological and biological properties of bone tissue, *Surf Eng* 29:300–305. doi: http://dx.doi.org/10.1179/1743294412Y.0000000095
150. Firouzi-Arani, M., Savaloni, H. and Ghoranneviss, M., 2010, Dependence of surface nano-structural modifications of Ti implanted by N^+ ions on temperature, *Appl Surf Sci* 256:4502–4511. doi: http://dx.doi.org/10.1016/j.apsusc.2010.01.083
151. Berberich, F., Matz, W., Kreissig, U.,E Richter, E., Schell, N. and Möller, W., 2001, Structural characterisation of hardening of Ti–Al–V alloys after nitridation by plasma immersion ion implantation, *Appl Surf Sci* 179:13–19. doi: http://dx.doi.org/10.1016/S0169-4332(01)00256-2
152. Gordin, D.M., Gloriant, T., Chane-Pane, V., Busardo, D., Mitran, V., Höche, D., Vasilescu, C., Drob, S.I. and Cimpean, A.J., 2012, Surface characterization and biocompatibility of titanium alloys implanted with nitrogen by Hardion+ technology, *J Mater Sci Mater Med* 23:2953–2966.
153. Leitão, E., Sa, C., Silva, R.A., Barbosa, M.A. and Ali, H., 1995, Electrochemical and surface modifications on N^+-ion implanted Ti–6A1–4V immersed in HBSS, *Corr Sci* 37:1861–1866. doi: http://dx.doi.org/10.1016/0010-938X(95)00091-W
154. Leitão, E., Silva, R.A. and Barbosa, M.A., 1997, Electrochemical and surface modifications on N^+-ION implanted Ti–5Al–2.5Fe immersed in HBSS, *Corr Sci* 39:377–383. doi: http://dx.doi.org/10.1016/S0010-938X(97)83352-5
155. Pye,D., 2004, Ion nitriding—basics, *Adv Mater Process* 162:41–43.

156. Xie, Y., Liu, X., Huang, A., Ding, C. and Chu, P.K., 2005, Improvement of surface bioactivity on titanium by water and hydrogen plasma immersion ion implantation, *Biomaterials* 26:6129–6135. doi: http://dx.doi.org/10.1016/j.biomaterials.2005.03.032
157. Rautray, T.R., Narayanan, R., Kwon, T-Y. and Kim, K-H., 2010, Surface modification of titanium and titanium alloys by ion implantation, *J Biomed Mater Res Part B* 93:581–591. doi: http://dx.doi.org/10.1002/jbm.b.31596
158. Liu, X.M., Wu, S.L., Chu, P.K., Chung, C.Y., Chu, C.L., Yeung, K.W.K., Lu, W.W., Cheung, K.M.C. and Luk, K.D.K., 2007, Effects of water plasma immersion ion implantation on surface electrochemical behavior of NiTi shape memory alloys in simulated body fluids, *Appl Surf Sci* 253:3154–3159. doi: http://dx.doi.org/10.1016/j.apsusc.2006.07.008
159. Ishikawa, J., Tsuji, H. and Gotoh, Y., 2009, Surface modification by negative-ion implantation, *Surf Coat Tech* 203:2351–2356. doi: http://dx.doi.org/10.1016/j.surfcoat.2009.02.023
160. Byon, E., Moon, S., Cho, S-B., Jeong, C-Y., Jeong, Y., Sul, Y-T., 2005, Electrochemical property and apatite formation of metal ion implanted titanium for medical implants, *Surf Coat Tech* 200:1018–1021. doi: http://dx.doi.org/10.1016/j.surfcoat.2005.02.133
161. Armitage, D.A., Mihoc, R., Tate, T.J., McPhail, D.S., Chater, R., Hobkirk, J.A., Shinawi, L. and F.H. Jones, F.H., 2007, The oxidation of calcium implanted titanium in water: A depth profiling study, *Appl Surf Sci* 253:4085–4093. doi: http://dx.doi.org/10.1016/j.apsusc.2006.09.006
162. Gallardo-Moreno, A.M., Multigner, M., Calzado-Martín, A., Méndez-Vilas, A., Saldaña, L., Galván, J.C., Pacha-Olivenza, M.A., Perera-Núñez, J., González-Carrasco, J.L., Braceras, I., Vilaboa, N. and González-Martín, M.L., 2011, Bacterial adhesion reduction on a biocompatible Si + ion implanted austenitic stainless steel, *Mater Sci Eng C* 31:1567–1576. doi: http://dx.doi.org/10.1016/j.msec.2011.07.008
163. Xue, W., Liu, X., Zheng, X-B. and Ding, C., 2005, In vivo evaluation of plasma-sprayed titanium coating after alkali modification, *Biomaterials* 26:3029–3037. doi: http://dx.doi.org/10.1016/j.biomaterials.2004.09.003
164. Azarmi, F., 2005, Vacuum plasma spraying, *Adv Mater Process* 163:37–39.
165. Fomin, A.A., Steinhauer, A.B., Lyasnikov, V.N., Wenig, S.B. and A. M. Zakharevich, A.M., 2012, Nanocrystalline structure of the surface layer of plasma-sprayed hydroxyapatite coatings obtained upon preliminary induction heat treatment of metal base, *Tech Phys Lett* 38:481–483. doi: http://dx.doi.org/10.1134/S1063785012050227
166. Latka, L., Goryachev, S.B., Kozerski, S. and Pawlowski, L., 200, Sintering of fine particles in suspension plasma sprayed coatings, *Materials 3:*3845–3866.
167. Montazeri, M., Dehghanian, C., Shokouhfar, M. and Baradaran, A., 2011, Investigation of the voltage and time effects on the formation of hydroxyapatite-containing titania prepared by plasma electrolytic oxidation on Ti–6Al–4V alloy and its corrosion behavior, *Appl Surf Sci* 257:7268–7275. doi: http://dx.doi.org/10.1016/j.apsusc.2011.03.103
168. Silva, M.A.M., Martinelli, A.E., Alves, C., Nascimento, R.M., Távora, M.P. and Vilar, C.D., 2006, Surface modification of Ti implants by plasma oxidation in hollow cathode discharge, *Surf Coat Tech* 200:2618–2626. doi: http://dx.doi.org/10.1016/j.surfcoat.2004.12.027
169. Huan, Z., Fratila-Apachitei, L.E., Apachitei, I. and Duszczyk, J., 2012, Porous NiTi surfaces for biomedical applications, *Appl Surf Sci* 258:5244–5249. doi: http://dx.doi.org/10.1016/j.apsusc.2012.02.002
170. Rie, K-T., Stucky, T., Silva, R.A., Leitao, E., Bordji, K., Jouzeau, J-Y. and Mainard, D., 1995, Plasma surface treatment and PACVD on Ti alloys for surgical implants, *Surf Coat Tech* 74/75:973–980. doi: http://dx.doi.org/10.1016/0257-8972(95)08316-2

171. Abd El-Rahman, A.M., Maitz, M.F., Kassem, M.A., El-Hossary, F.M., Prokert, F., Reuther, H., Pham, M.T. and Richter, E., 2007, Surface improvement and biocompatibility of $TiAl_{24}Nb_{10}$ intermetallic alloy using rf plasma nitriding, *Appl Surf Sci* 253:9067–9072. doi: http://dx.doi.org/10.1016/j.apsusc.2007.05.021
172. Fouquet, V., Pichon, L., Drouet, M. and Sraboni, A., 2004, Plasma assisted nitridation of Ti-6Al-4V, *Appl Surf Sci* 221:248–258. doi: http://dx.doi.org/10.1016/S0169-4332(03)00889-4
173. Chrzanowski, W., Szade, J., Hart, A.D., Knowles, J.C. and Dalby, M.J., 2012, Biocompatible, smooth, plasma-treated nickel–titanium surface—An adequate platform for cell growth, *J Biomater Appl* 26:707–731. doi: http://dx.doi.org/10.1177/0885328211416023
174. Fu, Y., Yan, B., Loh, N.L., Sun, C.O. and Hing, P., 1999, Deposition of diamond coating on pure titanium using micro-wave plasma assisted chemical vapor deposition, *J Mater Sci* 34:2269–2283. doi: http://dx.doi.org/10.1023/A:1004430311364
175. Bazaka, K., Jacob, M.V., Crawford, R.J. and Ivanova, E.P., 2011, Plasma-assisted surface modification of organic biopolymers to prevent bacterial attachment, *Acta Biomater* 7:2015–2028. doi: http://dx.doi.org/10.1016/j.actbio.2010.12.024
176. Chen, Y., Sun, Y., Zhao, B., Wan, H. and Wu, D., 2011, Surface modification of titanium by using plasma-induced graft-polymerization, *Surf Interf Anal* 43:1566–1574. doi: http://dx.doi.org/10.1002/sia.3750
177. Sawase, T., Jimbo, R., Wennerberg, A., Suketa, N., Tanaka, Y. and Atsuta, M., 2007, A novel characteristic of porous titanium oxide implants, *Clin Oral Implants Res* 18:680–685. doi: http://dx.doi.org/10.1111/j.1600-0501.2007.01404.x
178. Stachowski, M.J., Medige, J. and Baier, R.E., 1987, Methodology for testing the mechanical properties of the bone/titanium implant interface, *Environ Degrad Eng Mater* 3:493–500.
179. Dutta Majumdar, J. and Manna, I., 2011, Laser material processing, *Int Mater Rev* 56:341–388. doi: http://dx.doi.org/10.1179/1743280411Y.0000000003
180. Dahotre, N.B., 2002, Laser surface engineering, *Adv Mater Process* 160:35–39.
181. Narayan, R.J., Jin, C., Patz, T., Doraiswamy, A., Modi, R., Chrisey, D.B., Su, Y-Y., Lin, S.J., Ovsianikov, A. and Chichkov, B., 2005, Laser processing of advanced biomaterials, *Adv Mater Process* 163:39–42.
182. Tian, Y.S., Chen, C.Z., Li, S.T. and Huo, Q.H., 2005, Research progress on laser surface modification of titanium alloys, *Appl Surf Sci* 242:177–184. doi: http://dx.doi.org/10.1016/j.apsusc.2004.08.011
183. Romanos, G.E., Gupta, B., Yunker, M., Romanos, E.B. and Malmstrom, H., 2013, Lasers use in dental implantology, *Implant Dent* 22:282–288. doi: http://dx.doi.org/10.1097/ID.0b013e3182885fcc
184. Bandyopadhyay, A., Balla, V.K., Roy, M. and Bose, S., 2011, Laser surface modification of metallic biomaterials, *JOM* 63:94–99.
185. Liu, X-B and Wang, H-M., 2006, Modification of tribology and high-temperature behavior of Ti–48Al–2Cr–2Nb intermetallic alloy by laser cladding, *Appl Surf Sci* 252:5735–5744. doi: http://dx.doi.org/10.1016/j.apsusc.2005.07.064
186. Trtica, M., Gakovic, B., Batani, D., Desai, T., Panjan, P. and Radak, B., 2006, Surface modifications of a titanium implant by a picosecond Nd:YAG laser operating at 1064 and 532 nm, *Appl Surf Sci* 253:2551–2556. doi: http://dx.doi.org/10.1016/j.apsusc.2006.05.024
187. Pető, G., Karacs, A., Pászti, Z., Guczi, L., Divinyi, T. and Joób, A., 2002, Surface treatment of screw shaped titanium dental implants by high intensity laser pulses, *Appl Surf Sci* 186:7–13. doi: http://dx.doi.org/10.1016/S0169-4332(01)00769-3
188. Roy, M., Bandyopadhyay, A. and Bose, S., 2008, Laser surface modification of electrophoretically deposited hydroxyapatite coating on titanium, *J Am Ceramic Soc* 91:3517–3521. doi: http://dx.doi.org/10.1111/j.1551-2916.2008.02698.x

189. Ciganovic, J., Stasic, J., Gakovic, B., Momcilovic, M., Milovanovic, D., Bokorov, M. and Trtica, M., 2012, Surface modification of the titanium implant using TEA CO_2 laser pulses in controllable gas atmospheres—Comparative study, *Appl Surf Sci* 258:2741–2748. doi: http://dx.doi.org/10.1016/j.apsusc.2011.10.125
190. Stübinger, S., Etter, C., Miskiewicz, M., Homann, F., Saldamli, B., Wieland, M. and Sader, R., 2010, Surface alterations of polished and sandblasted and acid-etched titanium implants after Er:YAG, carbon dioxide, and diode laser irradiation, *Int J Oral Maxillofac Implants* 25:104–111.
191. Vorobyev, A.Y. and Guo, C., 2007, Femtosecond laser structuring of titanium implants, *Appl Surf Sci* 253:7272–7280. doi: http://dx.doi.org/10.1016/j.apsusc.2007.03.006
192. Landis, E.C., Phillips, K.C., Mazur, E. and Friend, C.M., 2012, Formation of nanostructured TiO2 by femtosecond laser irradiation of titanium in O2, *J Appl Phys* 112. doi: http://dx.doi.org/10.1063/1.4752276
193. Tian, Y.S., Chen, C.Z., Wang, D.Y., Huo, Q.H. and Lei, T.Q., 2005, Laser surface alloying of pure titanium with TiN–B–Si–Ni mixed powders, *Appl Surf Sci* 250:223–227. doi: http://dx.doi.org/10.1016/j.apsusc.2005.01.001
194. Gu, D. D., Meiners, W., Wissenbach, K. and Poprawe, R., 2012, Laser additive manufacturing of metallic components: Materials, processes and mechanisms, *Int Mater Rev* 57:133–164. doi: http://dx.doi.org/10.1179/1743280411Y.0000000014
195. Waugh, D. and Lawrence, J., 2013, Laser surface processing of polymers for biomedical applications, *In Laser-Assisted Fabrication of Materials*, Springer Series in Materials Science, 161:275–318. doi: http://dx.doi.org/10.1007/978-3-642-28359-8_7
196. Witek, L., Marin, C., Granato, R., Bonfante, E.A., Campos, F., Bisinotto, J., Suzuki, M. and Coelho, P.G., 2012, Characterization and *in vivo* evaluation of laser sintered dental endosseous implants in dogs, *J Biomed Mater Res Part B* 100:1566–1573. doi: http://dx.doi.org/10.1002/jbm.b.32725
197. Walczak, M., Papadopoulou, E.L., Sanz, M., Manousaki, A., Marco, J.F. and Castillejo, M., 2009, Structural and morphological characterization of TiO_2 nanostructured films grown by nanosecond pulsed laser deposition, *Appl Surf Sci* 255:5267–5270. doi: http://dx.doi.org/10.1016/j.apsusc.2008.07.098
198. Sanz, M., Walczak, M., de Nalda, R., Oujja, M., Marco, J.F., Rodriguez, J., Izquierdo, J.G., Bañares, L. and Castillejo, M., 2009, Femtosecond pulsed laser deposition of nanostructured TiO_2 films, *Appl Surf Sci* 255:5206–5210. doi: http://dx.doi.org/10.1016/j.apsusc.2008.07.148
199. Nikolov, A.S., Atanasov, P.A., Milev, D.R., Stoyanchov, T.R., Deleva, A.D. and Peshev, Z.Y., 2009, Synthesis and characterization of TiO_x nanoparticles prepared by pulsed-laser ablation of Ti target in water, *Appl Surf Sci* 255:5351–5354. doi: http://dx.doi.org/10.1016/j.apsusc.2008.09.007
200. Kurland, H-D., Stötzel, C., Grabow, J., Zink, I., Müller, E., Staupendahl, G. and Müller, F.A., 2010, Preparation of spherical titania nanoparticles by CO_2 laser evaporation and process-integrated particle coating, *J Am Ceramic Soc* 93:1282–1289.
201. Mihailescu, I.N., Ristoscu, C., Bigi, A. and Mayer, I., 2010, laser-surface interactions for new materials production, in *Advanced Biomimetic Implants Based on Nanostructured Coatings Synthesized by Pulsed Laser Technologies*, Springer Series in Materials Science 130:235–260. doi: http://dx.doi.org/10.1007/978-3-642-03307-0_10
202. Cotell, C.M., Chrisey, D.B., Grabowski, K.S., Sprague, J.A. and Gossett, C.R., 1992, Pulsed laser deposition of hydroxylapatite thin films on Ti–6Al–4V, *J Appl Biomater* 3:87–93. doi: http://dx.doi.org/10.1002/jab.770030204
203. Liang, C.Y., Yang, X.J., Wei, Q. and Cui, Z.D., 2008, Comparison of calcium phosphate coatings formed on femtosecond laser-induced and sand-blasted titanium, *Appl Surf Sci* 255:515–518. doi: http://dx.doi.org/10.1016/j.apsusc.2008.06.054

204. Lavisse, L., Grevey, D., Langlade, C. and Vannes, B., 2002, The early stage of the laser-induced oxidation of titanium substrates, *Appl Surf Sci* 186:150–155. doi: http://dx.doi.org/10.1016/S0169-4332(01)00761-9
205. Höche, D., Rapin, G. and Schaaf, P., 2007, FEM simulation of the laser plasma interaction during laser nitriding of titanium, *Appl Surf Sci* 254:888–892. doi: http://dx.doi.org/10.1016/j.apsusc.2007.08.079
206. Carpene, E., Shinn, M. and Schaaf, P., 2005, Free-electron laser surface processing of titanium in nitrogen atmosphere, *Appl Surf Sci* 247:307–312. doi: http://dx.doi.org/10.1016/j.apsusc.2005.01.059
207. György, E., del Pino, A.P., Serra, P. and Morenza, J.L., 2002, Surface nitridation of titanium by pulsed Nd:YAG laser irradiation, *Appl Surf Sci* 186:130–134. doi: http://dx.doi.org/10.1016/S0169-4332(01)00612-2
208. Yue, T.M., Yu, J.K., Mei, Z. and Man, H.C., 2002, Excimer laser surface treatment of Ti–6Al–4V alloy for corrosion resistance enhancement, *Mater Lett* 52:206–212. doi: http://dx.doi.org/10.1016/S0167-577X(01)00395-0
209. Man, H.C., Bai, M. and Cheng, F.T., 2011, Laser diffusion nitriding of Ti–6Al–4V for improving hardness and wear resistance, *Appl Surf Sci* 258:436–441. doi: http://dx.doi.org/10.1016/j.apsusc.2011.08.114
210. Dahotre, S.N., Vora, H.D., Pavani, K. and Banerjee, R., 2013, An integrated experimental and computational approach to laser surface nitriding of Ti–6Al–4V, *Appl Surf Sci* 271:141–148. doi: http://dx.doi.org/10.1016/j.apsusc.2013.01.151
211. Queiroz, T.P., Souza, F. Á., Guastaldi, A.C., Margonar, R., Garcia-Júnior, I.R. and Hochuli-Vieira, E., 2012, Commercially pure titanium implants with surfaces modified by laser beam with and without chemical deposition of apatite. Biomechanical and topographical analysis in rabbits, *Clin Oral Implants Res* 24:896–903. doi: http://dx.doi.org/10.1111/j.1600-0501.2012.02471.x
212. Duty, C., Jean, D. and Lackey, W.J., 2001, Laser chemical vapour deposition: Materials, modelling, and process control, *Int Mater Rev* 46:271–287. doi: http://dx.doi.org/10.1179/095066001771048727
213. Paun, I.A., Moldovan, A., Luculescu, C.R. and Dinescu, M., 2013, Antibacterial polymeric coatings grown by matrix assisted pulsed laser evaporation, *Appl Phy A* 110:895–902. doi: http://dx.doi.org/10.1007/s00339-012-7193-y
214. Mishra, V.K., Srivastava, S.K., Asthana, B.P. and Kumar, D., 2012, Structural and spectroscopic studies of hydroxyapatite nanorods formed via microwave-assisted synthesis route, *J Am Ceramic Soc* 95:2709–2715. doi: http://dx.doi.org/10.1111/j.1551-2916.2012.05134.x
215. Balasubramanian, S., Ramadoss, A., Kobayashi, A. and Muthirulandi, J., 2012, Nanocomposite Ti–Si–N coatings deposited by reactive dc magnetron sputtering for biomedical applications, *J Am Ceramic Soc* 95:2746–2752. doi: http://dx.doi.org/10.1111/j.1551-2916.2011.05029.x
216. Yoshinari, M., Oda, Y., Inoue, T. and Shimono. M., 2002, Dry-process surface modification for titanium dental implants, *Metallurg Mater Trans A* 33:511–519. doi: http://dx.doi.org/10.1007/s11661-002-0113-6
217. Noorakma, A.C.W., Zuhailawati, H., Aishvarya, V. and Dhindaw, B.K., 2013, Hydroxyapatite-coated magnesium-based biodegradable alloy: Cold spray deposition and simulated body fluid studies, *J Mater Eng Perform* 22:2997-3004. doi: http://dx.doi.org/10.1007/s11665-013-0589-9
218. Cai, K., Rechtenbach, A., Hao, J., Bossert, J. and Klaus D. Jandt, K.D., 2005, Polysaccharide-protein surface modification of titanium via a layer-by-layer technique: Characterization and cell behaviour aspects, *Biomaterials* 26:5960–5971. doi: http://dx.doi.org/10.1016/j.biomaterials.2005.03.020

219. Ai, H., Jones, S.A. and Lvov,Y.M., 2003, Biomedical applications of electrostatic layer-by-layer nano-assembly of polymers, enzymes, and nanoparticles, *Cell Biochem Biophys* 39:23–43. doi: http://dx.doi.org/10.1385/CBB:39:1:23
220. Zhang, Y., Kong, D., Yokogawa, Y., Feng, X., Tao, Y. and Tai Qiu, T., 2012, Fabrication of porous hydroxyapatite ceramic scaffolds with high flexural strength through the double slip-casting method using fine powders, *J Am Ceram Soc* 95:147–152. doi: http://dx.doi.org/10.1111/j.1551-2916.2011.04859.x
221. Turner, M.W., Crouse, P.L. and Li, L., 2006, Comparison of mechanisms and effects of Nd:YAG and CO_2 laser cleaning of titanium alloys, *Appl Surf Sci* 252:4792–4797. doi: http://dx.doi.org/10.1016/j.apsusc.2005.06.050
222. Turner, M.W., Crouse, P.L., Li, L. and Smith, A.J.E., 2006, Investigation into CO_2 laser cleaning of titanium alloys for gas-turbine component manufacture, *Appl Surf Sci* 252:4798–4802. doi: http://dx.doi.org/10.1016/j.apsusc.2005.06.061
223. Kamath, K.R. and Park, K., 1994, Surface modification of polymeric biomaterials by albumin grafting using γ-irradiation, *J Appl Biomater* 5:163–173. doi: http://dx.doi.org/10.1002/jab.770050210
224. Li, S., Ni, J., Liu, X., Zhang, X., Yin, S., Rong, M., Guo, Z. and Zhou, L., 2012, Surface characteristics and biocompatibility of sandblasted and acid-etched titanium surface modified by ultraviolet irradiation: An *in vitro* study, *J Biomed Mat Res Part B* 100:1587–1598. doi: http://dx.doi.org/10.1002/jbm.b.32727
225. Sultana, R., Kon, M., Hirakata, L.M., Fujihara, E., Asaoka, K. and Ichikawa, T., 2006, Surface modification of titanium with hydrothermal treatment at high pressure, *Dent Mater J* 25:470–479. doi: http://dx.doi.org/10.4012/dmj.25.470
226. Park, J-W., TsutsumiY., Lee, C.S., Park, C.H., Kim, Y-J., Jang, J-H., Khang, D., Im, Y-M., Doi, H., Nomura, N. and Hanawa, T., 2011, Surface structures and osteoblast response of hydrothermally produced $CaTiO_3$ thin film on Ti–13Nb–13Zr alloy, *Appl Surf Sci* 257:7856–7863. doi: http://dx.doi.org/10.1016/j.apsusc.2011.04.054
227. Drnovšek, N., Daneu, N., Rečnik, A., Mazaj, M., Kovač, J. and Novak, S., 2009, Hydrothermal synthesis of a nanocrystalline anatase layer on Ti6A4V implants, *Surf Coat Tech* 203:1462–1468. doi: http://dx.doi.org/10.1016/j.surfcoat.2008.11.031
228. Valanezhad, A., Tsuru, K., Maruta, M., Kawachi, G., Matsuya, S. and Ishikawa, K., 2012, A new biocompatible coating layer applied on titanium substrates using a modified zinc phosphatizing method, *Surf Coat Tech* 206:2207–2212. doi: http://dx.doi.org/10.1016/j.surfcoat.2011.09.064
229. Dorfman, M.R., 2002, Thermal spray—Basics, *Ad Mater Process* 160:47–50.
230. Puerta, D.G., 2013, Thermal spray coating—characterization and evaluation, *Adv Mater Process* 171:16–19.
231. Gruner, H., 2001, *Thermal Spray Coatings on Titanium Titanium in Medicine*, Engineering Materials, pp. 375–416. doi: http://dx.doi.org/10.1007/978-3-642-56486-4_12
232. Scott, K.T. and Kingswell, R., 1991,Thermal praying, in D.S.Rickerby ed. *Advanced Surface Coatings: A Handbook of Surface Engineering*, Spinger-Science, New York, NY, pp. 217–243.
233. Haman, J.D., Boulware, A.A., Lucas, L.C. and Crawmer, D.E., 1995, High-velocity oxy-fuel thermal spray coatings for biomedical applications, *J Thermal Spray Tech* 4:179–184. doi: http://dx.doi.org/10.1007/BF02646110
234. Lima, R.S., Dimitrievska, S., Bureau, M.N., Marple, B.R., Petit, A., Mwale, F. and Antoniou, J., 2010, HVOF-sprayed nano TiO_2-HA coatings exhibiting enhanced biocompatibility, *J Thermal Spray Tech* 19:336–343. doi: http://dx.doi.org/10.1007/s11666-009-9442-y
235. Siva, D., Krishna, R. and Sun, Y., 2005, Thermally oxidised rutile-TiO_2 coating on stainless steel for tribological properties and corrosion resistance enhancement, *Appl Surf Sci* 252:1107–1116. doi: http://dx.doi.org/10.1016/j.apsusc.2005.02.046

236. Petrovicova, E. and Schadler, L. S., 2002, Thermal spraying of polymers, *Int Materials Rev* 47:169–190. doi: http://dx.doi.org/10.1179/095066002225006566
237. Li, J-G. and Hashida, T., 2006, In situ formation of hydroxyapatite-whisker ceramics by hydrothermal hot-pressing method, *J Am Ceram Soc* 89:3544–3546. doi: http://dx.doi.org/10.1111/j.1551-2916.2006.01149.x
238. Tang, Y.J., Tang, Y.F., Lv, C.T. and Zhou, Z.H., 2008, Preparation of uniform porous hydroxyapatite biomaterials by a new method, *Appl Surf Sci* 254:5359–5362. doi: http://dx.doi.org/10.1016/j.apsusc.2008.02.059
239. Lee, W.H. and Hyun, C.Y., 2007, Surface characteristics of self-assembled microporous Ti–6Al–4V compacts fabricated by electro-discharge-sintering in air, *Appl Surf Sci* 253:4649–4651. doi: http://dx.doi.org/10.1016/j.apsusc.2006.10.021
240. Seah, K.H.W., Thampuran, R., Chen, X. and Teoh, S.H., 1995, A comparison between the corrosion behaviour of sintered and unsintered porous titanium, *Corr Sci* 37:1333–1340. doi: http://dx.doi.org/10.1016/0010-938X(95)00033-G
241. Dewidar, M.M. and Lim, J.K., 2008, Properties of solid core and porous surface Ti–6Al–4V implants manufactured by powder metallurgy, *J Alloys Compd* 454:442–446. doi: http://dx.doi.org/10.1016/j.jallcom.2006.12.143
242. T.Okazumi, K.Ueda, K.Tajima, N.Umetsu, T.Narushima; Anatase formation on titanium by two-step thermal treatment. *J Mater Sci.*, 2011;46:2998–3005. doi: http://dx.doi.org/10.1007/s10853-010-5177-x
243. Rodionov, I.V., 2012, Steam-thermal oxide coatings for titanium medical implants, *Biomed Eng* 46:58–61. doi: http://dx.doi.org/10.1007/s10527-012-9267-8
244. Lee, W.H., Kim, S.J., Lee, W.J., Byun, C.S., Kim, D.K., Kim, J.Y., Hyun, C.Y., Lee, J.G. and Park, J.W., 2001, Mechanism of surface modification of a porous-coated Ti-6Al-4V implant fabricated by electrical resistance sintering, *J Mater Sci* 36:3573–3577. doi: http://dx.doi.org/10.1023/A:1004814002344
245. Shenhar, A., Gotman, I., Gutmanas, E.Y. and Ducheyne, P., 1999, Surface modification of titanium alloy orthopaedic implants via novel powder immersion reaction assisted coating nitriding method, *Mater Sci Eng A* 268:40–46. doi: http://dx.doi.org/10.1016/S0921-5093(99)00111-2
246. Zhang, P., Zhang, Z., Li, W. and Zhu, M., 2013, Effect of Ti-OH groups on microstructure and bioactivity of TiO$_2$coating prepared by microarc oxidation, *Appl Surf Sci* 268:381–386. doi: http://dx.doi.org/10.1016/j.apsusc.2012.12.105
247. Nie, X., Leyland, A. and Matthews, A., 2000, Deposition of layered bioceramic hydroxyapatite/TiO$_2$ coatings on titanium alloys using a hybrid technique of microarc oxidation and electrophoresis, *Surf Coat Tech* 125:407–414. doi: http://dx.doi.org/10.1016/S0257-8972(99)00612-X
248. Liu, F., Wang, F., Shimizu, T., Igarashi, K. and Zhao, L., 2005, Formation of hydroxyapatite on Ti–6Al–4V alloy by microarc oxidation and hydrothermal treatment, *Surf Coat Tech* 199:220–224. doi: http://dx.doi.org/10.1016/j.surfcoat.2004.10.146
249. Martines , R.T., Sendyk , W.R., Gromatzky, A. and Cury, P.R., 2008, Sandblasted/acid-etched vs smooth-surface implants: Implant mobility and clinical reaction to experimentally induced peri-implantitis in beagle dogs, *J Oral Implant* 34:185–189. doi: http://dx.doi.org/10.1563/0.880.1
250. Wei, Q., Cui, Z-D., Yang, X-J. and Shi, J. 2008, Improving the bioactivity of NiTi shape memory alloy by heat and alkali treatment, *Appl Surf Sci* 255:462–465. doi: http://dx.doi.org/10.1016/j.apsusc.2008.06.069
251. Nishiguchi, S., Kato, H., Neo, M., Oka, M., Kim, H-M., Kokubo, T. and Nakamura, T., 2001, Alkali- and heat-treated porous titanium for orthopedic implants, *J Biomed Mat Res* 54:198–208. doi: http://dx.doi.org/10.1002/1097-4636(200102)54:2<198::AID-JBM6>3.0.CO;2-7

252. Juodzbalys, G., Sapragoniene, M., Wennerberg, A. and Baltrukonis, T., 2007, Titanium dental implant surface micromorphology optimization, *J Oral Implant* 33:177-185. doi: http://dx.doi.org/10.1563/1548-1336(2007)33[177:TDISMO]2.0.CO;2
253. Ishizawa, H. and Ogino, M., 1996, Thin hydroxyapatite layers formed on porous titanium using electrochemical and hydrothermal reaction, *J Mater Sci* 31:6279–6284. doi: http://dx.doi.org/10.1007/BF00354450
254. Ribeiro, A.A., Marques, R.F.C., Guastaldi, A.C. and Sinézio, J.C.C., 2009, Hydroxyapatite deposition study through polymeric process on commercially pure Ti surfaces modified by laser beam irradiation, *J Mater Sci* 44:4056–4062. doi: http://dx.doi.org/10.1007/s10853-009-3585-6
255. Shtansky, D.V., Batenina, I.V., Yadroitsev, I.A., Ryashin, N.S., Kiryukhantsev-Korneev, P.V., Kudryashov, A.E., Sheveyko, A,N., Zhitnyak, I.Y., Gloushankova, N.A., Smurov, I.Y. and Levashov, E.A., 2012, A new combined approach to metal-ceramic implants with controllable surface topography, chemistry, blind porosity, and wettability, *Surf Coat Tech* 208:14–23. doi: http://dx.doi.org/10.1016/j.surfcoat.2012.07.008
256. Sun, Y., 2004,Tribological rutile-TiO_2 coating on aluminium alloy, *Appl Surf Sci* 233:328–335. doi: http://dx.doi.org/10.1016/j.apsusc.2004.03.241
257. Sun, T. and Wang, M., 2008, Mechanical performance of apatite/TiO_2 composite coatings formed on Ti and NiTi shape memory alloy, *Appl Surf Sci* 255:404–408. doi: http://dx.doi.org/10.1016/j.apsusc.2008.06.123
258. Xie, Y., Zheng, X., Huang, L. and Ding, C., 2011, Influence of hierarchial hybrid micro/nano-structured surface on biological performance of titanium coating, *J Mater Sci* 2011; DOI 10.1007/s10853-011-5921-x. doi: http://dx.doi.org/10.1007/s10853-011-5921-x
259. Zheng, C.Y., Nie, F.L., Zheng, Y.F., Cheng, Y., Wei, S.C. and Valiev, R.Z., 2011, Enhanced in vitro biocompatibility of ultrafine-grained titanium with hierarchical porous surface, *Appl Surf Sci* 257:5634–5640. doi: http://dx.doi.org/10.1016/j.apsusc.2011.05.105
260. Jiang, W., Wang,W.D., Shi, X.H., Chen, H.Z., Zou, W., Guo, Z., Luo, J.M., Gu, Z.W. and Zhang, X.D., 2008,The effects of hydroxyapatite coatings on stress distribution near the dental implant–bone interface, *Appl Surf Sci* 255:273–275. doi: http://dx.doi.org/10.1016/j.apsusc.2008.06.165
261. Suska, F., Svensson, S., Johansson, A., Emanuelsson, L., Karlholm, H., Ohrlander, M. and Thomsen, P., 2010, In vivo evaluation of noble metal coatings, *J Biomed Mater Res B Appl Biomater* 92:86–94. doi: http://dx.doi.org/10.1002/jbm.b.31492
262. Chen, Y., Zheng, X., Xie, Y., Ji, H. and Ding, C., 2009, Antibacterial properties of vacuum plasma sprayed titanium coatings after chemical treatment, *Surf Coat Tech* 204:685–690. doi: http://dx.doi.org/10.1016/j.surfcoat.2009.09.010
263. Yao, C., Storey, D. and Webster, T., 2007, Nanostructured metal coatings on polymers increase osteoblast attachment, *Int J Manomed* 2:487–492.
264. Young, L., Soon, K., Doo, S. and Yong, K., 2011, Enhanced biocompatibility of stainless steel implants by titanium coating and microarc oxidation, *Clin Orthop Relat Res* 469:330–338. doi: http://dx.doi.org/10.1007/s11999-010-1613-0
265. Mwenifumbo, S., Li, M., Chen, J., Beye, A. and Soboyejo, W., 2007, Cell/surface interactions on laser micro-textured titanium-coated silicon surfaces, *J Mater Sci Mater Med* 18:9–23. doi: http://dx.doi.org/10.1007/s10856-006-0658-9
266. Neumeister, A., Bartke, D., Bärsch, N., Weingärtner, T., Guetaz, L., Montani, A., Compagnini, G. and Barcikowski, S., 2012, Interface of nanoparticle-coated electropolished stents, *Langmuir* 28:12060–12066. doi: http://dx.doi.org/10.1021/la300308w
267. Fallah, V., Corbin, S.F and Khajepour, A., 2010, Process optimization of Ti–Nb alloy coatings on a Ti–6Al–4V plate using a fiber laser and blended elemental powders, *J Mater Process Tech* 210:2081–2087. doi: http://dx.doi.org/10.1016/j.jmatprotec.2010.07.030

268. Sonoda, T., Saito, T., Watazu, A., Katou, K. and Asahina, T., 2006, Coating of Ti–6Al–4V alloy with pure titanium film by sputter-deposition for improving biocompatibility, *Surf Interf Analy* 38:797–800. doi: http://dx.doi.org/10.1002/sia.2357
269. Devine, D.M., Hahn, J., Richards, R.G., Gruner, H., Wieling, R. and Pearce, S.G., 2013, Coating of carbon fiber-reinforced polyetheretherketone implants with titanium to improve bone apposition, *J Biomed Mater Res B Appl Biomater* 101:591–598. doi: http://dx.doi.org/10.1002/jbm.b.32861
270. Kovacs, P. and Davidson, J.A., 1996, Medical applications of titanium and its alloys: the material and biological issues, In S.A.Brown, J.E.Lemons ed., *Chemical, Electrochemical Aspects of the Biocompatibility of Titanium and its Alloys*. Philadelphia, PA, pp. 163–165.
271. Jaschke, W., Klose, K.J. and Strecker, E.P., 1992, A new balloon-expandable tantalum stent (Strecker-Stent) for the biliry system: Preliminary Experince, *Cardiovasc Intervent Radiol* 15:356–359. doi: http://dx.doi.org/10.1007/BF02734118
272. Johasson, C.B., Hansson, H.A. and Albreksson, T., 1990, Qualitative interfacial study between bone and tantalum, niobium or commercially pure titanium, *Biomaterials* 11:277–280. doi: http://dx.doi.org/10.1016/0142-9612(90)90010-N
273. Matsuno, H., Yokoyama, A., Watari, F., Uno, M. and Kawasaki, T., 2001, Biocompatibility and osteogenesis of refractory metal implants, titanium, hafnium, niobium, tantalum and rhenium, *Biomaterials* 22:1253–1262. doi: http://dx.doi.org/10.1016/S0142-9612(00)00275-1
274. Dolatshahi-Pirouz, A., Jensen, T., Kraft, D.C., Foss, M., Kingshott, P., Hansen, J.L., Larsen, A.N., Chevallier, J. and Besenbacher, F., 2010, Fibronectin adsorption, cell adhesion, and proliferation on nanostructured tantalum surfaces, *ACS Nano 4:*2874–2882. doi: http://dx.doi.org/10.1021/nn9017872
275. Lee, S.L., Cipollo, M., Windover, D. and Rickard, C., 1999, Analysis of magnetron-sputtered tantalum coatings versus electrochemically deposited tantalum from molten salt, *Surf Coat Tech* 120/121:44–52. doi: http://dx.doi.org/10.1016/S0257-8972(99)00337-0
276. Sartwell, S.D., Natishan, P.N., Donovan, E.P., Bunker, S.N. and Armini, A.J., 1996, Composition and corrosion properties of reactive-oxygen tantalum and niobium-implanted 52100 steel and aluminum, *Surf Coat Tech* 83:183–188. doi: http://dx.doi.org/10.1016/0257-8972(95)02842-0
277. Macionczyk, R., Gerold, B. and Thull, R., 2001, Repassivating tantalum/tantalum oxide surface modification on stainless steel implants, *Surf Coat Tech* 142/144:1084–1087. doi: http://dx.doi.org/10.1016/S0257-8972(01)01096-9
278. Cheng, Y., Cai, W., Li, H.T. and Zheng, Y.F., 2006, Surface modification of NiTi alloy with tantalum to improve its biocompatibility and radiopacity, *J Mater Sci* 41:4961–4964. doi: http://dx.doi.org/10.1007/s10853-006-0096-6
279. Spriano, S., Vernè, E., Guala, C., Faga, M.G. and Eitel, F., 2009, Surface modification of cobalt alloys for articular prostheses, *J Bone Joint Surg Br* 91:265–266.
280. Pham, V-H., Lee, S-H., Li, Y., Kim, H-E., Shin, K-H. and Koh, Y-H., 2012, Utility of tantalum (Ta) coating to improve surface hardness *in vitro* bioactivity and biocompatibility of Co–Cr, *Thin Solid Films* 536:269–274. doi: http://dx.doi.org/10.1016/j.tsf.2013.03.042
281. Levine, B.R., Sporer, S., Poggie, R.A., Della Valle, C.J. and Jacobs, J.J., 2006, Experimental and clinical performance of porous tantalum in orthopedic surgery, *Biomaterials* 27:4671–4681. doi: http://dx.doi.org/10.1016/j.biomaterials.2006.04.041
282. Macheras, G.A., Papagelopoulos, P.J., Kateros, K., Kostakos, A.T., Baltas, D. and Karachalios, T.S., 2006, Radiological evaluation of the metal–bone interface of a porous tantalum monoblock acetabular component, *J Bone Joint Surg Br* 88:304–309. doi: http://dx.doi.org/10.1302/0301-620X.88B3.16940

283. Balla, V.K., Bodhak, S., Bose, S. and Bandyopadhyay, A., 2010, Porous tantalum structures for bone implants: Fabrication, mechanical and in vitro biological properties, *Acta Biomater* 6:3349–3359. doi: http://dx.doi.org/10.1016/j.actbio.2010.01.046
284. Olivares-Navarrete, R., Olaya, J.J., Ramírez, C. and Rodil, S.E., 2011, Biocompatibility of niobium coatings, *Coatings* 1:72–87. doi: http://dx.doi.org/10.3390/coatings1010072
285. Ramírez, G., Rodil, S.E., Arzate, H., Muhl, S. and Olaya, J.J., 2011, Niobium based coatings for dental implants, *Appl Surf Sci* 257:2555–2559. doi: http://dx.doi.org/10.1016/j.apsusc.2010.10.021
286. Liu, B.T., Yan, X.B., Zhang, X., Zhou, Y., Guo, Y.N., Bian, F., Zhang, X.Y., 2009, Investigation of oxidation resistance of Ni–Ti film used as oxygen diffusion barrier layer, *Appl Surf Sci* 255:6179–6182. doi: http://dx.doi.org/10.1016/j.apsusc.2009.01.081
287. Liu, X., Wu, S., Yeung, K.W.K., Chan, Y.L., Hu, T., Xu, Z., Liu, X., Chung, J.C.Y., Cheung, K.M.C. and Chu, P.K., 2011, Relationship between osseointegration and superelastic biomechanics in porous NiTi scaffolds, *Biomaterials* 32:330–338. doi: http://dx.doi.org/10.1016/j.biomaterials.2010.08.102
288. Bansiddhi, A., Sargeant, T.D., Stupp, S.I. and Dunand, D.C., 2008, Porous NiTi for bone implants: A review, *Acta Biomater* 4:773–782. doi: http://dx.doi.org/10.1016/j.actbio.2008.02.009
289. Salunke, P., Shanov, V. and Witte, F., 2011, High purity biodegradable magnesium coating for implant application, *Mater Sci Eng B* 176:1711–1717. doi: http://dx.doi.org/10.1016/j.mseb.2011.07.002
290. Yang, J., Cui, F. and Lee, I.S., 2011, Surface modifications of magnesium alloys for biomedical applications, *Annals of Biomed Eng* 39:1857–1871. doi: http://dx.doi.org/10.1007/s10439-011-0300-y
291. Kirkland, N.T., Birbilis, N. and Staiger, M.P., 2012, Assessing the corrosion of biodegradable magnesium implants: A critical review of current methodologies and their limitations, *Acta Biomater* 8:925–936. doi: http://dx.doi.org/10.1016/j.actbio.2011.11.014
292. Virtanen, S., 2011, Biodegradable Mg and Mg alloys: Corrosion and biocompatibility, *Mater Sci Eng B* 176:1600–1608. doi: http://dx.doi.org/10.1016/j.mseb.2011.05.028
293. Yuen, C.K. and Ip, W.Y., 2010, Theoretical risk assessment of magnesium alloys as degradable biomedical implants, *Acta Biomater* 6:1808–1812. doi: http://dx.doi.org/10.1016/j.actbio.2009.11.036
294. Li, Y., Wen, C., Mushahary, D., Sravanthi, R., Harishankar, N., Pande, G. and Hodgson, P., 2012, Mg–Zr–Sr alloys as biodegradable implant materials, *Acta Biomater* 8:3177–3188. doi: http://dx.doi.org/10.1016/j.actbio.2012.04.028
295. Yang, X., Li, M., Lin, X., Tan, L., Lan, G., Li, L., Yin, Q., Xia, H., Zhang, Y. and Yang, K., 2013, Enhanced in vitro biocompatibility/bioactivity of biodegradable Mg–Zn–Zr alloy by microarc oxidation coating contained Mg_2SiO_4, *Surf Coat Tech* 233:65–73. doi: http://dx.doi.org/10.1016/j.surfcoat.2013.01.052
296. Li, M., Cheng, Y., Zheng, Y.F., Zhang, X., Xi, T.F. and S.C. Wei, S.C., 2012, Plasma enhanced chemical vapor deposited silicon coatings on Mg alloy for biomedical application, *Surf Coat Tech* 228:S262-S265. doi: http://dx.doi.org/10.1016/j.surfcoat.2012.05.128
297. Krishna, B.V., Xue, W., Bose, S. and Bandyopadhyay, A., 2008, Functionally graded Co–Cr–Mo coating on Ti–6Al–4V alloy structures, *Acta Biomater* 4:697–706. doi: http://dx.doi.org/10.1016/j.actbio.2007.10.005
298. Holinka, J., Pilz, M., Kubista, B., Presterl, E. and Windhager, R., 2013, Effects of selenium coating of orthopaedic implant surfaces on bacterial adherence and osteoblastic cell growth, *Bone Joint J* 95:678–682. doi: http://dx.doi.org/10.1302/0301-620X.95B5.31216

299. Gomes, M.E. and Reis, R.L., 2004, Biodegradable polymers and composites in biomedical applications: from catgut to tissue engineering. Part 1: Available systems and their properties, *Int Mater Rev* 49:261–273. doi: http://dx.doi.org/10.1179/095066004225021918
300. Gomes, M.E. and Reis, R.L., 2004, Biodegradable polymers and composites in biomedical applications: from catgut to tissue engineering. Part 2: Systems for temporary replacement and advanced tissue regeneration, *Int Mater Rev* 49:274–285. doi: http://dx.doi.org/10.1179/095066004225021918
301. Wong, H.M., Yeung, K.W.K., Lam, K.O., Tam, V., Chu, P.K., Luk, K.D.K. and Cheung, K.M.C., 2010, A biodegradable polymer-based coating to control the performance of magnesium alloy orthopaedic implants, *Biomaterials* 31:2084–2096. doi: http://dx.doi.org/10.1016/j.biomaterials.2009.11.111
302. Tepe, G., Schmehl, J., Wendel, H.P., Schaffner, S., Heller, S., Gianotti, M., Claussen, C.D. and Duda, S.H., 2006, Reduced thrombogenicity of nitinol stents—In vitro evaluation of different surface modifications and coatings, *Biomaterials* 27:643–650. doi: http://dx.doi.org/10.1016/j.biomaterials.2005.06.004
303. Bakhshi, R., Darbyshire, A., Evans, J.E., You, Z., Lu, J. and Seifalian, A.M., 2011, Polymeric coating of surface modified nitinol stent with POSS-nanocomposite polymer, *Colloids Surf B: Biointerfaces* 86:93–105. doi: http://dx.doi.org/10.1016/j.colsurfb.2011.03.024
304. Ye, S.H., Carl A. Johnson, Jr. J., Woolley, R., Oh, H-I., Gamble, L.J., Ishihara, K. and Wagner, W.R., 2009, Surface modification of a titanium alloy with a phospholipid polymer prepared by a plasma-induced grafting technique to improve surface thromboresistance; *Colloids Surf B: Biointerfaces* 74:96–102. doi: http://dx.doi.org/10.1016/j.colsurfb.2009.06.032
305. Nakahira, A., Tamai, M., Miki, S. and Pezzotti, G., 2002, Fractrure behavior and biocompatibility evaluation of nylon-infiltrated porous hydroxyapatite, *J Mater Sci* 37:4425–4430. doi: http://dx.doi.org/10.1023/A:1020681309572
306. Ahmed W., 2007, Titanium dioxide coatings in medical device applications, In: M.J.Jackson ed., *Surface Engineered Surgical Tools and Medical Devices*, Springer-Verlag, Berlin, Germany, pp. 49–63.
307. Oshida, Y., 2007, *Bioscience and Bioengineering of Titanium Materials*, Elsevier, London, UK, p. 91.
308. Saito, T., Takemoto, M., Fukuda, A., Kuroda, Y., Fujibayashi, S., Neo, M., Honjoh, D., Hiraide, T., Kizuki, T., Kokubo, T. and Nakamura, T., 2011, Effect of titania-based surface modification of polyethylene terephthalate on bone–implant bonding and peri-implant tissue reaction, *Acta Biomater* 7:1558–1569. doi: http://dx.doi.org/10.1016/j.actbio.2010.11.018
309. Xie, D., Wan, G., Maitz, M.F., Sun, H. and Huang, N., 2013, Deformation and corrosion behaviors of Ti–O film deposited 316L stainless steel by plasma immersion ion implantation and deposition, *Surf Coat Tech* 214:117–123. doi: http://dx.doi.org/10.1016/j.surfcoat.2012.11.012
310. Siu, H.T. and Man, H.C., 2013, Fabrication of bioactive titania coating on nitinol by plasma electrolytic oxidation, *Appl Surf Sci* 274:181–187. doi: http://dx.doi.org/10.1016/j.apsusc.2013.03.008
311. Liu, J-X., Yang, D-Z., Shi, F. and Cai, Y-J., 2003, Sol–gel deposited TiO_2 film on NiTi surgical alloy for biocompatibility improvement, *Thin Solid Films* 429:225–230. doi: http://dx.doi.org/10.1016/S0040-6090(03)00146-9
312. Wang, H.R., Liu, F., Zhang, Y.P., Yu, D.Z. and F.P. Wang, F.P., 2011, Preparation and properties of titanium oxide film on NiTi alloy by microarc oxidation, *Appl Surf Sci* 257:5576–5580. doi: http://dx.doi.org/10.1016/j.apsusc.2011.01.047

313. Sugita, Y., Ishizaki, K., Iwasa, F., Ueno, T., Minamikawa, H., Yamada, M., Suzuki, T. and Ogawa, T., 2011, Effects of pico-to-nanometer-thin TiO_2 coating on the biological properties of microroughened titanium, *Biomaterials* 32:8374–8384. doi: http://dx.doi.org/10.1016/j.biomaterials.2011.07.077
314. Ou, J., Wang, J., Zhang, D., Zhang, P., Liu, S., Yan, P., Liu, B. and Yang, S., 2010, Fabrication and biocompatibility investigation of TiO_2 films on the polymer substrates obtained via a novel and versatile route, *Colloids Surf B: Biointerfaces* 76:123–127. doi: http://dx.doi.org/10.1016/j.colsurfb.2009.10.024
315. Kim, H-K., Jang, J-W. and Chang-Hee Lee, C-H., 2004, Surface modification of implant materials and its effect on attachment and proliferation of bone cells, *J Mater Sci Mater Med* 15:825–830. doi: http://dx.doi.org/10.1023/B:JMSM.0000032824.62866.a1
316. Oshida, Y., 2007, *Bioscience and Bioengineering of Titanium Materials*, Elsevier, London, UK, pp. 87–89.
317. György, E., Socol, G., Axente, E., Mihailescu, I.N., Ducu, C. and Ciuca, S., 2005, Anatase phase TiO_2 thin films obtained by pulsed laser deposition for gas sensing applications, *Appl Surf Sci* 247:429–433. doi: http://dx.doi.org/10.1016/j.apsusc.2005.01.074
318. Grigal, I.P., Markeev, A.M., Gudkova, S.A., Chernikova, A.G., Mityaev, A.S. and Alekhin, A.P., 2012, Correlation between bioactivity and structural properties of titanium dioxide coatings grown by atomic layer deposition, *Appl Surf Sci* 258:3415–3419. doi: http://dx.doi.org/10.1016/j.apsusc.2011.11.082
319. Hiratani, M., Kadoshima, M., Hirano, T., Shimamoto, Y., Matsui, Y., Nabatame, T., Torii, K. and Kimura, S., 2003, Ultra-thin titanium oxide film with a rutile-type structure, *Appl Surf Sci* 207:13–19. doi: http://dx.doi.org/10.1016/S0169-4332(02)01228-X
320. Ou, K-L., Shih, Y-H., Huang, C-F., Chen, C-C. and Liu, C-M., 2008, Preparation of bioactive amorphous-like titanium oxide layer on titanium by plasma oxidation treatment, *Appl Surf Sci* 255:2046–2051. doi: http://dx.doi.org/10.1016/j.apsusc.2008.06.189
321. Acik, I.O., Junolainen, A., Mikli, V., Danilson, M. and Krunks, M., 2009,Growth of ultra-thin TiO_2 films by spray pyrolysis on different substrates, *Appl Surf Sci* 256:1391–1394. doi: http://dx.doi.org/10.1016/j.apsusc.2009.08.101
322. Rawat, R.S., Aggarwal, V., Hassan, M., Lee, P., Springham, S.V., Tan, T.L. and Lee, S., 2008, Nano-phase titanium dioxide thin film deposited by repetitive plasma focus: Ion irradiation and annealing based phase transformation and agglomeration, *Appl Surf Sci* 255:2932–2941. doi: http://dx.doi.org/10.1016/j.apsusc.2008.08.055
323. Advincula, M., Fan, X., Lemons, J. and Advincula, R., 2005, Surface modification of surface sol–gel derived titanium oxide films by self-assembled monolayers (SAMs) and non-specific protein adsorption studies, *Colloids Surf B: Biointerfaces* 42:29–43. doi: http://dx.doi.org/10.1016/j.colsurfb.2004.12.009
324. Fu, T., Liu, B.G., Zhou, Y.M. and Wu, X.M., 2011, Sol–gel titania coating on NiTi alloy with a porous titania film as interlayer, *J Sol-Gel Sci Technol* 58:307–311. doi: http://dx.doi.org/10.1007/s10971-010-2392-5
325. Shirkhanzadeh, M., 1998, Nanoporous alkoxy-derived titanium oxide coating: a reactive overlayer for functionalizing titanium surface, *J Mater Sci Mater Med* 9:355–362. doi: http://dx.doi.org/10.1023/A:1008883704269
326. Lai, Y.K., Sun, L., Chen, C., Nie, C.G., Zuo, J. and Lin, C.J., 2005, Optical and electrical characterization of TiO_2 nanotube arrays on titanium substrate, *Appl Surf Sci* 252:1101–1106. doi: http://dx.doi.org/10.1016/j.apsusc.2005.02.035
327. Yun, H., Lin, C., Li, J., Wang, J. and Chen, H., 2008, Low-temperature hydrothermal formation of a net-like structured TiO_2 film and its performance of photogenerated cathode protection, *Appl Surf Sci* 255:2113–2117. doi: http://dx.doi.org/10.1016/j.apsusc.2008.06.194

328. Lim, J.I., Yu, B., Woo, K.M. and Lee, Y-K., 2008, Immobilization of TiO_2 nanofibers on titanium plates for implant applications, *Appl Surf Sci* 255:2456–2460. doi: http://dx.doi.org/10.1016/j.apsusc.2008.07.146
329. Shi, X., Tsuru, K., Xu, L., Kawachi, G. and Ishikawa, K., 2013, Effects of solution pH on the structure and biocompatibility of Mg-containing TiO_2 layer fabricated on titanium by hydrothermal treatment, *Appl Surf Sci* 270:445–451. doi: http://dx.doi.org/10.1016/j.apsusc.2013.01.046
330. Park, J-W., Kim, Y-J., Jang, J-H. and An, C-H., 2010, *In vitro* biocompatibility of magnesium- incorporated submicro-porous titanium oxide surface produced by hydrothermal treatment, *Appl Surf Sci* 257:925–931. doi: http://dx.doi.org/10.1016/j.apsusc.2010.07.092
331. Czarnowska, E., Wierzchoń, T. and Maranda-Niedbała, A., 1999, Properties of the surface layers on titanium alloy and their biocompatibility in vitro tests, *J Mater Process Tech* 92/93:190–194. doi: http://dx.doi.org/10.1016/S0924-0136(99)00228-9
332. Huang, F., Xie, B., Wu, B., Shao, L., Li, M., Wang, H., Jiang, Y. and Song, Y., 2009, Enhancing the crystallinity and surface roughness of sputtered TiO_2 thin film by ZnO underlayer, *Appl Surf Sci* 255:6781–6785. doi: http://dx.doi.org/10.1016/j.apsusc.2009.02.060
333. Hang, R., Huang, X., Tian, L., He, Z. and Tang, B., 2012, Preparation, characterization, corrosion behavior and bioactivity of Ni_2O_3-doped TiO_2 nanotubes on NiTi alloy, *Electrochimica Acta* 70:382–393. doi: http://dx.doi.org/10.1016/j.electacta.2012.03.085
334. Zhu, S., Huang, N., Xu, L., Zhang, Y., Liu, H., Lei, Y., Sun, H. and Yao, Y., 2009, Biocompatibility of Fe–O films synthesized by plasma immersion ion implantation and deposition, *Surf Coat Tech* 203:1523–1529. doi: http://dx.doi.org/10.1016/j.surfcoat.2008.11.033
335. Arnould, C., Volcke, C., Lamarque, C., Thiry, P.A., Delhalle, J. and Mekhalif, Z., 2009, Titanium modified with layer-by-layer sol–gel tantalum oxide and an organodiphosphonic acid: A coating for hydroxyapatite growth, *J Colloid Interf Sci* 336:497–503. doi: http://dx.doi.org/10.1016/j.jcis.2009.03.092
336. Maho, A., Linden, S., Arnould, C., Detriche, S., Delhalle, J. and Mekhalif, Z., 2012, Tantalum oxide/carbon nanotubes composite coatings on titanium, and their functionalization with organophosphonic molecular films: A high quality scaffold for hydroxyapatite growth, *J Colloid Interf Sci* 371:150–158. doi: http://dx.doi.org/10.1016/j.jcis.2011.12.066
337. Sollazzo, V., Pezzetti, F., Scarano, A., Piattelli, A., Bignozzi, C.A., Massari, L., Brunelli, G. and Carinci, F., 2008, Zirconium oxide coating improves implant osseointegration in vivo, *Dent Mater* 24:357–361. doi: http://dx.doi.org/10.1016/j.dental.2007.06.003
338. Yan, Y., Han, Y. and Lu, C., 2008, The effect of chemical treatment on apatite-forming ability of the macroporous zirconia films formed by microarc oxidation, *Appl Surf Sci* 254:4833–4839. doi: http://dx.doi.org/10.1016/j.apsusc.2008.01.117
339. Li, J., Hermansson, L. and Söremark, R., 1993, Joining of ceramics of different biofunction by hot isostatic pressing, *J Am Ceramic Soc* 76:2685–2686. doi: http://dx.doi.org/10.1111/j.1151-2916.1993.tb04002.x
340. Balla, V.K., Xue, W., Bose, S. and Bandyopadhyay, A., 2009, Laser-assisted Zr/ZrO_2 coating on Ti for load-bearing implants, *Acta Biomater* 5:2800–2809. doi: http://dx.doi.org/10.1016/j.actbio.2009.03.032
341. Emadi, R., Tavangarian, F., Esfahani, S.I.R., Sheikhhosseini, A. and Kharaziha, M., 2010, Nanostructured forsterite coating strengthens porous hydroxyapatite for bone tissue engineering, *J Am Ceram Soc* 93:2679–2683. doi: http://dx.doi.org/10.1111/j.1551-2916.2010.03817.x
342. Arcos, D. and Vallet-Regí, M., 2010, Sol–gel silica-based biomaterials and bone tissue regeneration, *Acta Biomater* 6:2874–2888. doi: http://dx.doi.org/10.1016/j.actbio.2010.02.012

343. Pérez, P., Haanappel, V.A.C. and Stroosnijder, M.F., 2001, Formation of an alumina layer on A FeCrAlY alloy by thermal oxidation for potential medical implant applications, *Surf Coat Tech* 139:207–215. doi: http://dx.doi.org/10.1016/S0257-8972(00)01169-5
344. Ezz, T., Crouse, P., Li, L, and Liu, Z., 2007, Synthesis of TiN thin films by a new combined laser/sol–gel processing technique, *Appl Surf Sci* 253:7903–7907. doi: http://dx.doi.org/10.1016/j.apsusc.2007.02.189
345. Shenhar, A., Gotman, I., Radin, S., Ducheyne, P. and Gutmanas, E.Y., 2000, Titanium nitride coatings on surgical titanium alloys produced by a powder immersion reaction assisted coating method: residual stresses and fretting behavior, *Surf Coat Tech* 126:210–218. doi: http://dx.doi.org/10.1016/S0257-8972(00)00524-7
346. Hübler, R., 1999, Hardness and corrosion protection enhancement behaviour of surgical implant surfaces treated with ceramic thin films, *Surf Coat Tech* 116/119:1111–1115. doi: http://dx.doi.org/10.1016/S0257-8972(99)00221-2
347. Xiao, L., Yan, D., He, J., Zhu, L., Dong, Y., Zhang, J. and Li, X., 2007, Nanostructured TiN coating prepared by reactive plasma spraying in atmosphere, *Appl Surf Sci* 253:7535–7539. doi: http://dx.doi.org/10.1016/j.apsusc.2007.03.062
348. Mutlu, I., 2013, Sinter-coating method for production of TiN coated titanium foam for biomedical implant applications, *Surf Coat Tech* 232:396–402. doi: http://dx.doi.org/10.1016/j.surfcoat.2013.05.041
349. Mao, Z., Ma, J., Wang, J. and Sun, B., 2007, The effect of powder preparation method on the corrosion and mechanical properties of TiN-based coatings by reactive plasma spraying, *Appl Surf Sci* 255:3784–3788. doi: http://dx.doi.org/10.1016/j.apsusc.2008.10.047
350. Flores, M., Huerta, L., Escamilla, R., Andrade, E. and Muhl, S., 2007, Effect of substrate bias voltage on corrosion of TiN/Ti multilayers deposited by magnetron sputtering, *Appl Surf Sci* 253:7192–7196. doi: http://dx.doi.org/10.1016/j.apsusc.2007.02.203
351. Hyde, G.K., McCullen, S.D., Jeon, S., Stewart, S.M., Jeon, H., Loboa, E.G. and G N Parsons, G.N., 2009, Atomic layer deposition and biocompatibility of titanium nitride nano-coatings on cellulose fiber substrates, *Biomed Mater* 4. doi: http://dx.doi.org/10.1088/1748-6041/4/2/025001
352. Balla, V.K., Bhat, A., Bose, S. and Bandyopadhyay, A., 2012, Laser processed TiN reinforced Ti6Al4V composite coatings, *J Mech Behav Biomed Mater* 6:9–20. doi: http://dx.doi.org/10.1016/j.jmbbm.2011.09.007
353. Rieder, P., Scherrer, S., Filieri, A., Wiskott, H.W.A. and Durual,S., 2012,TiNOx coatings increase human primary osteoblasts proliferation independenty of the substrate—A short report, *Bio-Med Mater Eng* 22:277–281.
354. Freemanm, C.O. and Brook, I.M., 2006, Bone response to a titanium aluminium nitride coating on metallic implants, *J Mater Sci Mater Med* 17:465–470. doi: http://dx.doi.org/10.1007/s10856-006-8474-9
355. Mukherjee, S., Maitz, M.F., Pham, M.T., Richter, E., Prokert, F. and Moeller, W., 2005, Development and biocompatibility of hard Ti-based coatings using plasma immersion ion implantation-assisted deposition, *Surf Coat Tech* 196:312–316. doi: http://dx.doi.org/10.1016/j.surfcoat.2004.08.202
356. García, G.L., Hernández, T.J., Flores, R.N., Argumedo, M.P., López,V.A., Araujo, L.D.J. and Courrech, A.A.M., 2013, Influence of nitrogen in TiAlNO coatings fabricated by co-sputtering, *IOP Conf Ser: Mater Sci Eng* 45. doi: http://dx.doi.org/10.1088/1757-899X/45/1/012024
357. Shtansky, D.V., Grigoryan, A.S., Toporkova, A.K., Arkhipov, A.V., Sheveyko, A.N. and Kiryukhantsev-Korneev, P.V., 2011, Modification of polytetrafluoroethylene implants by depositing TiCaPCON films with and without stem cells, *Surf Coat Tech* 206:1188–1195. doi: http://dx.doi.org/10.1016/j.surfcoat.2011.08.029

358. Brama, M., Rhodes, N., Hunt, J., Ricci, A., Teghil, R., Migliaccio, S., Rocca, C.D., Leccisotti, S., Lioi, A., Scandurra, M., De Maria, G., Ferro, D., Pu, F., Panzini, G., Politi, L. and Scandurra, R., 2007, Effect of titanium carbide coating on the osseointegration response in vitro and in vivo, *Biomaterials* 28: 595–608. doi: http://dx.doi.org/10.1016/j.biomaterials.2006.08.018
359. Tian, Y.S., Chen, C.Z., Chen, L.B. and Chen, L.X., 2006, Study on the microstructure and wear resistance of the composite coatings fabricated on Ti–6Al–4V under different processing conditions, *Appl Surf Sci* 253:1494–1499. doi: http://dx.doi.org/10.1016/j.apsusc.2006.02.026
360. Levashov, E.A., Petrzhik, M.I., Kiryukhantsev-Korneev, F.V., Shtansky, D.V., Prokoshkin, S.D., Gunderov, D.V., Sheveiko, A.N., Korotitsky, A.V. and R. Z. Valiev, R.Z., 2012, Structure and mechanical behavior during indentation of biocompatible nanostructured titanium alloys and coatings, *Metallurgist* 56:395–407. doi: http://dx.doi.org/10.1007/s11015-012-9589-5
361. Rogers, K.D., Etok, S.E. and R.Scott, R., 2004, Structural characterization of apatite coatings, *J Mater Sci* 39:5747–5754. doi: http://dx.doi.org/10.1023/B:JMSC.0000040085.43633.8a
362. Jaffe, W.L. and Scott, D.F., 1996, Current concepts review—Total hip arthroplasty with hydroxyapatite-coated prostheses, *J Bone Joint Surg Am* 78:1918–1934.
363. Ong, J.L. and Daniel C. N. Chan, D.C.N., 2000, Hydroxyapatite and their use as coatings in dental implants: A review, *Crit Rev Biomed Eng* 28:667–707. doi: http://dx.doi.org/10.1615/CritRevBiomedEng.v28.i56.10
364. Arias, J.L., Mayor, M.B., Pou, J., León, B. and Pérez-Amor, M., 2002, Transport of ablated material through a water vapor atmosphere in pulsed laser deposition of hydroxylapatite, *Appl Surf Sci* 186:448–452. doi: http://dx.doi.org/10.1016/S0169-4332(01)00734-6
365. Stiegler, N., Bellucci, D., Bolelli, G., Cannillo, V., Gadow, R., Killinger, A., Lusvarghi, L. and Sola, A., 2012, High-velocity suspension flame sprayed (HVSFS) hydroxyapatite coatings for biomedical applications, *J Therm Spray Tech* 21:275–287. doi: http://dx.doi.org/10.1007/s11666-011-9724-z
366. Guo, C.Y., Tang, A.T.H. and Jukka Pekka Matinlinna, J.P., 2012, Insights into surface treatment methods of titanium dental implants, *J Adhes Sci Technol* 26:189–205.
367. Hirai, S., Nishinaka, K., Shimakage, K., Uo, M. and Watari, F., 2004, Hydroxyapatite Coating on Titanium Substrate by the Sol-Gel Process, *J Amer Ceramic Soc* 87:29–34. doi: http://dx.doi.org/10.1111/j.1151-2916.2004.tb19940.x
368. Hahn, B-D., Park, D-S., Choi, J-J., Ryu, J., Yoon, W-H., Kim, K-H., Park, C. and Kim, H-E., 2009, Dense nanostructured hydroxyapatite coating on titanium by aerosol deposition, *J Am Ceramic Soc* 92:68–687. doi: http://dx.doi.org/10.1111/j.1551-2916.2008.02876.x
369. Mansur, M.R., Wang, J. and Berndt, C.C., 2013, Microstructure, composition and hardness of laser assisted hydroxyapatite and Ti–6Al–4V composite coatings, *Surf Coat Tech* 232:482–488. doi: http://dx.doi.org/10.1016/j.surfcoat.2013.06.006
370. Parast, S.Y., Jauhari, I. and Zaeem, M.A., 2011, Implantation of HA into superplastic Ti-6Al-4V: Kinetics and mechanical behaviors of implanted layer, *Metallurg Mater Trans A* 42:219–226. doi: http://dx.doi.org/10.1007/s11661-010-0504-z
371. Hung, K-Y., Lo, S-C., Shih, C-S., Yang, Y-C., Feng, H-P. and Lin, Y-C., 2012, Titanium surface modified by hydroxyapatite coating for dental implants, *Surf Coat Tech* 231:337–345. doi: http://dx.doi.org/10.1016/j.surfcoat.2012.03.037
372. Luo, R., Liu, Z., Yan, F., Kong, Y. and Zhang, Y., 2013, The biocompatibility of hydroxyapatite film deposition on microarc oxidation Ti6Al4V alloy, *Appl Surf Sci* 266:57–61. doi: http://dx.doi.org/10.1016/j.apsusc.2012.11.074

373. Maleki-Ghaleh, H., Khalili, V., Khalil-Allafi, J. and Javidi, M., 2012, Hydroxyapatite coating on NiTi shape memory alloy by electrophoretic deposition process, *Surf Coat Tech* 208:57–63. doi: http://dx.doi.org/10.1016/j.surfcoat.2012.08.001
374. Gopi, D., Indira, J., Kavitha, L. and J. M. F. Ferreira, J.M.F., 2013, Hydroxyapatite coating on selectively passivated and sensitively polymer-protected surgical grade stainless steel, *J Appl Electroch* 43:331–345., doi: http://dx.doi.org/10.1007/s10800-012-0508-z
375. Kar, A., Raja, K.S. and M. Misra, M., 2006, Electrodeposition of hydroxyapatite onto nanotubular TiO_2 for implant applications, *Surf Coat Tech* 201:3723–3731. doi: http://dx.doi.org/10.1016/j.surfcoat.2006.09.008
376. Cao, N., Dong, J., Wang, Q., Q., Ma, Xue, C. and Li, M., 2010, An experimental bone defect healing with hydroxyapatite coating plasma sprayed on carbon/carbon composite implants, *Surf Coat Tech* 205:1150–1156. doi: http://dx.doi.org/10.1016/j.surfcoat.2010.05.008
377. Kong, Y-M., Bae, C-J., Lee, S-H., Kim, H-W. and Kim, H-E., 2005, Improvement in biocompatibility of by addition of HA, *Biomaterials* 26:509–517. doi: http://dx.doi.org/10.1016/j.biomaterials.2004.02.061
378. Nelea, V., Morosanu, C., Iliescu, M. and Mihailescu, I.N., 2004, Hydroxyapatite thin films grown by pulsed laser deposition and radio-frequency magnetron sputtering: Comparative study, *Appl Surf Sci* 228:346–356. doi: http://dx.doi.org/10.1016/j.apsusc.2004.01.029
379. Nelea, V., Pelletier, H., Müller, D., Broll, N., Mille, P., Ristoscu, C. and Mihailescu, I. N., 2002, Mechanical properties improvement of pulsed laser-deposited hydroxyapatite thin films by high energy ion-beam implantation, *Appl Surf Sci* 186:483–489. doi: http://dx.doi.org/10.1016/S0169-4332(01)00754-1
380. Grigorescu, S., Carradò, A., Ulhaq, C., Faerber, J., Ristoscu, C., Dorcioman, G., Axente, E., Werckmann, J. and Mihailescu, I.N., 2007,Study of the gradual interface between hydroxyapatite thin films PLD grown onto Ti-controlled sublayers, *Appl Surf Sci* 254:1150–1154. doi: http://dx.doi.org/10.1016/j.apsusc.2007.09.056
381. Yang, S., Xing, W. and Man, H.C., 2009, Pulsed laser deposition of hydroxyapatite film on laser gas nitriding NiTi substrate, *Appl Surf Sci* 255:9889–9892. doi: http://dx.doi.org/10.1016/j.apsusc.2009.04.113
382. Lee, K., Choe, H-C., Kim, B-H. and Ko, Y-M., 2010, The biocompatibility of HA thin films deposition on anodized titanium alloys, *Surf Coat Tech* 205:S267-S270. doi: http://dx.doi.org/10.1016/j.surfcoat.2010.08.015
383. Jeong, Y-H., Choe, H-C., Brantley, W.A. and Sohn, I-B., 2013, Hydroxyapatite thin film coatings on nanotube-formed Ti–35Nb–10Zr alloys after femtosecond laser texturing, *Surf Coat Tech* 217:13–22. doi: http://dx.doi.org/10.1016/j.surfcoat.2012.11.066
384. Lee, S-H., Kim, H-E. and Kim, H-W., 2007, Nano-sized hydroxyapatite coatings on Ti substrate with TiO_2 buffer layer by E-beam deposition, *J Am Ceram Soc* 90:50–56. doi: http://dx.doi.org/10.1111/j.1551-2916.2006.01351.x
385. Khalid, H.M., Jauhari, I. and Dom, A.H.M., 2012, Development of nanolayer hydroxyapatite (HA) on titanium alloy *via* superplastic deformation method, *Metall Mater Trans A* 43:3776–3785. doi: http://dx.doi.org/10.1007/s11661-012-1185-6
386. Roy, M., Bandyopadhyay, A. and Bose, S., 2011, Induction plasma sprayed nano hydroxyapatite coatings on titanium for orthopaedic and dental implants, *Surf Coat Tech* 205:2785–2792. doi: http://dx.doi.org/10.1016/j.surfcoat.2010.10.042
387. Duta, L., Oktar, F.N., Stan, G.E., Popescu-Pelin, G., Serban, N., Luculescu, C. and Mihailescu, I.N., 2013, Novel doped hydroxyapatite thin films obtained by pulsed laser deposition, *Appl Surf Sci* 265:41–49. doi: http://dx.doi.org/10.1016/j.apsusc.2012.10.077
388. Mohammadi Zahrani, E., Fathi, M.H. and Alfantazi, A.M., 2011, Derived nanocrystalline fluoridated hydroxyapatite powders and nanostructured coatings for tissue engineering

applications, *Metall Mater Trans A* 42:3291–3309. doi: http://dx.doi.org/10.1007/s11661-010-0465-2

389. Tredwin, C.J., Georgiou, G., Kim, H-W. and Knowles, J.C., 2013, Hydroxyapatite, fluor-hydroxyapatite and fluorapatite produced via the sol–gel method: Bonding to titanium and scanning electron microscopy, *Dent Mater* 29:521–529. doi: http://dx.doi.org/10.1016/j.dental.2012.11.008
390. Miao, S., Lin, N., Cheng, K., Yang, D., Huang, X., Han, G., Weng, W. and Ye, Z., 2011, Zn-Releasing FHA coating and its enhanced osseointegration ability, *J Am Ceramic Soc* 94:255–260. doi: http://dx.doi.org/10.1111/j.1551-2916.2010.04038.x
391. Balani, K., Anderson, R., Laha, T., Andara, M., Tercero, J., Crumpler, E. and Agarwal, A., 2007, Plasma-sprayed carbon nanotube reinforced hydroxyapatite coatings and their interaction with human osteoblasts in vitro, *Biomaterials* 28:618–624. doi: http://dx.doi.org/10.1016/j.biomaterials.2006.09.013
392. Zhou, H., Lawrence, J,G., Touny, A.H. and Bhaduri, S.B., 2011, Biomimetic coating of bisphosphonate incorporated CDHA on Ti6Al4V, *J Mater Sci Mater Med* 23:365–374. doi: http://dx.doi.org/10.1007/s10856-011-4524-z
393. Hayakawa, T., Takahashi, K., Okada, H., Yoshinari, M., Hara, H., Mochizuki, C., Yamamoto, H. and Sato, M., 2008, Effect of thin carbonate-containing apatite (CA) coating of titanium fiber mesh on trabecular bone response, *J Mater Sci Mater Med* 19:2087–2096. doi: http://dx.doi.org/10.1007/s10856-007-3293-1
394. Li, H., Zhao, X., Cao, S., Li, K., Chen, M., Xu, Z., Lu, J. and Zhang, L., 2012, Na-doped hydroxyapatite coating on carbon/carbon composites: Preparation, in vitro bioactivity and biocompatibility, *Appl Surf Sci* 263:163–173. doi: http://dx.doi.org/10.1016/j.apsusc.2012.09.022
395. Thian, E.S., Huang, J., Barber, Z.H., Best, S.M. and Bonfield, W., 2011, Surface modification of magnetron-sputtered hydroxyapatite thin films via silicon substitution for orthopaedic and dental applications, *Surf Coat Tech* 205:3472–3477. doi: http://dx.doi.org/10.1016/j.surfcoat.2010.12.012
396. Guo, D.G., Wang, A.H., Han, Y. and Xu, K.W., 2009, Characterization, physicochemical properties and biocompatibility of La-incorporated apatites, *Acta Biomater* 5:3512–3523. doi: http://dx.doi.org/10.1016/j.actbio.2009.05.026
397. Li, Y., Li, Q., Zhu, S., Luo, E., Li, J., Feng, G., Liao, Y. and Hu, J., 2010,The effect of strontium-substituted hydroxyapatite coating on implant fixation in ovariectomized rats, *Biomaterials* 31:9006–9014. doi: http://dx.doi.org/10.1016/j.biomaterials.2010.07.112
398. Bornapour, M., Muja, N., Shum-Tim, D., Cerruti, M. and Pekguleryuz, M., 2013, Biocompatibility and biodegradability of Mg–Sr alloys: The formation of Sr-substituted hydroxyapatite, *Acta Biomater* 9:5319–5330. doi: http://dx.doi.org/10.1016/j.actbio.2012.07.045
399. Ji X., , Lou, W., Wang, Q., Ma, J., Xu, H., Bai, Q., Liu, C. and Jinsong Liu, J., 2012, Sol-gel- derived hydroxyapatite-carbon nanotube/titania coatings on titanium substrates, *Int. J. Mol. Sci 13:*5242–5253. doi: http://dx.doi.org/10.3390/ijms13045242
400. Damia, C., Sarda, S., Deydier, E. and Sharrock, P., 2006, Study of two hydroxyapatite/poly(alkoxysilane) implant coatings, *Surf Coat Tech* 201:3008–3015. doi: http://dx.doi.org/10.1016/j.surfcoat.2006.06.025
401. Tkalcec, E., Sauer, M., Nonninger, R. and Schmidt, H., 2001, Sol-gel-derived hydroxyapatite powders and coatings, *J Mater Sci* 36:5253–5263. doi: http://dx.doi.org/10.1023/A:1012462332440
402. Wang, L. and Luo, J., 2011, Formation of hydroxyapatite coating on anodic titanium dioxide nanotubes *via* an efficient dipping treatment, *Metall Mater Trans A* 42:3255–3264. doi: http://dx.doi.org/10.1007/s11661-010-0484-z

403. Chou, B-Y. and Chang, E., 2003, Influence of deposition temperature on mechanical properties of plasma-sprayed hydroxyapatite coating on titanium alloy with ZrO_2 intermediate layer, *J Therm Spray Technol* 12:199–207. doi: http://dx.doi.org/10.1361/105996303770348302
404. Leem, J.M. and Lim, Y.J., 2010, In vitro investigation of anodization and CaP deposited titanium surface using MG63 osteoblast-like cells, *Appl Surf Sci* 256:3086–3092. doi: http://dx.doi.org/10.1016/j.apsusc.2009.11.078
405. Junker, R., Manders, P.J.D., Wolke, J., Borisov, Y., Braceras, I. and Jansen, J.A., 2010, Loaded microplasma-sprayed CaP-coated implants in vivo, *J Dent Res* 89:1489–1493. doi: http://dx.doi.org/10.1177/0022034510384621
406. Maitz, M.F., Pham, M.T., Matz, W., Reuther, H. and Steiner, G., 2002, Promoted calcium-phosphate precipitation from solution on titanium for improved biocompatibility by ion implantation, *Surf Coat Tech* 158/159:151–156. doi: http://dx.doi.org/10.1016/S0257-8972(02)00189-5
407. Xiropaidis, A.V., Qahash, M., Lim, W.H., Shanaman, R.H., Rohrer, M.D., Wikesjö, U.M.E. and Hall, J., 2005, Bone–implant contact at calcium phosphate-coated and porous titanium oxide (TiUnite™)-modified oral implants, *Clin Oral Implants Res* 16:532–539. doi: http://dx.doi.org/10.1111/j.1600-0501.2005.01126.x
408. Zhang, B., Lu, J., Chen, J., Zhang, X., Gu, Z. and Yang, X., 2010, Biomimetic Ca–P coating on pre-calcified Ti plates by electrodeposition method, *Appl Surf Sci* 256:2700–2704. doi: http://dx.doi.org/10.1016/j.apsusc.2009.11.004
409. Ribeiro, A.A., Balestra, R.M., Rocha, M.N., Peripolli, S.B., Andrade, M.C., Pereira, L.C. and Oliveira. M.V., 2013, Dense and porous titanium substrates with a biomimetic calcium phosphate coating, *Appl Surf Sci* 265:250–256. doi: http://dx.doi.org/10.1016/j.apsusc.2012.10.189
410. Narayanan, R., Seshadri, S.K., Kwon, T.Y. and Kim, K.H., 2008, Calcium phosphate-based coatings on titanium and its alloys, *J Biomed Mater Res B Appl Biomater* 85:279–299. doi: http://dx.doi.org/10.1002/jbm.b.30932
411. Paital, S.R., Bunce, N., Nandwana, P., Honrao, C., Nag, S., He, W., Banerjee, R. and Dahotre, N.B., 2011, Laser surface modification for synthesis of textured bioactive and biocompatible Ca–P coatings on Ti–6Al–4V, *J Mater Sci Mater Med* 22:1393–1406. doi: http://dx.doi.org/10.1007/s10856-011-4321-8
412. Durdu, S., Deniz, Ö.F., Kutbay, I. and Usta, M., 2013, Characterization and formation of hydroxyapatite on Ti6Al4V coated by plasma electrolytic oxidation, *J Alloys Compd* 551:422–429. doi: http://dx.doi.org/10.1016/j.jallcom.2012.11.024
413. Symietz, C., Lehmann, E., Gildenhaar, R., Koter, R., Berger, G. and Krüger, J., 2011, Fixation of bioactive calcium alkali phosphate on Ti6Al4V implant material with femtosecond laser pulses, *Appl Surf Sci* 257:5208–5212. doi: http://dx.doi.org/10.1016/j.apsusc.2010.10.046
414. Yu, S., Yu, Z., Wang, G., Han, J., Ma, X. and Dargusch, M.S., 2011, Biocompatibility and osteoconduction of active porous calcium–phosphate films on a novel Ti–3Zr–2Sn–3Mo–25Nb biomedical alloy, *Colloids and Surf B: Biointerfaces* 85:103–115;. doi
415. Wang, Y., Khor, K.A. and Cheang, P., 1998, Thermal spraying of functionally graded calcium phosphate coatings for biomedical implants, *J Therm Spray Technol* 7:50–57. doi: http://dx.doi.org/10.1361/105996398770351034
416. Chen, D., Bertollo, N., Lau, A., Taki, N., Nishino, T., Mishima, H., Kawamura, H. and Walsh, W.R., 2011, Osseointegration of porous titanium implants with and without electrochemically deposited DCPD coating in an ovine model, *J Orthopaedic Surg Res* **6.** doi: http://dx.doi.org/10.1186/1749-799X-6-56

417. Lin, K., Yuan, W., Wang, L., Lu, J., Chen, L. and Jiang, Z.W., 2011, Evaluation of host inflammatory responses of β-tricalcium phosphate bioceramics caused by calcium pyrophosphate impurity using a subcutaneous model, *J Biomed Mater Res B Appl Biomater* 99:350–358. doi: http://dx.doi.org/10.1002/jbm.b.31906
418. Roy, M., Krishna, B.V., Bandyopadhyay, A. and Bose, S., 2008, Laser processing of bioactive tricalcium phosphate coating on titanium for load-bearing implants, *Acta Biomater* 4:324–333. doi: http://dx.doi.org/10.1016/j.actbio.2007.09.008
419. Mo, A., Liao, J., Xu, W., Xian, S., Li, Y. and Bai, S., 2008, Preparation and antibacterial effect of silver–hydroxyapatite/titania nanocomposite thin film on titanium, *Appl Surf Sci* 255:435–438. doi: http://dx.doi.org/10.1016/j.apsusc.2008.06.083
420. Sima, F., Socol, G., Axente, E., Mihailescu, I.N., Zdrentu, L., Petrescu, S.M. and Mayer, I., 2007, Biocompatible and bioactive coatings of Mn^{2+}-doped β-tricalcium phosphate synthesized by pulsed laser deposition, *Appl Surf Sci* 254:1155–1159. doi: http://dx.doi.org/10.1016/j.apsusc.2007.08.053
421. Mirhosseini, N., Crouse, P.L., Li, L. and Garrod, D., 2007, Combined laser/sol–gel synthesis of calcium silicate coating on Ti–6Al–4V substrates for improved cell integration, *Appl Surf Sci* 253:7998–8002. doi: http://dx.doi.org/10.1016/j.apsusc.2007.02.172
422. Wu, C., Ramaswamy, Y., Gale, D., Yang, W., Xiao, K., Zhang, L., Yin, Y. and Zreiqat, H., 2008, Novel sphene coatings on Ti–6Al–4V for orthopedic implants using sol–gel method, *Acta Biomater* 4:569–576. doi: http://dx.doi.org/10.1016/j.actbio.2007.11.005
423. Ng, B.S., Annergren, I., Soutar, A.M., Khor, K.A. and Jarfors, A.E.W., 2005, Characterisation of a duplex TiO_2/CaP coating on Ti6Al4V for hard tissue replacement, *Biomaterials* 26:1087–1095. doi: http://dx.doi.org/10.1016/j.biomaterials.2004.04.022
424. Bedi, R.S., Beving, D.E., Zanello, L.P. and Yan, Y., 2009, Biocompatibility of corrosion-resistant zeolite coatings for titanium alloy biomedical implants, *Acta Biomater* 5:3265–3271. doi: http://dx.doi.org/10.1016/j.actbio.2009.04.019
425. Yao, Z., Jiang, Y., Jia, F., Jiang, Z. and Wang, F., 2008, Growth characteristics of plasma electrolytic oxidation ceramic coatings on Ti–6Al–4V alloy, *Appl Surf Sci* 254:4084–4091. doi: http://dx.doi.org/10.1016/j.apsusc.2007.12.062
426. Moskalewicz, T., Seuss, S. and Boccaccini, A.R., 2013, Microstructure and properties of composite polyetheretherketone/Bioglass® coatings deposited on Ti–6Al–7Nb alloy for medical applications, *Appl Surf Sci* 273:62–67. doi: http://dx.doi.org/10.1016/j.apsusc.2013.01.174
427. Peddi, L., Brow, R.K. and Brown, R.F., 2008, Bioactive borate glass coatings for titanium alloys, *J Mater Sci Mater Med* 19:3145–3152. doi: http://dx.doi.org/10.1007/s10856-008-3419-0
428. Stan, G.E., Popa, A.C., Galca, A.C., Aldica, G. and Ferreira, J.M.F., 2013, Strong bonding between sputtered bioglass–ceramic films and Ti-substrate implants induced by atomic inter-diffusion post-deposition heat-treatments, *Appl Surf Sci* 280:530–538. doi: http://dx.doi.org/10.1016/j.apsusc.2013.05.022
429. Lee, C-K., 2012, Fabrication, characterization and wear corrosion testing of bioactive hydroxyapatite/nano-TiO_2 composite coatings on anodic Ti–6Al–4V substrate for biomedical applications, *Mater Sci Eng B*, 177:810–818. doi: http://dx.doi.org/10.1016/j.mseb.2012.03.034
430. He, G., Hu, J., Wei, S.C., Li, J.H., Liang, X.H. and Luo, E., 2008, Surface modification of titanium by nano-TiO_2/HA bioceramic coating, *Appl Surf Sci* 255:442–445. doi: http://dx.doi.org/10.1016/j.apsusc.2008.06.088
431. Han, J.Y., Yu, Z.T. and Zhou, L., 2008, Hydroxyapatite/titania composite bioactivity coating processed by sol–gel method, *Appl Surf Sci* 255:455–458. doi: http://dx.doi.org/10.1016/j.apsusc.2008.06.072

432. Wei, D., Zhou, Y., Jia, D. and Wang, Y., 2008, Chemical treatment of TiO_2-based coatings formed by plasma electrolytic oxidation in electrolyte containing nano-HA, calcium salts and phosphates for biomedical applications, *Appl Surf Sci* 254:1775–1782. doi: http://dx.doi.org/10.1016/j.apsusc.2007.07.144
433. Sarao, T.P.S., Sidhu, H.S. and Singh, H., 2012, Characterization and *in vitro* corrosion investigations of thermal sprayed hydroxyapatite and hydroxyapatite-titania coatings on Ti alloy, *Metall Mater Trans A* 43:4365–4376. doi: http://dx.doi.org/10.1007/s11661-012-1175-8
434. Evis, Z. and Doremus, R.H., 2007, Hot-pressed hydroxyapatite/monoclinic zirconia comnposites with improved mechanical properties, *J Mater Sci* 42:2426–2431. doi: http://dx.doi.org/10.1007/s10853-006-1299-6
435. Evis, Z., Ergun, C. and Doremus, R.H., 2005, Hydroxyapatite-zirconia composites: Thermal stability of phases and sinterability as related to the Cao-ZrO_2 phase diagram, *J Mater Sci* 40:127–1134. doi: http://dx.doi.org/10.1007/s10853-005-6928-y
436. Tanaskovic, D., Jokic, B., Socol, G., Popescu, A., Mihailescu, I.N., Petrovic, R. and Janackovic, D., 2007, Synthesis of functionally graded bioactive glass-apatite multistructures on Ti substrates by pulsed laser deposition, *Appl Surf Sci* 254:1279–1282. doi: http://dx.doi.org/10.1016/j.apsusc.2007.08.009
437. Lee, E-J., Chae, S-Y., Kim, H-E. and Kim, H-W., 2006, Improvement in biocompatibility of fluoridated apatite with addition of resorbable glass, *J Am Ceramic Soc* 89:1748–1751. doi: http://dx.doi.org/10.1111/j.1551-2916.2006.00952.x
438. Pei, X., Wang, J., Wan, Q., Kang, L., Xiao, M. and Bao, H., 2011, Functionally graded carbon nanotubes/hydroxyapatite composite coating by laser cladding, *Surf Coat Tech* 205:4380–4387. doi: http://dx.doi.org/10.1016/j.surfcoat.2011.03.036
439. Facca, S., Lahiri, D., Fioretti, F., Messadeq, N., Mainard, D., Benkirane-Jessel, N. and Agarwal, A., 2011, *In vivo* osseointegration of nano-designed composite coatings on titanium implants, *ACS Nano* 5:4790–4799. doi: http://dx.doi.org/10.1021/nn200768c
440. Lin, K., Zhang, M., Zhai, W., Qu, H. and Chang, J., 2011, Fabrication and characterization of hydroxyapatite/wollastonite composite bioceramics with controllable properties for hard tissue repair, *J Am Ceramic Soc* 94:99–105. doi: http://dx.doi.org/10.1111/j.1551-2916.2010.04046.x
441. Takatsuka, K., Yamamuro, T., Kitsugi, T., Nakamura, T., Shibuya, T. and Goto, T., 1993, A new bioactive glass–ceramic as a coating material on titanium alloy, *J Appl Biomater* 4:317–329. doi: http://dx.doi.org/10.1002/jab.770040406
442. Pattanayak, D.K., Prasad, R.C., Rao, B.T. and Mohan, T.R.R., 2006, Apatite wollastonite–titanium biocomposites: Synthesis and in vitroevaluation, *J Am Ceramic Soc* 89:2172–2176.
443. Pang, S.X. and Zhitomirsky, I., 2009, Electrophoretic deposition of composite hydroxyapatite– chitosan–heparin coatings, *J Mater Process Technol* 209:1597–1606. doi: http://dx.doi.org/10.1016/j.jmatprotec.2008.04.007
444. Rath, P.C., Singh, B.P., Besra, L. and Bhattacharjee, S., 2012, Multiwalled carbon nanotubes reinforced hydroxyapatite-chitosan composite coating on Ti metal: Corrosion and mechanical properties, *J Am Ceramic Soc* 95:2725–2731. doi: http://dx.doi.org/10.1111/j.1551-2916.2012.05195.x
445. Tang, X-J., Gui, L. and Xiao-Ying Lü, X-Y., 2008, Hard tissue compatibility of natural hydroxyapatite/chitosan composite, *Biomed Mater* 3. doi: http://dx.doi.org/10.1088/1748-6041/3/4/044115
446. Yang, C-C., Huang, C-Y., Lin, C-C. and Yen, S-K., 2011, Electrolytic deposition of collagen/HA composite on post HA/TiO_2 coated Ti6Al4V implant alloy electrochemical synthesis and engineering, *J Electrochem Soc 158:*E13-E20. doi: http://dx.doi.org/10.1149/1.3525604

447. Xia, Z., Yu, X. and Wei, M., 2012, Biomimetic collagen/apatite coating formation on Ti6Al4V substrates, *J Biomed Mater Res B Appl Biomater* 100:871–881.
448. Sugata, Y., Sotome, S., Yuasa, M., Hirano, M., Shinomiya, K. and Okawa, A., 2011, Effects of the systemic administration of alendronate on bone formation in a porous hydroxyapatite/collagen composite and resorption by osteoclasts in a bone defect model in rabbits, *J Bone Joint Surg* 93-B:510–516.
449. Du, C., Schneider, G.B., Zaharias, R., Abbott, C., Seabold, D., Stanford, C. and Moradian-Oldak, J., 2005, Apatite/amelogenin coating on titanium promotes osteogenic gene expression, *J Dent Res* 84:1070–1074. doi: http://dx.doi.org/10.1177/154405910508401120
450. Wang, G., Yang, H., Li, M., Lu, S., Chen, X. and Cai, X., 2010, The use of silk fibroin/hydroxyapatite composite co-cultured with rabbit bone-marrow stromal cells in the healing of a segmental bone defect, *J Bone Joint Surg* 92-B:320–325. doi: http://dx.doi.org/10.1302/0301-620X.92B2.22602
451. Zhang, Z., Gu, B., Zhang, W., Kan, G. and Sun, J., 2012, The enhanced characteristics of osteoblast adhesion to porous zinc–TiO_2 coating prepared by plasma electrolytic oxidation, *Appl Surf Sci* 258:6504–6511. doi: http://dx.doi.org/10.1016/j.apsusc.2012.03.067
452. Dastjerdi, R., Montazer, M. and Shahsavan, S., 2010, A novel technique for producing durable multifunctional textiles using nanocomposite coating, *Colloids Surf B: Biointerfaces* 81:32–41. doi: http://dx.doi.org/10.1016/j.colsurfb.2010.06.023
453. Cho, J., Schaab, S., Roether, J.A. and Boccaccini, A.R., 2008, Nanostructured carbon nanotube/TiO2 composite coatings using electrophoretic deposition (EPD), *J Nanopart Res* 10:99–105. doi: http://dx.doi.org/10.1007/s11051-007-9230-x
454. Cheng, S., Wei, D. and Zhou, Y., 2011, Formation and structure of sphene/titania composite coatings on titanium formed by a hybrid technique of microarc oxidation and heat-treatment, *Appl Surf Sci* 257:3410 3411. doi: http://dx.doi.org/10.1016/j.apsusc.2010.11.034
455. Wang, X., Wu, G., Zhou B. and Jun Shen, J., 2013, Thermal annealing effect on optical properties of binary TiO_2-SiO_2 sol-gel coatings, *Materials* 6:76–84. doi: http://dx.doi.org/10.3390/ma6010076
456. Hu, H., Qiao, Y., Meng, F., Liu, X. and Ding, C., 2013, Enhanced apatite-forming ability and cytocompatibility of porous and nanostructured TiO_2/$CaSiO_3$ coating on titanium, *Colloids Surf B: Biointerfaces* 101:83–90. doi: http://dx.doi.org/10.1016/j.colsurfb.2012.06.021
457. Pardun, K., Treccani, L., Volkmann, E., Li Destri, G., Marletta, G., Streckbein, P., Heiss, C. and Rezwan, K., 2013, Characterization of wet powder-sprayed zirconia/calcium phosphate coating for dental implants, *Clin Implant Dent Relat Res.* doi:10.1111/cid,12071
458. Kumar, A.M. and Rajendran, N., 2012, Influence of zirconia nanoparticles on the surface and electrochemical behaviour of polypyrrole nanocomposite coated 316L SS in simulated body fluid, *Surf Coat Tech* 213:155–166. doi: http://dx.doi.org/10.1016/j.surfcoat.2012.10.039
459. Gazia, R., Mandracci, P., Mussano, F. and Stefano Carossa, S., 2011, AlN_x and a-SiO_x coatings with corrosion resistance properties for dental implants, *Surf Coat Tech* 206:1109–1115. doi: http://dx.doi.org/10.1016/j.surfcoat.2011.07.091
460. Sokołowska, A., Rudnicki, J., Niedzielski, P., Boczkowska, A., Bogusławski, G., Wierzchoń, T. and Mitura, S., 2005, TiN–NCD composite coating produced on the Ti6Al4V alloy for medical applications, *Surf Coat Tech* 200:87–89. doi: http://dx.doi.org/10.1016/j.surfcoat.2005.02.037
461. Gurappa, I., 2002, Development of appropriate thickness ceramic coatings on 316 L stainless steel for biomedical applications, *Surf Coat Tech* 161:70–78. doi: http://dx.doi.org/10.1016/S0257-8972(02)00380-8

462. Martorana, S., Fedele, A., Mazzocchi, M. and Bellosi, A., 2009, Surface coatings of bioactive glasses on high strength ceramic composites, *Appl Surf Sci* 255:6679–6685. doi: http://dx.doi.org/10.1016/j.apsusc.2009.02.069
463. Nelson, G.M., Nychka, J.A. and McDonald, A.G., 2011, Flame spray deposition of titanium alloy-bioactive glass composite coatings, *J Therm Spray Technol* 20:1339–1351. doi: http://dx.doi.org/10.1007/s11666-011-9674-5
464. Avila, G., Misch, K., Galindo-Moreno, P. and Wang, H-Lay., 2009, Implant surface treatment using biomimetic agents, *Implant Dent* 18:17–26. doi: http://dx.doi.org/10.1097/ID.0b013e318192cb7d
465. Bougas, K., Jimbo, R., Xue, Y., Mustafa, K. and Wennerberg, A., 2012, Novel implant coating agent promotes gene expression of osteogenic markers in rats during early osseointegration, *Int J Biomater* 2012. doi: http://dx.doi.org/10.1155/2012/579274
466. Jemt T. and Johansson, J., 2006, Implant treatment in the edentulous maxillae: A 15-year follow-up study on 76 consecutive patients provided with fixed prostheses, *Clinical Implant Dent Relat Res* 8:61–69. doi: http://dx.doi.org/10.1111/j.1708-8208.2006.00003.x
467. Jemt, T., 2008, Single implants in the anterior maxilla after 15 years of follow-up: Comparison with central implants in the edentulous maxilla, *Int J Prosthodont* 21:400–408.
468. Åstrand, P., Ahlqvist, J., Gunne, J. and H. Nilson, H., 2008, Implant treatment of patients with edentulous jaws: A 20-year follow-up, *Clinic Implant Dent Relat Res* 10:207–217.
469. Oshida, Y., 2007, *Bioscience and Bioengineering of Titanium Materials*, Elsevier, London, UK, pp.185–193.
470. Fröjd, V., de Paz, L.C., Andersson, M., Wennerberg, A., Davies, J.R. and Svensäter, G., 2011, In situ analysis of multispecies biofilm formation on customized titanium surfaces, *Molec Oral Microbiol* 26:241–252. doi: http://dx.doi.org/10.1111/j.2041-1014.2011.00610.x
471. Wikesjö, U.M.E., Huang, Y.H., Xiropaidis, A.V., Sorensen, R.G., Rohrer, M.D., Prasad, H.S., Wozney, J.M. and Hall, J., 2008, Bone formation at recombinant human bone morphogenetic protein-2-coated titanium implants in the posterior maxilla (Type IV bone) in non-human primates, *J Clinical Periodontol* 35:992–1000. doi: http://dx.doi.org/10.1111/j.1600-051X.2008.01322.x
472. Thorey, F., Menzel, H., Lorenz, C., Gross, G., Hoffmann, A. and Windhagen, H., 2011, Osseointegration by bone morphogenetic protein-2 and transforming growth factor beta2 coated titanium implants in femora of New Zealand white rabbits, *Indian J Orthop* 45:57–62. doi: http://dx.doi.org/10.4103/0019-5413.73659
473. Abtahi, J., Tengvall, P. and Aspenberg, P., 2012, A bisphosphonate-coating improves the fixation of metal implants in human bone: A randomized trial of dental implants, *Bone* 50:1148–1151. doi: http://dx.doi.org/10.1016/j.bone.2012.02.001
474. Dorozhkin, S.V., 2012, Calcium orthophosphate coatings, films and layers, *Progress in Biomat* 1. doi: http://dx.doi.org/10.1186/2194-0517-1-1
475. Ruckenstein, E. and Gourisankar, S.V., 1986, Preparation and characterization of thin film surface coatings for biological environments, *Biomaterials* 7:403–422. doi: http://dx.doi.org/10.1016/0142-9612(86)90028-1
476. He, H.W., Liu, M.L., Zhu, Z.L., Yang, M.Z., Li, Q.L. and Chen, Z.Q., 2008, Influence of surface morphology of cpTi on the adsorption and attachment of collagen/chitosan, *Appl Surf Sci* 255:509–511. doi: http://dx.doi.org/10.1016/j.apsusc.2008.06.063
477. Patino , M.G., Neiders, M.E., Andreana, S., Noble, B. and Cohen, R.E., 2002, Collagen as an implantable material in medicine and dentistry, *J Oral Implant* 28:220–225. doi: http://dx.doi.org/10.1563/1548-1336(2002)028<0220:CAAIMI>2.3.CO;2
478. Müller, R., Abke, J., Schnell, E., Scharnweber, D., Kujat, R., Englert, C., Taheri, D., Nerlich, M. and Angele, P., 2006, Influence of surface pretreatment of titanium—and

cobalt-based biomaterials on covalent immobilization of fibrillar collagen, *Biomaterials* 27:4059–4068. doi: http://dx.doi.org/10.1016/j.biomaterials.2006.03.019

479. Morra, M., Cassinelli, C., Cascardo, G., Cahalan, P., Cahalan, L., Fini, M. and Giardino, R., 2003, Surface engineering of titanium by collagen immobilization; surface characterization and in vitro and in vivo studies, *Biomaterials* 24:4639–4654. doi: http://dx.doi.org/10.1016/S0142-9612(03)00360-0
480. Rammelt, S., Illert, T., Bierbaum, S., Scharnweber, D., Zwipp, H. and Schneiders, W., 2006, Coating of titanium implants with collagen, RGD peptide and chondroitin sulfate, *Biomaterials* 27:5561–5571. doi: http://dx.doi.org/10.1016/j.biomaterials.2006.06.034
481. Müller, R., Abke, J., Schnell, E., Macionczyk, F., Gbureck, U., Mehrl, R., Ruszczak, Z., Kujat, R., Englert, C., Nerlich, M. and Angele, P., 2005, Surface engineering of stainless steel materials by covalent collagen immobilization to improve implant biocompatibility, *Biomaterials* 26:6962–6972. doi: http://dx.doi.org/10.1016/j.biomaterials.2005.05.013
482. Glattauer, V., Briggs, K.L., Zappe, S., Ramshaw, J.A.M. and Truong, Y.B., 2012, Collagen-based layer-by-layer coating on electrospun polymer scaffolds, *Biomaterials* 33:9198–9204. doi: http://dx.doi.org/10.1016/j.biomaterials.2012.09.012
483. Yang, X., Jiang, B., Huang, Y., Tian, Y., Chen, H., Chen, J. and Yang, B., 2009 Collagen nanofilm immobilized on at surfaces by electrodeposition method, *J Biomed Mater Res B Appl Biomater* 90:608–613. doi: http://dx.doi.org/10.1002/jbm.b.31323
484. Miyamoto, S., Katz, B.Z., Lafrenie, R.M. and Yamada, K.M., 1998, Fibronectin and integrins in cell adhesion, signaling, and morphogenesis, *Ann N Y Acad Sci* 857:119–129. doi: http://dx.doi.org/10.1111/j.1749-6632.1998.tb10112.x
485. Elias, C.N., Gravina, P.A., de Filho, C.S. and Pedro Augusto de Paula Nascente, P.A., 2012, Preparation of bioactive titanium surfaces via fluoride and fibronectin retention, *Int J Biomater* 2012. doi: http://dx.doi.org/10.1155/2012/290179
486. Petrie, T.A., Raynor, J.E., Reyes, C.D., Burns, K.L, Collard, D.M., and García, A.J., 2008, The effect of integrin-specific bioactive coatings on tissue healing and implant osseointegration, *Biomaterials* 29:2849–2857. doi: http://dx.doi.org/10.1016/j.biomaterials.2008.03.036
487. Ku, Y., Chung, C.P. and Jang, J-H., 2005, The effect of the surface modification of titanium using a recombinant fragment of fibronectin and vitronectin on cell behavior, *Biomaterials* 26:5153–5157. doi: http://dx.doi.org/10.1016/j.biomaterials.2005.01.060
488. Erli, H-J., Rüger, M., Ragoß, C., Jahnen-Dechent, W., Hollander, D.A., Paar, O. and von Walter, M., 2006, The effect of surface modification of a porous TiO_2/perlite composite on the ingrowth of bone tissue in vivo, *Biomaterials* 27:1270–1276. doi: http://dx.doi.org/10.1016/j.biomaterials.2005.08.001
489. von Walter, M., Rüger, M., Ragoß, C., Steffens, G.C.M., Hollander, D.A., Paar, O., Maier, H.R., Jahnen-Dechent, W., Bosserhoff, A.K. and Erli, H-J., 2005, In vitro behavior of a porous TiO_2/perlite composite and its surface modification with fibronectin, *Biomaterials* 26:2813–2826. doi: http://dx.doi.org/10.1016/j.biomaterials.2004.07.066
490. Haruyama, T., Sakai, T. and Matsuno, K., 2005, Protein layer coating method on metal surface by electrochemical process through genetical introduced tag, *Biomaterials* 26:4944–4947. doi: http://dx.doi.org/10.1016/j.biomaterials.2005.01.027
491. Simon, Z., Deporter, D. A., Pilliar, R. M. and Clokie, C.M., 2006, Heterotopic bone formation around sintered porous-surfaced Ti–6Al–4V implants coated with native bone morphogenetic proteins, *Implant Dent* 15:265–274. doi: http://dx.doi.org/10.1097/01.id.0000226754.71828.6b
492. Guillot, R., Gilde, F., Becquart, P., Sailhan, F., Lapeyrere, A., Logeart-Avramoglou, D. and Picart, C., 2013, The stability of BMP loaded polyelectrolyte multilayer coatings

on titanium, *Biomaterials* 34:5737–5746. doi: http://dx.doi.org/10.1016/j.biomaterials.2013.03.067

493. Nayak, S., Dey, T., Naskar, D. and Kundu, S.C., The promotion of osseointegration of titanium surfaces by coating with silk protein sericin, *Biomaterials* 34:2855–2864. doi: http://dx.doi.org/10.1016/j.biomaterials.2013.01.019
494. Allenstein, U., Ma, Y., Arabi-Hashemi, A., Zink, M. and Mayr, S.G., 2013, Fe–Pd based ferromagnetic shape memory actuators for medical applications: Biocompatibility, effect of surface roughness and protein coatings, *Acta Biomater* 9:5845–5853. doi: http://dx.doi.org/10.1016/j.actbio.2012.10.040
495. Waterhouse, A., Yin, Y., Wise, S.G., Bax, D.V., McKenzie, D.R., Bilek, M.M.M., Weiss, A.S. and Ng, M.K.C., 2010, The immobilization of recombinant human tropoelastin on metals using a plasma-activated coating to improve the biocompatibility of coronary stents, *Biomaterials* 31:8332–8340. doi: http://dx.doi.org/10.1016/j.biomaterials.2010.07.062
496. Kazemzadeh-Narbat, M., Lai, B.F.L., Ding, C., Kizhakkedathu, J.N., Hancock, R.E.W. and Wang, R., 2013, Multilayered coating on titanium for controlled release of antimicrobial peptides for the prevention of implant-associated infections, *Biomaterials* 34:5969–5977. doi: http://dx.doi.org/10.1016/j.biomaterials.2013.04.036
497. Meyers, S.R., Khoo, X., Huang, X., Walsh, E.B., Grinstaff, M.W. and Kenan, D.J., 2009, The development of peptide-based interfacial biomaterials for generating biological functionality on the surface of bioinert materials, *Biomaterials* 30:277–286. doi: http://dx.doi.org/10.1016/j.biomaterials.2008.08.042
498. Yazici, H., Fong, H., Wilson, B., Oren, E.E., Amos, F.A., Zhang, H., Evans, J.S., Snead, M.L., Sarikaya, M. and Tamerler, C., 2013, Biological response on a titanium implant-grade surface functionalized with modular peptides, *Acta Biomater* 9:5341–5352. doi: http://dx.doi.org/10.1016/j.actbio.2012.11.004
499. Werner, S., Huck, O., Frisch, B., Vautier, D., Elkaim, R., Voegel, J-C., Brunel, G. and Tenenbaum, H., 2009, The effect of microstructured surfaces and laminin-derived peptide coatings on soft tissue interactions with titanium dental implants, *Biomaterials* 30:2291–2301. doi: http://dx.doi.org/10.1016/j.biomaterials.2009.01.004
500. Schuler, M., Owen, G.R., Hamilton, D.W., de Wild, M., Textor, M., Brunette, D.M. and Tosatti, S.G.P., 2006, Biomimetic modification of titanium dental implant model surfaces using the RGDSP-peptide sequence: A cell morphology study, *Biomaterials* 27:4003–4015. doi: http://dx.doi.org/10.1016/j.biomaterials.2006.03.009
501. Kazemzadeh-Narbat, M., Kindrachuk, J., Duan, K., Jenssen, H., Hancock, R.E.W. and Wang, R., 2010, Antimicrobial peptides on calcium phosphate-coated titanium for the prevention of implant-associated infections, *Biomaterials* 31:9519–9526. doi: http://dx.doi.org/10.1016/j.biomaterials.2010.08.035
502. Busscher, H.J., Rinastiti, M., Siswomihardjo, W. and van der Mei, H.C., 2010, Biofilm formation on dental restorative and implant materials, *J Dent Res* 89:657–665. doi: http://dx.doi.org/10.1177/0022034510368644
503. Zhao, L., Chu, P.K., Zhang, Y. and Wu, Z., 2009, Antibacterial coatings on titanium implants, *J Biomed Mater Res B Appl Biomater* 91:470–480. doi: http://dx.doi.org/10.1002/jbm.b.31463
504. Reyes, C.D., Petrie, T.A., Burns, K.L., Schwartz, Z. and García, A.J., 2007, Biomolecular surface coating to enhance orthopaedic tissue healing and integration, *Biomaterials* 28:3228–3235. doi: http://dx.doi.org/10.1016/j.biomaterials.2007.04.003
505. Leedy, M.R., Martin, H.J., Norowski, P.A., Jennings, J.A., Haggard, W.O. and Bumgardner, J.D., 2011, Use of Chitosan as a Bioactive Implant Coating for Bone-Implant Applications; Chitosan for Biomaterials II, *Adv Polym Sci* 244:129–165. doi: http://dx.doi.org/10.1007/12_2011_115

506. Darder, M., Aranda, P. and Eduardo Ruiz-Hitzky, E., 2012, Chitosan-Clay Bio-Nanocomposites, In: Luc Avérous, Eric Pollet ed. *Environmental Silicate Nano-Biocomposites* Springer-Verlag London, pp.365–391. doi: http://dx.doi.org/10.1007/978-1-4471-4108-2_14
507. Bumgardner, J.D., Chesnutt, B.M., Yuan, Y., Yang, Y., Appleford, M., Oh, S., McLaughlin, R., Elder, S.H. and Ong, J.L., 2007, The integration of chitosan-coated titanium in bone: An in vivo study in rabbits, *Implant Dent* 16:66–79. doi: http://dx.doi.org/10.1097/ID.0b013e3180312011
508. Frosch, K-H., Drengk, A., Krause, P., Viereck, V., Miosge, N., Werner, C., Schild, D., Stürmer, E.K. and Stürmer, K.M., 2006, Stem cell-coated titanium implants for the partial joint resurfacing of the knee, *Biomaterials* 27:2542–2549. doi: http://dx.doi.org/10.1016/j.biomaterials.2005.11.034
509. Hu, Y., Cai, K., Luo, Z., Zhang, R., Yang, L., Deng, L. and Jandt, K.D., 2009, Surface mediated *in situ* differentiation of mesenchymal stem cells on gene-functionalized titanium films fabricated by layer-by-layer technique, *Biomaterials* 30:3626–3635. doi: http://dx.doi.org/10.1016/j.biomaterials.2009.03.037
510. Achneck, H.E., Jamiolkowski, R.M., Jantzen, A.E., Haseltine, J.M., Lane, W.O., Huang, J.K., Galinat, L.J., Serpe, M.J., Lin, F-H., Li, M., Parikh, A., Ma, L., Chen, T., Sileshi, B., Milano, C.A.,. Wallace, C.S., Stabler, T.V., Allen, J.D., Truskey, G.A. and Lawson, J.H., 2011, The biocompatibility of titanium cardiovascular devices seeded with autologous blood-derived endothelial progenitor cells: EPC-seeded antithrombotic Ti Implants, *Biomaterials* 32:10–18. doi: http://dx.doi.org/10.1016/j.biomaterials.2010.08.073
511. Guo, K-T., Scharnweber, D., Schwenzer, B., Ziemer, G. and Wendel, H.P., 2007, The effect of electrochemical functionalization of Ti-alloy surfaces by aptamer-based capture molecules on cell adhesion, *Biomaterials* 28:468–474. doi: http://dx.doi.org/10.1016/j.biomaterials.2006.09.021
512. Siegel, J., Khalili, R., Slepičková-Kasálková, N. and Švorčík, V., 2013, Carbon coatings on polymers and their biocompatibility, *Appl Surf Sci* 275:43–48. doi: http://dx.doi.org/10.1016/j.apsusc.2013.01.127
513. Harris, P.J.F., 2004, Carbon nanotube composites, *Int Mater Rev* 49:31–43. doi: http://dx.doi.org/10.1179/095066004225010505
514. Gopi, D., Shinyjoy, E., Sekar, M., Surendiran, M., Kavitha, L. and Sampath, T.S., 2013, Development of carbon nanotubes reinforced hydroxyapatite composite coatings on titanium by electrodeposition method, *Corr Sci* 73:321–330. doi: http://dx.doi.org/10.1016/j.corsci.2013.04.021
515. Yang, X.F. and Lu, J., 2013, A new way to synthesize carbon nanofiber film on bulk titanium via hybrid surface mechanical attrition treatment, *Appl Surf Sci* 264:191–196. doi: http://dx.doi.org/10.1016/j.corsci.2013.04.021
516. Narayan, R.J., 2006, Laser processing of diamondlike carbon thin films for medical prostheses, *Int Mater Rev* 51:127–143. doi: http://dx.doi.org/10.1179/174328406X79432
517. Dearnaley, G. and Arps, J.H., 2005, Biomedical applications of diamond-like carbon (DLC) coatings, *Surf Coat Tech* 200:2518–2524. doi: http://dx.doi.org/10.1016/j.surfcoat.2005.07.077
518. Hinsworth, S.V. and Uhure, N.J., 2007, Diamond like carbon coatings for tribology: production techniques, characterization methods and applications, *Int Mater Rev* 52:153–174. doi: http://dx.doi.org/10.1179/174328007X160272
519. Jiang, S-W., Jiang, B., Li, Y., Li, Y-R., Yin, G-F. and Zheng, C-Q., 2004, Friction and wear study of diamond-like carbon gradient coatings on Ti6Al4V substrate prepared by plasma source ion implant-ion beam enhanced deposition, *Appl Surf Sci* 236:285–291. doi: http://dx.doi.org/10.1016/j.apsusc.2004.04.032

520. Liu, Y., Fu, X., Bu, Y., Zhang, J., Zhang, J. and Wu, L., 2012, Photochemical grafting of fluorinate alkenes on DLC coated Ti6Al4V to improve in vitro cytocompatibility, friction and corrosion resistance, *Surf Coat Tech* 208:51–56. doi: http://dx.doi.org/10.1016/j.surfcoat.2012.07.084
521. Heinrich, G., Grögler, T., Rosiwal, S.M. and Singer, R.F., 1997, CVD diamond coated titanium alloys for biomedical and aerospace applications, *Surf Coat Tech* 94/95:514–520. doi: http://dx.doi.org/10.1016/S0257-8972(97)00459-3
522. Batory, D., Czerniak-Reczulska, M., Kolodziejczyk, L. and Szymanski, W., 2013, Gradient titanium and silver based carbon coatings deposited on AISI316L, *Appl Surf Sci* 275:303–310. doi: http://dx.doi.org/10.1016/j.apsusc.2012.12.088
523. Koistinen, A., Santavirta, S.S., Kröger, H. and Lappalainen, R., 2005, Effect of bone mineral density and amorphous diamond coatings on insertion torque of bone screws, *Biomaterials* 26:5687–5694. doi: http://dx.doi.org/10.1016/j.biomaterials.2005.02.003
524. Liu, D.G., Tu, J.P., Chen, R. and Gu, C.D., 2011, Microstructure, corrosion resistance and biocompatibility of titanium incorporated amorphous carbon nitride films, *Surf Coat Tech* 206:165–171. doi: http://dx.doi.org/10.1016/j.surfcoat.2011.07.007
525. Tsuchiya, H., Shirai, T., Nishida, H., Murakami, H., Kabata, T., Yamamoto, N., Watanabe, K. and Nakase, J., 2012, Innovative antimicrobial coating of titanium implants with iodine, *J Orthop Sci* 17:595–604. doi: http://dx.doi.org/10.1007/s00776-012-0247-3
526. Shirai, T., Shimizu, T., Ohtani, K., Zen, Y., Takaya, Y.M. and Tsuchiya, H., 2011, Antibacterial iodine-supported titanium implants, *Acta Biomater* 7:1928–1933. doi: http://dx.doi.org/10.1016/j.actbio.2010.11.036
527. Zhu, S., Huang, N., Shu, H., Wu, Y. and Xu, L., 2009, Corrosion resistance and blood compatibility of lanthanum ion implanted pure iron by MEVVA, *Appl Surf Sci* 256:99–104. doi: http://dx.doi.org/10.1016/j.apsusc.2009.07.082
528. Fonner, J.M., Forciniti, L., Nguyen, H., Byrne, J.D., Kou, Y-F., Syeda-Nawaz, J. and Schmidt, C.E., 2008, Biocompatibility implications of polypyrrole synthesis techniques, *Biomed Mater* 3. doi: http://dx.doi.org/10.1088/1748-6041/3/3/034124
529. Khan, W., Kapoor, M. and Kumar, N., 2007, Covalent attachment of proteins to functionalized polypyrrole-coated metallic surfaces for improved biocompatibility, *Acta Biomater* 3:541–549. doi: http://dx.doi.org/10.1016/j.actbio.2007.01.006
530. Taxt-Lamolle, S.F., Rubert, M., Haugen, H.J., Lyngstadaas, S.P., Ellingsen, J.E. and Monjo, M., 2010, Controlled electro-implementation of fluoride in titanium implant surfaces enhances cortical bone formation and mineralization, *Acta Biomater* 6:1025–1032. doi: http://dx.doi.org/10.1016/j.actbio.2009.09.014
531. Park, J-W., Kim, H-K., Kim, Y-J., Jang, J-H., Song, H. and Hanawa, T., 2010, Osteoblast response and osseointegration of a Ti–6Al–4V alloy implant incorporating strontium, *Acta Biomater* 6:2843–2851. doi: http://dx.doi.org/10.1016/j.actbio.2010.01.017

Chapter 6

Evaluation and Characterization of Modified Surfaces

Prior to clinical applications, engineered surfaces are needed to be characterized and evaluated in terms of its bonding strength, surface roughness, chemical composition and impurity inclusion, surface energy, or, in some cases, depth profile in hardness and residual stress distribution. In this section, these surface characterizations and various evaluations will be reviewed.

6.1. Introduction

The science of surface engineering is of vital importance in advancing the field of implantology. This is evident, as shown in previous chapters, from the increased biocompatibility, bioactivity, and biofunctionality of surface engineered implants. Surface engineering techniques have also enhanced implants' mechanical (including biotribological) and biological actions, and led to better osseointegration. However, in the pursuit of these positive effects, the potential hazard (s) a foreign material may pose to a biological entity can't be overlooked. As ISO-10993 dictates, biological and chemical testing must be done to ensure that device materials are compatible with biological tissues, cells, and body fluids [1]. As an offshoot of surface engineering, coating technology applications should also undergo careful testing. Coatings are used to endow a biomaterial with various beneficial properties, among them are corrosion resistance, biotribology, and adherence strength, so it is particularly important to also evaluate their biocompatibility. This chapter will address these and other aspects that directly or indirectly relate to the biocompatibility, bioactivity, and biofunctionality of modified surfaces.

DOI 10.5643/9781606506288/ch6

6.2. Safety Concerns and Testing

Safety concerns should not be limited to implants but to all dental and medical devices. Specifications and standards have been developed to aid producers, users, and consumers in the evaluation of the safety and effectiveness of dental products. However, product compliance testing to meet national and international standards is not compulsory for manufacturers; it is purely voluntary [2]. Until the passage of the Medical Device Amendments to the Food and Drug Act in 1976, materials and devices intended for use in medicine and dentistry were not regulated by any agency of the U.S. government. The only exception was for materials for which therapeutic claims were made, which allowed the Food and Drug Administration (FDA) to consider them a drug. The Medical Device Amendments of 1976 gave the FDA jurisdiction over all materials, devices, and instruments used in the diagnosis, cure, mitigation, treatment, or prevention of disease in man. This includes materials used professionally and the over-the-counter products sold directly to the public. The FDA's Dental Products Panel places an item in one of three classes: Class I—materials posing minimum risk, these are subject only to good manufacturing and record keeping procedures; Class II—materials for which safety, efficacy, and adherence to published performance standards need to be demonstrated; and Class III—materials that pose significant risk and for which performance standards have not been formulated. Class III materials are subject to premarket approval by the FDA for safety and efficacy, in much the same manner as a new drug [3].

According to ISO specifications [4], implant devices are required to evaluate several tests: Group I (cytotoxicity tests: ISO 7405, 6.1 and 6.2, and cytotoxicity tests: ISO 10993.5), Group II (subchronic systemic toxicity—Oral application: ISO 10993.11.6.7.1, skin irritation and intracutaneous reactivity: ISO 10993-11.5.2, sensitization systemic toxicity—application by inhalation: ISO 10993.11.6.7.3, genotoxicity: ISO 10993.3, and local effects after implantation: ISO 10993.6), and Group III tests (pulp capping and pulpotomy: ISO 7405.6.4 and endodontic usage test: ISO 7405.6.5).

Surface engineering opens up very many exciting opportunities for the design of new biomedical implant devices, like total joint replacements (TJRs). However, the development of these new bearing surfaces for such devices is a very slow process. This is due to the time consumed by *in vitro* wear tests, biocompatibility studies, clinical trials, and final adoption. Given the diversity of new bearing surface materials that modern surface engineering makes possible, there is a clear need to develop valid and rapid screening tests. The tests would be designed to evaluate their tolerance to: (a) mechanical (third-body abrasion) damage, (b) corrosion, and (c) corrosion-wear. It has been shown that for a given TJR surface engineering design, both the mechanical and chemical attributes are important to the realization of the overall goal of improving bearing surfaces [5].

The *in vitro* biocompatibility of novel materials has to be proven before a material can be used as a component of a medical device. This must be done in cell culture tests, according to internationally recognized standard protocols. Subsequently, preclinical and clinical tests must be performed to verify the safety of the new material and device. The present chapter focuses on the first step, the *in vitro* testing according to ISO 10993-5, and critically discusses its limited significance [1]. Biomedical testing allows the performance and compatibility of new materials and medical devices to be proven *in vitro*, without putting patients at risk, and for the evaluation of critical and complex issues in a controlled and repeatable manner. In addition to helping new products meet essential regulations, biomedical testing allows the quality of medical products to be verified in a production line, and the development of new and innovative solutions in the laboratory [6].

Although dental implants exhibit limited failure rates, their fracture is associated with major modifications of the prosthetic treatment and complex surgery for the removal of the remaining embedded implant part. Hence, the stress fields in the bone–implant interface during the mastication and the failure modes of the oral implants are needed to be assessed [7, 8]. Michailidis et al. [9] had reverse-engineered the FEM model of an implant and virtually loaded at the top of the crown for a force spectrum ranging from 75 to 225 N in vertical, horizontal, and oblique occlusal directions. It was reported that obtained results were verified by comparing the simulated stress fields to fractured implants (clinically retrieved) and the correlation affirmed the bio-realistic stress development, as the predicted critical regions calculated by the model cohere to the fracture site of the prosthesis [9].

6.3. Magnetic Resonance Imaging Safety and Image Compatibility

Magnetic resonance imaging (MRI) is probably the most innovative and revolutionary imaging technology, with the exception of computed tomography. MRI is a three-dimensional (3D) imaging technique used to image the protons of the body by employing magnetic fields, radio frequencies, electromagnetic detectors, and computers [10]. For millions of patients worldwide, MRI examinations provide essential and potentially life-saving information. Some devices, such as pacemakers and neurostimulators, have limitations related to MRI safety and may be contraindicated for use with MRI. Other internal devices such as stents, vena cava filters, and some types of catheters and guidewires, are safe for use with MRI but have limited MRI image compatibility. Some of these devices are simply not well-imaged under MRI. Others have properties that interfere with the MRI image by causing an image artifact (distortion) in the area in and around the device, limiting the effectiveness of MRI for assisting placement or diagnostic follow up on these implants. It may be contraindicated in certain situations because the magnetic field present in the MRI environment may, under certain circumstances, result in movement or heating of a metallic orthopedic implant device. Further, metals that exhibit magnetic attraction in the MRI setting may be subject to movement (deflection) during the procedure. Both magnetic and nonmagnetic metallic devices of certain geometries may be subjected to heating caused by interactions with the magnetic field.

There are currently several researchers and an ASTM (American Society for Testing and Materials) committee exploring methods for accurately assessing the MRI compatibility of implant devices. The primary focus of their research has been the measurement of implant movement in response to a magnetic field. Shellock and co-workers [11–13] conducted several studies in which the movement/deflection of various orthopedic implants was measured in the high magnetic field (0.3–1.5 Tesla) region of MRI units. The results of these studies show no measurable movement of implants fabricated from cobalt, titanium, and stainless steel alloys [14].

Ferromagnetic metal will cause a magnetic field inhomogeneity, which, in turn, causes a local signal void, often accompanied by an area of high signal intensity, as well as a distortion of the image. They create their own magnetic fields and dramatically alter precession frequencies of protons in the adjacent tissues. Tissues adjacent to ferromagnetic components become influenced by the induced magnetic field of the metal hardware rather than the parent field and, therefore, either fail to process or do so at a different frequency and hence do not generate useful signal. Two components contribute to the susceptibility artifact: induced magnetism in the ferromagnetic component itself and induced magnetism in protons adjacent to the component. Artifacts from metal may have varied appearances on MRI scans due to different types of metal or configuration of the piece of metal. In relation to MRI, titanium alloys are less ferromagnetic than both cobalt and stainless steel, induce less susceptibility artifacts, and result in less marked image degradation [14–16].

MRI use is contraindicated for the following devices (except where noted) [17]:

- **Cardiac pacemakers**—are absolutely contraindicated; however, MRI compatible pacemakers are being developed. A few pacemaker patients have been scanned for life-threatening situations or inadvertently. Subsequently, their pacemakers must be meticulously checked for function. Some deaths have been reported.
- **Intracranial aneurysm clips**—are contraindicated, unless the specific type of MRI-compatible clip can be absolutely documented.
- **Neurostimulators/spinal-fusion stimulators**—generally are contraindicated. There are two manufacturers that are seeking FDA approval for usage of their product in MRI, but under strict guidelines.
- **Drug infusion pumps**—generally are contraindicated. There are two models Synchro Med and Synchro Med EL that are currently FDA approved with specific guidelines.
- **Metallic foreign bodies**—may or may not preclude MRI scanning depending on type, size, and location. These patients must be screened by X-ray. Detection should also target possible orbital metallic foreign bodies.
- **Cochlear implants**—contraindicated.
- **Other otologic implants**—generally, these are non-ferromagnetic and MRI compatible. The exception is the McGee stapedectomy piston prosthesis—it is not MRI compatible.
- **Dental implants**—generally are compatible, except for those that contain magnetically activated components.
- **Ocular implants**—some are MRI compatible.
- **Intravascular stents, filters, and coils**—most of these are compatible 6–8 weeks following placement, unless they are made of nonferrous metal, for example, titanium, in which case they can be imaged right after placement. Drug-eluting stents must be cleared by the implanting physician if they have been in less than 3 months.
- **Vascular access ports and catheters**—are compatible, excluding the Swan Ganz Catheter.

- **Penile implants**—these are of mixed compatibility and should be checked.
- **Orthopedic implants/prosthesis**—are compatible, though MRI may cause local heating and MRI will cause local image artifact.
- **Heart valve prosthesis**—is compatible, but there is a prototype electromagnetically controlled heart valve that is being developed, which is contraindicated.
- **Pacer wires (without pacemaker)**—the compatibility is controversial, but they are probably fine at low MR fields but questionable at high field imaging. All patients must have a chest X-ray prior to having an MRI to ensure that the wires are not looped or crossed.
- **Holter monitor**—contraindicated.
- **Ventricular-peritoneal shunts**—compatible, except SOPHY® adjustable pressure valve type.
- **Swan Ganz catheter**—contraindicated. The thermal dilutor may melt.
- **Dermal patches**—can cause burns during MRI study and should be removed.
- **Pessary, and diaphragm**—compatible, but will produce local image artifact.
- **Hearing aids**—must be removed.
- **Permanent eyeliner/tattoos**—can cause local burns.
- **Body rings/spikes**—can cause local burns, dislodgment, or artifacts. It is suggested to remove these devices under normalMRI or the use under low field MR.
- **Breast tissue expanders**—not compatible.
- **Bullets, shrapnel, and pellets**—depends on the foreign body's location and duration of the MRI. An X-ray is required before an MRI can be done.

6.4. Hydrophilicity and Hydrophobicity

The interaction between an implant's metal surface and the host's cells/tissues are important parameters for the biocompatibility, in particular, for materials used in either dental or orthopedic implants. Hydrophilicity, or surface wettability, is a function of surface energy. It plays an important role in the biological response to an implant, as it controls the adsorption of proteins. These proteins promote and greatly influence whether cells attach to the implant's surface and the subsequent cell spreading [18].

Many techniques and methods have been reported and proposed to increase surface hydrophilicity. Polymer nanofibers were surface-functionalized by sputter coating with TiO_2. It was reported that the surface wettability of TiO_2 sputter-coated nanofibers was significantly improved after UV irradiation [19]. Similarly, TiO_2 coating resulted in increasing surface wettability [20,21]. Surface hydrophilicity can also be improved by surface texturing [22–25]. Fleming et al. [23] treated the titanium surface by sandblasting and dip-coating it with colloidal silica nanoparticles in order to produce superhydrophilicity. It was reported that the treated surface was suitable for the potential use in a variety of applications, such as prosthetic dentistry and other biomedical fields [23]. The Ti–6Al–4V surface was modified using a combination of various techniques such as cold spray, selective laser sintering, pulsed electro-erosion treatment, and magnetron sputtering to control surface topography (roughness and blind porosity), surface chemistry, and wettability, that is the characteristics which affect osseointegration. It was concluded that the combination of high surface roughness, blind porosity, hydrophilicity, and biocompatibility makes fabricated metal-ceramic materials promising candidates for applications involving tissue regeneration [25]. Nano- or microstructured materials composed of TiO_2 [26], Y_2O_3 [27], and Ti [28,29] showed improving surface wettability. The hydroxyapatite (HA) coating increases the surface hydrophilicity of Ti–6Al–4V [30,31]. Another study that demonstrated an increase in surface hydrophilicty showed that when TiO_2 was incorporated with strontium (Sr) and P elements, the treated surfaces showed significantly higher wettability and surface energy. Also, after immersion in Hank's balanced salt solution (HBSS), considerable apatite deposition was observed on the Sr- and P-doped surfaces, suggesting that Sr- and P-incorporated Ti oxide surfaces may improve implant bone healing by enhancing attachment, viability, and differentiation of osteoblastic cells [32]. Tsuji et al. [33] employed an Ar-ion implantation technique on a polystyrene surface and reported that atomic bonds of C–O, C=O, and O=C–O endowed hydrophilicity to the polystyrene surface. It was also observed that human umbilical vascular endothelial cells, cultured on traT surfaces, only exhibited cell growth and attachment on Ag-implanted surfaces [33].

Lin et al. deposited a TiO_x film by an electron-beam evaporation system and then treated it with ultraviolet or visible light irradiation [34]. It was reported that the ultraviolet irradiation treated TiO_x film became highly hydrophilic and returned to its original hydrophobic state by visible-light irradiation. This demonstrates the responsiveness and plasticity of TiO_x: its wettability is dependent on exposure to light irradiation. Wu et al. deposited the TiO_2 film on unheated glass substrates by using a twin DC magnetron sputtering system [35]. After irradiating the oxide film surface with UV, the water contact angle of the freshly TiO_2 film was found to be within 100°–112°. However, within 60 minutes of UV irradiation, the film became highly hydrophilic; the water contact angle was nearly zero. Also, the surface of the film with 12.6–14.5 nm was relatively rough. Hence, it was concluded that high hydrophobicity and photo-induced hydrophilicity can be attributed to fully oxidized chemical composition and higher roughness on the film surface [35]. In some tribological orthopedic implants, high hydrophobicity is required. There are reports about the superhydrophobic effect perfluoropolyether [36] and perfluorooctyltrichlorosilane [37] bestow when deposited on Ti surfaces.

Increased wettability may be an important factor for re-osseointegration. Duske et al. [38] applied cold atmospheric pressure gas-discharge plasma to titanium disks with different surface topography in order to reduce water contact angles and to improve the spreading of osteoblastic cells. It was reported that the contact angle of the titanium disks (baseline values: 68°–117°) were significantly reduced, close to 0°, irrespective of surface topography after the application of argon plasma with 1.0% oxygen admixture for 60 or 120 seconds. Also, the cell size of osteoblastic cells grown on argon–oxygen plasma-treated titanium disks was significantly larger than on non-treated surfaces irrespective of surface topography, indicating that the application of cold plasma may be supportive in the treatment of peri-implant lesions and may improve the process of re-osseointegration [38].

Functionalizing implant surfaces implies the increasing surface energy (with improved wettability). Schliephake et al. [39] hypothesized that organically coating titanium screw implants provides binding sites for integrin receptors that can enhance peri-implant bone formation. Ten adult female foxhounds received experimental titanium screw implants in the mandible 3 months after removal of all premolar teeth. Four types of implants were evaluated in each animal: (i) implants with machined titanium surfaces, (ii) implants coated with collagen I, (iii) implants with collagen I and cyclic RGD (Arg-Gly-Asp) peptide coating with low RGD concentrations (100 μmol/mL), and (iv) implants with collagen I and RGD coating with high RGD concentrations (1000 μmol/mL). Peri-implant bone regeneration was assessed histomorphometrically after 1 and 3 months, in five dogs per interval, by measuring bone implant contact (BIC) and the bone volume density (BVD) of the newly formed peri-implant bone. It was found that after 1 month, BIC was significantly enhanced only in the group of implants coated with the higher concentration of RGD peptides and that the volume density of the newly formed peri-implant bone was significantly higher in all implants with organic coatings—no significant difference was found between collagen coating and RGD coatings. Furthermore, after 3 months, BIC was significantly higher in all implants with organic coating than in implants with machined surfaces. The peri-implant BVD was significantly increased in all coated implants in comparison to machined surfaces. It was therefore concluded that the organic coating of machined screw implant surfaces provided binding sites for integrin receptors and enhanced both BIC and peri-implant bone formation [39].

6.5. Blood Compatibility

Layers of pure Ti, Ti oxynitrides ($TiN_{1-x}O_x$ with $x = 0.25$, 0.50, and 0.75), and Ti oxides were plasma deposited on oxidized Si by cathodic arc evaporation, in the presence of N_2- or O_2-enriched, or both, ambient air near the substrate in order to evaluate the suitability of Ti-based coatings for blood-contacting implants [40]. It was reported that (i) TiN and oxynitrides showed the longest clotting time compared to rutile TiO_2, (ii) minimum platelet adhesion was observed for pure TiO_2, (iii) contrasting tendencies in the dependence of clotting time and platelet adhesion on the microstructure were found, and (iv) for P^+-doped rutile, both enhanced clotting time and improved platelet adhesion were observed [40]. In an effort to improve the blood compatibility of titanium, its surface was coated with heparin and collagen using a layer-by-layer self-assembly technique [41]. The *in vitro* platelet adhesion and activation were investigated by using a static platelet adhesion assay to test for the presence of lactate dehydrogenase released from adherent platelets. Clotting time was examined by activated partial thromboplastin time and prothrombin time assays. It was reported that treated film significantly decreased platelet adhesion and activation, and prolonged clotting time of thromboplastin time and prothrombin time compared to untreated titanium film. Additionally, the heparin-collagen-treated titanium films displayed greater anti-coagulation performance than untreated titanium surfaces [41]. Surface modification with extracellular matrix (ECM) components, including fibronectin, laminin, and collagen (type IV), have been recognized as a promising method for improving cardiovascular material hemocompatibility [42]. Xue et al. [42] cultured human umbilical vein endothelial cells to produce a native ECM on a pure titanium surface and reported that the ECM produced by human umbilical vein endothelial cells improved the adhesion and proliferation ability of endothelial cells, and inhibited the adhesion and activation of platelets—suggesting that this approach may provide a basis for the preparation of modified surfaces in cardiovascular implant applications [42].

The titanium bone plate was treated by plasma discharge oxidation to produce a nanostructural oxide layer. During the process, the oxygen phase transition, ($\alpha \rightarrow (\alpha + TiO) \rightarrow (\alpha + TiO + \gamma\text{-}TiO_2)$ transformation, was observed. Based on this phenomenon, Huang et al. investigated the feasibility of using oxygen plasma discharging on titanium for forming a biocompatible layer between the bone plate and bone tissue [43]. It was reported that (i) nano-rutile-TiO_2(γ-TiO_2) can be used to enhance the osseointegration of implants, such as orthopedic and dental implants, and (ii) the formation of a nanostructural rutile-TiO_2 on the oxidation layer is related with the cell and blood reaction and distribution selectivity, promoting hemocompatibility, and protein binding as well as osseointegration, suggesting that surface oxidation by plasma discharging improves the biocompatibility and tissue healing [43]. The surface of 316L stainless steels with different wettabilities and similar topographies were treated by the sol–gel process. The proportions of tetraethoxysilane and methyltriethoxysilane were manipulated in order to evaluate the adhesion and proliferation of vascular endothelial and smooth muscle cells. Data was collected on cell number, cell morphology, and the expression of cytoskeletal protein [44]. It was found that (i) endothelial cells and smooth muscle cells responded differently to the coated surfaces, and (ii) moderate hydrophilic coating (contact angle 45.3°) enhanced the endothelialization of bare 316L, which exhibited effective inhibition of smooth muscle cell and negligible influence on endothelial cells [44].

6.6. Cell Adhesion and Adhesive Strength

It is widely accepted that implant surface factors affect the quality of the bone-to-implant interface via enhancement of osteoblast cell adhesion. Hyperhydrophilic sandblasted and acid-etched (SBA) titanium surfaces were prepared by alkali treatment and their responses to partially heparinized whole human blood were analyzed [45]. Results indicate that the alkali-treated SBA Ti surfaces perform better in terms of osseointegration; a continuous and structured layer of blood components on the blood-facing surface supports later tissue integration of an endosseous implant [45]. Similarly, the sandblasted, large-grit, and acid-etched (SLA) implants were studied and it was concluded that significant bone apposition was found for the SLA surface at the early stage of healing, indicating that the SLA surface may enhance bone apposition in coronal circumferential defects in non-submerged implants [46]. The morphology generated by TiO_2 particle blasting on CpTi and the attachment of cells were investigated after CpTi surfaces were blasted with 45 μm (standard), 45–63 μm, and 63–90 μm TiO_2 particles [47]. It was reported that (i) the cells had spread well on all titanium surfaces, indicating good attachment to both smooth and rough surfaces, and (ii) after 24 hours the surfaces blasted with 63–90 μm particles had a higher rate of cell attachment than all the other surfaces including the controls, concluding that attachment and growth of cells originating from human mandibular bone *in vitro* are influenced by the microtexture of the implant surface [47].

Ti–24Nb–4Zr–8Sn was anodically oxidized in NH_4F containing electrolyte to produce nanotubes consisting of the amorphous mixed oxides of TiO_2, Nb_2O_5, SnO_2, and ZrO_2 [48]. Then, *in vitro* studies of the oestoblast-like MG-63 cells were performed to evaluate their biological behavior in nanotubes of varied outer diameter (30,50,70, and 90 nm). This was compared to MG-63 cells exposed to polished CpTi and untreated Ti–24Nb–4Zr–8Sn. It was reported that the smallest diameter, 30 nm, promoted cell adhesion, proliferation, and differentiation, whereas the largest diameter of 90 nm had the worst cell viability with small spreading area of cytoskeletal actin—suggesting that the topography of the amorphous nanotube plays an important role on cell response [48].

Resorbable blast media treated or anodized CpTi surfaces were subjected to MG63 osteoblast-like cell culture tests. It was concluded that surface treatment by anodization may improve initial attachment of cells, proliferation ability, and differentiation activity, which play important roles in providing better osseointegration of implants. It was suggested that quicker and stronger implant osseointegration may yield the best anchorage outcomes and shorten the healing time required prior to functional loading [49]. Similarly, anodized Ti plates were subjected to MG-63 osteoblast-like cell culture tests and it was mentioned that superior cell adhesion was observed on anodized, hydrothermically treated Ti plates [50]. There is a report indicating that the presence of a TiO_2 nano-mesh layer on the anodized Ti surface increased the corrosion potential and decreased the corrosion rate and passive current in simulated body fluid (SBF). The TiO_2 nano-mesh layer caused better cell adhesion and spreading, as well as faster cell proliferation and initial differentiation [51]. MC3T3-E1 cell adhesion to TiO_2-grit blasted CpTi and to TiO_2 grit blasted, hydrofluoric (HF)-treated CpTi was compared. The increased levels of RUNX-2 in cells adherent to the TiO_2/HF-treated surfaces suggested that the addition of the HF treatment to the TiO_2 grit blasting resulted in surface properties that support adherent cell osteoinduction [52]. Similarly, different surface treatments (machined, anodized, or anodized and calcium phosphate-enriched) of CpTi grade 4 and grade 5 were subjected to MC3T3 cell culture tests [53]. It was reported that although the grade 4 titanium enriched with calcium phosphate had the highest level of differentiation *in vitro*, grade 5 titanium machined surfaces supported cell proliferation and matrix synthesis and induced high expression of early differentiation markers. The increased mechanical resistance of grade 5 titanium makes it a potential candidate for orthodontic mini-implants [53].

Wang et al. investigated the effect of the interaction between modified implant surface structures and their susceptibility to bacteria [54]. CpTi surfaces were sandblasted, microarc oxidized, and SBF coated. *Staphylococcus aureu*, a major pathogen often found in the percutaneous implant-associated infections, was chosen for the *in vitro* study. It was reported that all surface coating treatments promoted *S. aureus* adhesion. It was suggested that the use of the tested coatings could lead to a higher occurrence of *in vivo* infection. The beneficial properties that coatings lend to osseointegration are well documented. However, given their susceptibility to bacterial infection, it is essential to perform further research on the selection of proper parameters for the implant surface coating techniques [54].

In order to improve human cell growth on dentally implanted titanium (Ti), Chiang et al. [55] created a nano-network surface oxide layer by electrochemical anodization treatment. Human bone marrow mesenchymal stem cells (hMSCs) were made to express a green fluorescent protein (GFP) by retroviral transduction. It was reported that (i) a multilayer TiO_2 nano-network was produced rapidly on Ti surfaces using a simple electrochemical anodization treatment, (ii) the TiO_2 nano-network layer on the anodized Ti surfaces significantly improved *in vitro* and *in vivo* hMSC growth, as assessed by measurement of GFP fluorescence, relative to hMSC growth on untreated Ti surfaces, (iii) the TiO_2 nano-network layer on the anodized Ti surfaces also induced the differentiation of hMSCs after 28 days *in vivo*, and (iv) the formation of the TiO_2 nano-network on the Ti surfaces increased hMSC growth *in vitro* and *in vivo* [55]. Zhang et al. [56] utilized several surface modification methods in their experiments that aimed to improve the seal between the neck portion of a dental implant and the surrounding soft tissue. Titanium surfaces were variously modified by (a) machining, (b) machining and acid etching, or (c) machining, acid etching, and depositing 4.5 collagen/hyaluronic acid (col/HA) polyelectrolyte bilayers. Human gingival fibroblasts were cultured on the different surfaces, and cell morphology and spreading were observed using fluorescence microscopy and a shape factor measurement. Cell proliferation was examined by fluorometric quantification of the amount of cellular DNA. It was found that (i) similar surface topology for these three groups was observable on a microscopic scale, and morphologic differences were apparent on the nanoscale, (ii) both acid etching and col/HA deposition improved the hydrophilicity of the titanium surface, in contrast to machining alone, (iii) the proliferation and differentiation of human gingival fibroblasts (HGF) were greatly stimulated when cultured on the surface treated with (c). It was, accordingly, concluded that in contrast to two control surfaces (a) and (b), the (c) surface treatment improved the attachment, spreading, proliferation, and differentiation of HGF on CpTi [56].

Although dental and orthopedic implants have achieved high success rates, two major complications may be encountered: the lack of bone tissue integration and implant-centered infection. The surface of the implant, through its interactions with proteins, bacteria, and tissue cells, plays a determining role in the success or failure of the implant. Neoh et al. [57] pointed out that in order to enhance the success of implants, implant surfaces should inhibit bacterial colonization and concomitantly promote osteoblast functions. Hence, tailoring implant surfaces to differentially affect the response of bacteria and osteoblasts is very crucial. Nevertheless, limitations still exist in the quest for an ideal implant surface. It was also mentioned that further advances in this field will require concurrent development in surface modification techniques and a better understanding of the complex and highly interrelated events occurring at the implant surface after implantation [57].

Dense and uniform fluoridated HA coating material was deposited on Ti–6Al–4V substrates using the sol–gel dip coating method. The load at which complete removal of the coating occurs is taken as an indication of the adhesion strength [58]. It was reported that adhesion strength increased with an increase of both fluorine concentration and firing temperature. Additionally, the coating-substrate interfacial failure mode changed from brittle to ductile [58], which suggested that the strain state might have changed. Glass was coated on Ti substrates that were previously treated by preoxidation or phosphatation combined with preoxidation [59]. It was reported that (i) the pull-off tests measured a maximum strength from 1.5 to 3 MPa, whatever the surface treatment, and (ii) measurement of transverse crack densities in the vitreous coatings yielded a higher values for phosphate than for preoxidized titanium, which indicated that better adhesion is obtained after phosphatation treatment [59].

The bond strength of an oxide film to a titanium substrate and its inherent structural characteristics are very important preconditions for the success of titanium implants. It was reported that (i) oxide films anodized in sulfuric acid consisted of anatase and rutile TiO_2, while TiP_2O_7 was predominantly formed on the Ti surfaces that were anodized using phosphoric acid as the electrolyte, (ii) those specimens which experienced initial spark deposition with a low current showed the highest bond strengths (34.2 MPa), (iii) the growth rates of the oxide film thicknesses, in relation to the electric current changes, varied according to the type of electrolyte, and (iv) oxide film thickness influenced the bond strength [60]. Bone-like apatite coatings were prepared on Ti substrates using a biomimetic method in a modified SBF. It was reported that the bonding strengths were 8.52 ± 2.41, 10.36 ± 2.78, and 17.23 ± 2.55 MPa for types I, II, and III apatite coatings, respectively. The failure analyses suggested that type III coating failed mostly at the interface between the coating and the substrate but type I and II coatings failed mostly within the apatite coating—cohesive debonding [61]. Three functional coatings (i.e., Al-C, Si-P-Al, and P-F-Al coatings) were fabricated by the microarc oxidation method and deposited on the Ti–6Al–4V alloy in different aqueous solutions. It was found that the coatings exhibit high adhesion strength by the quantitative shearing test, registering as 110, 70, and 40 MPa for Al–C, Si–P–Al, and P–F–Al coatings, respectively [62]. HA coatings were deposited on Ti–6Al–4V substrates by laser ablation with a KrF excimer laser and the bond strength was evaluated through the scratch-test technique. By prolonging heating time, an interface layer was formed between HA and Ti–6Al–4V, which attributes higher bond strength due to the presence of interdiffused oxygen. The failure mode was adhesive [63].

Scratch testing has been used to assess the adhesion of thin hard coatings [64]. However, the scratch test possesses some crucial problems because the stress state around a moving indenter scratching a coating/substrate system is very complex and it is difficult to determine the stresses which lead to detachment. Also, it is unclear which material parameters, such as work of adhesion or interfacial toughness, are appropriate for modeling the coating-substrate system's stress state [64,65].

6.7. Osseointegration

The surface of an implant ultimately determines its ability to integrate into the surrounding tissue. The composite effect of surface energy, composition, roughness, and topography plays a major role during the initial phases of the biological response to the implant, such as protein adsorption and cellular adherence, as well as during the later and more chronic phases of the response. For bone, the successful incorporation (and hence rigid fixation) of an alloplastic material within the surrounding bony bed is called ossteointegration. The exact surface characteristics that lead to optimal osseointegration, however, remain to be elucidated. This review will focus on how surface characteristics, such as composition and roughness, affect cellular responses to implant materials. Data from two different culture systems suggest that surface characteristics play a significant role in the recruitment and maturation of cells along relevant differentiation pathways. In the case of osseointegration, if the implant surface is inappropriate or less than optimal, cells will be unable to produce the appropriate complement of autocrine and paracrine factors required to adequately stimulate osteogenesis at the implant site. In contrast, if the surface is appropriate, cells at the implant surface will stimulate interactions between cells at the surface and those in distal tissues. This, in turn, will initiate a timely sequence of events which include cell proliferation, differentiation, matrix synthesis, and local factor production, thereby resulting in the successful incorporation of the implant into the surrounding bony tissue [66]. The characteristics of high-quality osseointegration are an accelerated healing process, high stability, and the durability of the dental implant. A major factor that determines the success of a dental implant is the stable anchorage of the implant in living bone [67,68]. In most cases osseointegration is incomplete. An analysis of retrieved titanium implants showed that bone-to-implant attachment averaged 70%–80%, with a minimum of 60%, even for successful implants that had lasted for up to 17 years [69]. This leaves much room for improvement. Bettering the surface quality of titanium dental implants may help bridge the gap.

The surface energy of a biomaterial is determined by the material's surface-charge density and the net polarity of the charge. Compared to an electrically neutral surface, a surface with net positive or negative charge may be more hydrophilic [70]. The surface-charge of a dental implant is known to be a key factor for bone cell adhesion and early-stage bone mineralization at the bone–implant interface. Thus, surface-charge modification seems to be a promising new direction for improving the osseointegration of titanium dental implants. Although surface-charge modification is a relatively new methodology, it has been rapidly gaining research attention in recent years. The main challenge, however, lies in effective modification of the surface charge of the dental implant material. The main objective, hence, is to develop effective and practical techniques that create a long-lasting electric field on the implant's surface, in order to promote the implant's osseointegration without incurring the drawbacks of existing surface-treatment methods. Implant stability and osseointegration are important factors in the success of treatment. Commercially pure titanium and its alloys were coated with HA and the healing response of various nanocoating surface implants by ion beam assisted deposition (IBAD) placed in surgically created circumferential gaps 12 weeks postplacement [71]. It was reported that calcium phosphate coatings improved the bone response; they may therefore be suitable for implant designs with complex surface geometries [71]. In order to improve fixation in bone, HA has been extensively coated on titanium implants [72–75] and Co–Cr implants [76]. Similar to the previous study, Ca–P compound was coated on implant surfaces to promote fixation [77,78]. Schiegnitz et al. [78] coated Ca–P compound onto SLA implants in a rabbit model and used the percentage of linear bone fill as well as bone–implant contact as osseointegration assessment. It was concluded that (i) the calcium phosphate-coated surfaces on supracrestal inserted implants have vertical osteoconductive characteristics and increase the bone–implant contact at the implant shoulder significantly in a rabbit model and (ii) in clinical long-term settings, these implants may contribute to a better vertical bone height [78].

Compounds that encourage osseointegration can be created by oxidizing titanium surfaces [79]. The β titanium was subjected to microarc oxidation, in order to create anatase-rich (A-TiO_2) and rutile-rich (R-TiO_2) titanium dioxide samples. It was found that osteoblasts adhered more tenaciously and grew more lamellipodia on R-TiO_2 than on either A-TiO_2 or raw β-Ti. The number of cells that adhered and proliferated on the R-TiO_2 surface was visually greater than that on the others. These results showed two things: the osteoblasts can grow into the porous structure of TiO_2 surfaces, and β-Ti alloys with rutile-rich surfaces may be ideal for orthopedic and dental implants [79]. Other studies have also reported similar beneficial results from titanium surface oxidation [80]; both TiO_2 [81] and ZrO_2 surfaces exhibited a similar effect on osseointegration [82].

Plecko et al. [83] evaluated Co–Cr alloy, Ti-coated Co–Cr, Ti/Zr-coated Co–Cr, CpTi and steel in terms of their osseointegration and biocompatibility in a pelvic implantation model in sheep. It was reported that the Co–Cr screws showed significantly lower removal torque values than CpTi screws and generally tended toward lower torque values than the other materials, with the exception of steel screws, which showed no significant difference. Histomorphometrically, there were no significant differences of bone area between the groups. Based on these findings, it was concluded that Co–Cr and steel show less osseointegration than the other tested materials. However, the osseointegration of Co–Cr was improved by zirconium-or titanium-based, or both, coatings; their osseointegrative behavior is similar to that of pure titanium [83]. A TiN coating also affects bone formation, as it was reported that the healing observed around TiN-coated implants was similar to uncoated surfaces, and that TiN coating demonstrated good biocompatibility [84]. It is important to acknowledge that not all coatings encourage osseointegration. Freeman et al. [85] evaluated the effect of titanium aluminum nitride (TiAlN) coating on osseointegration and on the biological response and reported that TiAlN coatings may result in reduced osseointegration between bone and implant.

Surface modification of Ti-based metals is an important issue in improving the bone cell responses and bone-implant integration [86]. Hacking et al. investigated whether the superimposition of a microtexture on a porous-coated Ti substrate affected the extent of bone ingrowth [87]. Cylindrical titanium intramedullary implants were coated with sintered titanium beads to form a porous finish using commercial sintering techniques. A control group of implants was left in the as-sintered condition. The test group was etched in a boiling acidic solution to create an irregular surface over the entire porous coating. The results showed that bone formation was positively affected by the microtextured implant surface [87].

Rough implant surfaces have been shown to improve osseointegration rates [88,89]. This phenomenon is commonly referred to as rugophilia. In the majority of dental implants, microrough surfaces are obtained by sand blasting or acid-etching, or both, (SLA—sandblasting with large grit and acid-etching-treatment). The surfaces with increasing roughness show more osteoblastic adhered cells and the combination of the grit-blasted and acid-etched accelerated lightly bone regeneration at the different periods of implantation in comparison with the grit-blasted implants [88]. The SLA technique offers good morphological and biological management on implant surfaces [90–92].

A study by Stadlinger et al. [94] tested whether ossification could be improved by coating titanium implants with ECM components. They coated the implants with collagen alone, collagen and chondriotin sulfate, or chondroitin sulfate and growth factor BMP4 [95]. Peri-implant bone formation was measured within a defined recess along the long axis of the implant. BIC and BVD were determined using histomorphometry and synchrotron radiation micro computed tomography. It was concluded that collagen and collagen/chondroitin sulfate implant coatings impart an advantage to peri-implant bone formation [94].

Titanium surface modifications that simultaneously prevent bacterial adhesion and promote bone-cell functions could be highly beneficial to improving implant osseointegration. Alcheikh et al. [95] studied the effect of sulfonate groups on titanium surfaces with respect to both *S. aureus* adhesion and osteoblast functions pertinent to new bone formation. Oxydized CpTi was covalently bonded with poly (sodium styrene sulfonate) groups via radical polymerization. It was reported that grafting poly (sodium styrene sulfonate) groups to CpTi simultaneously inhibited bacteria adhesion and promoted osteoblast functions pertinent to new bone formation. Such modified titanium surfaces offer a promising strategy for preventing biofilm-related infections and enhancing osseointegration of implants in orthopedic and dental applications [95].

Titanium and its alloys represent the gold standard for orthopedic and dental prosthetic devices because of their good mechanical properties and biocompatibility. Recent research has focused on surface treatments designed to promote the rapid osseointegration of titanium implants, even when bone quality of the implant site is poor. Ferraris et al. [96] investigated a new surface treatment designed to improve the tissue integration of titanium-based implants. The surface treatment was able to induce bioactive behavior (without the introduction of a coating) and preserved the mechanical properties of Ti–6Al–4V substrates (e.g., fatigue resistance). The technique created a complex surface topography that was characterized by a combination of micro-roughness and nanotexture. Further surface texture was created by coupling this technique with conventional macro-roughness blasting. The modified metallic surfaces were rich in hydroxyl groups—this feature is extremely important for inorganic bioactivity (*in vitro* and *in vivo* apatite precipitation) and also for further functionalization procedures, such as the grafting of biomolecules. Modified Ti6–Al4–V induced HA precipitation after 15 days soaking in SBF. It was reported that the process was optimized in order to not induce cracks or damages on the surface and the surface oxide layer presents high scratch resistance [96].

Pham et al. [97] investigated the effect of fluoride on the surface chemistry of polycrystalline ceramic titanium dioxide (TiO_2) and metallic titanium (Ti), as well as its effect on the proliferation and differentiation of primary human osteoblasts. The osteoblasts were exposed to fluoride-modified and unmodified samples for 1, 3, 7, 14, and 21 days. It was reported that cell differentiation, with regard to gene expression, showed no significant difference between fluoride-modified and unmodified samples and less effect on protein release for all groups. Primary human osteoblast cells did not differ on fluoride-treated Ti and TiO_2 surfaces, indicating that fluoride is not the unique factor for the bioactivity of Ti and TiO_2surfaces [97].

Osseointegration was examined using titanium implants that had hydrophilic phosphate ion-incorporated oxide surfaces [98]. The implants were grit blasted and assessed in rabbit cancellous bone. Bone healing was compared between these samples and commercially available microarc oxidized, phosphate-incorporated clinical implants (TiUnite, TU implant). The hydrophilic phosphate-incorporated Ti surface (P implant) was produced by hydrothermal treatment on grit-blasted, moderately rough-surfaced clinical implants. The TU implant was used as a control. Thirty-two threaded implants (16 P implants and 16 TU implants), 10 mm in length × 3.3 mm in diameter, were placed in the femoral condyles of 16 New Zealand White rabbits. Histomorphometric analysis, removal torque tests, and surface analysis of the torque-tested implants were performed 4 weeks after implantation. It was found that the P and TU implants displayed micro-rough surface features. Torque-tested P and TU implants had a considerable amount of bone attached to their surfaces, yet P implants exhibited significantly higher bone–implant contact percentages, both in the thread region and the total lateral length of the implants, as compared to the TU implants. However, no statistical difference was found for the removal torque values. This suggested that the phosphate incorporated Ti oxide surface obtained by hydrothermal treatment achieves rapid osseointegration in cancellous bone by increasing the degree of bone–implant contact [98].

Sul [99] fabricated TiO_2 nanotubes on TiO_2grit-blasted, screw-shaped rough titanium (CpTi Grade IV) implants (3.75 × 7 mm) using potentiostatic anodization at 20 V in 1 M H_3PO_4 + 0.4 wt.% HF. The resulting nanotunes were vertically aligned and approximately 700 nm in length, and highly ordered; the structures were spaced ≈40 nm apart and had a wall thickness of ≈15 nm. It was found that the fluorinated chemistry of the nanotubes of F–TiO_2, $TiOF_2$, and F Ti–O with F ion incorporation of ≈5 at.%, and their amorphous structure was the same regardless of reaction time, while the average roughness gradually decreased and the developed surface area slightly increased with reaction time. The results of studies on animals show that, despite their low roughness values, after six weeks the fluorinated TiO_2nanotube implants in rabbit femurs demonstrate significantly increased osseointegration strengths (41 vs 29 Ncm) and new bone formation (57.5% vs 65.5%). It was indicated that the method provided potential applications of the TiO_2 nanotubes in the field of bone implants and bone tissue engineering [99].

6.8. Biomimetic Coating

HA can be prepared by chemical synthesis or biomimetically using SBF. HA produced from SBF can be used for a range of applications such as improved fixation of fine- and complex-shaped orthopedic and dental implants, tissue engineering scaffolds, and localized and sustained drug delivery. McLeod et al. [100] investigated the SBF-grown HA coatings with respect to growth kinetics over short deposition periods, and possible differences between the coatings deposited with and without periodic SBF replenishment. It was reported that a continuous, stable HA coating fully covered the titanium substrate after a growth period of 13 hours without SBF replenishment, and that thicker HA coatings of about 1 μm resulted after a growth period of 21 days, both with and without SBF replenishment. The Ca/P ratio at the surface of the HA coating was significantly lower than that in its bulk, and no significant difference was observed between

HA grown with and without periodic replenishment of SBF [100]. Vidigal et al. conducted a similar study that compared two different HA coatings preparation processes on CpTi, namely the modified bomimetric process and the plasma spray process [101]. It was reported that the plasma spray process generated a typical rough topography mainly consisting of HA, while the HA coating produced by the biomimetic process was partially dissolved in water and only a very thin layer of calcium titanate plus calcium phosphate. Although *in vitro* tests showed that both coatings can be considered bioactive, the modified biomimetic process seems to be a simple and low-cost alternative, with high potential for *in vitro* applications [101]. It was also reported that biomimetic HA coatings can be used to enhance bone ingrowth on a cubic surface structure (porosity 77%) [102]. Similarly, Ca-P coatings can be prepared biomimetrically by immersing an anodized Ti sample in HBSS and modified SBF solution for 2 weeks at physiologic conditions of 37 °C, initial pH of 7.4, and p(CO_2) of 0.05 atm [103].

The ability of chitosan coating to support bone formation and osseointegration was investigated [104]. Chitosan-coated Ti pins were implanted unilaterally in the tibia of 16 adult male New Zealand white rabbits. At 2, 4, 8, and 12 weeks, undecalcified sections were histologically evaluated for healing and bone formation. It was concluded that the chitosan-coatings enabled the development of close, bony apposition (osteointegration), of dental/craniofacial and orthopedic implants [104]. Kim et al. [105] investigated the biologic function of recombinant human bone morphorgentic protein-2 (rhBMP-2) immobilized on a heparin-grafted Ti surface. The biological activity of MG-63 cells on pristine and functionalized Ti surfaces was investigated by cell proliferation assays. It was reported that Ti surfaces with immobilized rhBMP-2 were more hydrophilic than pristine Ti. Furthermore, rhBMP-2 immobilized on Ti promoted significantly higher alkaline phosphate activity and calcium deposition by MG-63 cells than pristine Ti. This suggested that by grafting heparin and immobilizing BMP-2 on Ti surfaces, inflammation can be inhibited and osteoblast function can be promoted [105]. Similar beneficial effects have been reported for a variety of protein coatings [106–108].

For improving the seal between the neck portion of Ti dental implant and the surrounding soft tissue, several surface modifications were prepared: machining, machining and acid etching, and machining, acid etching, and depositing 4.5 collagen/hyaluronic acid polyelectrolyte bilayers [56]. Human gingival fibroblasts were cultured on the different surfaces, and cell morphology, spreading, and proliferation were observed. It was reported that all three sample types showed a similar, microscopic surface topology. However, morphologic differences were apparent at the nanoscale: both acid etching and collagen/hyaluronic acid deposition improved the hydrophilicity of the titanium surface, cell attachment and the spreading of HGF was better on collagen/hyaluronic acid coating, and the proliferation and differentiation of fibroblasts were greatly stimulated when cultured on collagen/hyaluronic acid-coated Ti. It was concluded that the collagen/hyaluronic acid treatment of Ti improved the attachment, spreading, proliferation, and differentiation of HGF [56]. Similarly, it was reported that a biofunctional protein coating accelerated autologous *in vivo* endothelialization and induced a significantly increased medial recellularization [109]. Since one of the key challenges in bone healing and regeneration is the engineering of an implant with surface properties that can enhance revascularization to meet the metabolic demands of recovery, successful implant integration into the surrounding tissue is highly dependent on the crucial role of blood supply in driving bone repair and development [110]. Poh et al. [110] investigated the effects of the immobilized vascular endothelial growth factor (VEGF) on titanium alloy substrates coated with a thin adherent polydopamine film. It was reported that the functionalized surfaces showed a significant increase in human dermal microvascular endothelial cell attachment, viability, and proliferation when compared to the pristine substrate. Additionally, the immobilized VEGF was able to induce the differentiation of human mesenchymal stem cells into endothelial cells, suggesting that utilizing the reactivity of polydopamine films to immobilize the vascular endothelial growth factor onto metal substrates may provide a promising approach for application in situations where revascularization around implants would be beneficial in improving bone healing and implant integration [110]. The Ca–P compound was biomimetrically deposited on the titanium substrate and the response of human mesenchymal stem cells was evaluated. It was concluded that biomimetic surface modification could lead to a substantial improvement in osteoinduction in titanium alloy implants [111].

Several studies have been performed to assess the effectiveness of antibacterial-coated biomaterials' ability to reduce surgical site infection. Such antibacterial coatings should include the chitosan-copper complex [112], carboxymethyl chitosan and bone morphogenetic protein 2 [113], Ag and $AgNO_3^-$ ion [114,115], surface-modified TiO_2 [116–118].

6.9. Measures Against Toxic Ion Elution

The release of Ni from biomedical NiTi materials [119–121] has stimulated a great deal of research on its surface modifications and coatings. The selective dissolution of the Ni ion from the NiTi alloy during the naturally occurring *in vivo* corrosion process could lead to potential danger [122–124]. There are basically two ways to prevent the release of Ni ions: selectively leach out Ni ions chemically or electrochemically, or entirely cover the Ni-containing surface with a noble species. The actual methods used to achieve these ends include etching in acids and alkaline solutions, electropolishing, heat and ion beam treatments, boiling in water and autoclaving, conventional and ion plasma implantations, laser melting and bioactive coating deposition [125–128]. It should be noted that electrochemical treatments run the risk of causing hydrogen embrittlement, depending on the extent of hydrogen overpotential [129–131].

The leaching of Ni ions from NiTi alloys was prevented by using plasma surface modification to form a hard surface layer of TiO_2 (from 4.6 to 23.0 GPa) [132]. Ni ion leaching was also prevented by Ta coating [130], Hafnium (Hf) ion implantation [133], or nitrogen implantation [134]. Potentially toxic Al and V elements from the Ti–6Al–4V alloy were suppressed by oxygen glow-discharge plasma oxidation [135].

6.10. Evaluation of Biocompatibility

As we discussed earlier, there is no concrete definition for the term biocompatibility. As we will demonstrate in this section, there are various methods to evaluate biocompatibility. Surface-treated titanium materials (CpTi, Ti–6Al–4V, or Ti–6Al–7Nb) were subjected to biocompatibility evaluation through electrochemical corrosion resistance, cell proliferation, adhesion, and viability [136–138]. MTT (3-(4,5-dimethylthiazol-2-yl)-2,5-diphenyltetrazolium bromide), cell apoptosis, and cell adhesion tests were conducted using (Ti, Al, V)N coating on Ti–6Al–4V [139], HA+TiO_2 deposited Ti–6Al–4V [140], porous Ti [141] and TiNi [142]. Moreover, MC3T3-E1 fibroblast or preosteoblast cellular responses were evaluated on HA coatings [143], HA+polyurethane composite coatings [144], TiO_2 coatings [145], SLA Ti [146], and plasma-nitrided ultrahigh-molecular-weight polyethylene (UHMWPE) [147]. Shim et al. evaluated the biocompatibility by examining the fibrous tissue surrounding the implant made of CpTi, Ti–6Al–4V, and Ti–6Al–7Nb alloys [148]. Similarly, cell attachment and proliferation of osteblast cell were tested on Ti–6Al–7Nb [149], fluoridated HA coatings [150], and Ca–P-coated oxidized Ti surface [151]. The reaction to human umbilical vein endothelial cells was used for biocompatibility evaluation on the Ti–6Al–4V alloy [152] and TiN/Ag composite-coated 317 stainless steel [153]. MG 63 (human osteosarcoma cell line) was used for F-ion-implanted CpTi [154] and CaP containing TiO_2 composite coatings [155].

For the improvement of surface roughness and mechanical interlocking with bone, titanium prostheses are grit-blasted with Al_2O_3particles during manufacturing. Oshida et al. [156] have pointed out that the blasting media may contaminate the implant surface, causing an adverse effect on subsequent processing. Rüger et al. [157] studied that the effect of the cleansing process reduces residual Al_2O_3 particles on the biocompatibility of the implants through histomorphometic tests at the bone–implant contact area and biomechanical push-out tests on the interface strength. It was reported that clinically, Al_2O_3-free titanium prostheses could lead to less mechanical wear of the articulating surfaces and ultimately result in less aseptic loosening and longer implant life [157].

6.11. Mechanical Properties

Vickers hardness was measured on cross sections and the top surface of high-velocity oxyfuel sprayed titania (TiO_2) coatings under 25, 50, 100, 300, 500, and 1000 g loads. The uniformity of the microstructure resulted in near isotropic behavior with regard to hardness [158]. Since orthopedic implants such as total hip replacement or knee joint systems involve biotribologial actions, evaluations on wear and friction become very crucial (wear debris toxicity is another important issue of concern). Friction and wear were evaluated on passivated CpTi and Ti–6Al–4V implants [159], wear of implants against UHMWPE [160,161], wear of TiN-coated Ti alloys against (WC–Co) steel [162], ceramic coatings on the Ti–6Al–4V alloy surface [163], SiO_2/TiO_2 coating on Ti–6Al–4V [164] and oxidized zirconium (Zr) on UHMWPE [165]. Combined wear-corrosion tests can provide more complete information about an implant's behavior in an aggressive body environment than separate wear and corrosion testing. The DLC (diamond-like-carbon)-coated Co–28Cr–6Mo alloy was tested in the wear-corrosion tests' performance in 0.9 wt% NaCl, at room temperature [166]. Various types of nitrided surfaces were subjected to wear testing: TiN-coated CpTi (grade II) [167], nitrided

Ti–3Nb–13Zr, nitride CpTi [168], nitrogen ion-implanted Ti–6Al–4V [169], nitrogen ion implanted Ti–6Al–4V and Co–28Cr–6Mo [170], and nitrided Co–28Cr–6Mo alloy [171].

In the area of orthodontic mechano-therapy, the friction between archwire and bracket is very important. NiTi orthodontic archwires were DLC coated and the friction between the samples and bracket surfaces were evaluated in a fluoride-containing environment. It was reported the DLC coating significantly decreased the fretting wear and the coefficient of friction, both in ambient air and artificial saliva [172].

Shot blasting or peening (which generates surface compressive residual stress and increases effective surface area) has a beneficial effect on fatigue strength and fatigue life [173]. Similar improvement of fatigue strength was reported on Ti materials [174,175]. It was also reported that a biodegradable Mg alloy's fatigue property was improved by HA coating [176].

During the ion implantation and IBAD processes, residual stress in the deposited film was created, depending on processing parameters. He et al. [177] reported that, while depositing Ti thin films on Si substrates, the residual stress was sensitive to film thickness and anneal temperature [177]. The effects of different thicknesses of HA coatings on bone stress distribution near the dental implant/bone interface are very important factors to HA-coated dental implant design and to the designs' clinical application [178]. Jiang et al. [178], using finite element analysis (FEA), calculated the bone stress distributions near dental implants coated with different thicknesses of HA, from 0 to 200 μm, under a 200 N chewing load. It was reported that the HA coatings weaken the stress concentration and improve the biomechanical property in the bone. However, in HA coating thicknesses in the 60–120 μm range, benefits are not obvious [178].

There are several studies on fatigue characteristics. Stráský et al. [179] prepared three different microstructures: equiaxed, bi-modal, and coarse lamellar forms of the Ti–6Al–4V alloy. Electric discharge machining (EDM) with a high peak current (29Å) was performed in order to impose surface roughness and modify the chemical composition of the surface. Rotating bending fatigue tests were undertaken for all three EDM-treated microstructures. The fatigue performance was found to be rather poor and not particularly dependent on the microstructure. The bi-modal microstructure showed a slightly superior high-cycle fatigue performance. This performance can be further improved by suitable heat treatment to an endurance limit of 200 MPa [179]. Many surface treatments used in cementless and endosseous implants modify the surfaces' topography and roughness to increase the implant-bone contact area, and thus favor bio-mechanical anchorage and shortening the period of osseointegration. Surprisingly, the effects that the surface treatments can have on the fatigue life of the material are not generally considered. In this sense, the superficial condition of the component is one of the features that have an effect on fatigue strength, especially on fatigue crack nucleation. Pazos et al. [180] studied the fatigue behavior of annealed CpTi grade IV. The surface treatments used were acid etching, shot blasting, and a dual treatment of blasting + acid etching. An as-machined surface was used as a control. Rotating-bending fatigue tests of each surface treatment were conducted at room temperature and a frequency of 33 Hz. Tested samples were also characterized to evaluate fatigue damage. Acid etching decreased fatigue endurance, while blasting and blasting + acid etching treatments showed a similar behavior with respect to the control. For acid etching, the modifications introduced stress raisers and appeared to accelerate the nucleation of cracks. Both blasting treatments generated stress raisers, and additionally introduced compressive residual stresses and superficial plastic deformation that tended to improve the fatigue endurance of the material [180].

There are several studies on effects of residual stress. Mode I edge delamination could be initiated due to the presence of the interfacial peeling stresses near the edges of the multilayered systems—this may arise because of material mismatches between adjacent layers. However, the exact peeling stress distributions could not be quantified using existing analytical and numerical models. It was recently proposed that the peeling moment, resulting from the localized peeling stresses, could be used to characterize mode I edge delamination. Zhang et al. [181] investigated the effect of the graded interlayer on the mode I edge delamination by thermal residual stresses in multilayer coating-based systems. In accordance with prior analytical approaches, the exact closed-form solutions for the peeling moments at individual interfaces and the curvatures for a bi-layered system were derived for both a typical thermal barrier coating (TBC) system and a TBC-based system with a graded interlayer inserted between the metallic and the ceramic layers. Case studies have shown that edge delamination by thermal stress can be impeded by properly selecting the coating materials and individual layer thicknesses. It was concluded that this study may provide some important insights for developing fail-safe design methodologies for multilayered systems [181].

Different thicknesses of HA coatings affect bone stress distribution near the dental implant-bone interface. As a result, HA thickness is a very important factor for HA-coated dental implant design and clinical application. The proximal bone stress distribution was calculated and analyzed under the 200 N chewing load for dental implants coated with different HA thicknesses (0–200 μm) was observed. In all cases, the greatest von Mises stresses in the bone were near the neck of dental implant on the lingual side. It was also shown that von Mises stresses decreased as HA coatings' thickness increased, HA coatings abate the stress concentration, and HA coating improved the biomechanical property in the bone. However, in HA coatings' thickness range of 60–120 μm, the distinctions of that benefit are not obvious. In addition, considering the technical intent of coating implants with HA, we conclude that thicknesses of HA coatings in the range of 60–120 μm would be a better choice for clinical applications [178]. Ti films with a thickness of 1.6 μm (group A) and 4.6 μm (group B) were prepared on the surface of the silicon crystal substrate by metal vapor vacuum arc (MEVVA) ion implantation, combined with IBAD. Different annealing temperatures ranging from 100 °C to 500 °C were used to investigate the effect of temperature on residual stress and the mechanical properties of the Ti films. The experimental results suggest that residual stress was sensitive to film thickness and annealing temperature. The critical temperatures, which the residual stress changed from compressive to tensile, were found to be 404 °C and 428 °C for groups A and B, respectively. The mean surface roughness and grain size of the annealed Ti films increased with increasing annealing temperature and Ti film's nanohardness and modulus values reached their maximum values near the surface, and then, reached corresponding values with increasing depth of the indentation [177].

6.12. Temperature Changes

Patel et al. [182] analyzed temperature changes along the surface of a dental implant to establish the abutment temperature that could cause the critical 47 °C/1 min threshold at the implant level. Eight thermocouples were attached at 1-mm intervals to an abutment/implant configuration. The model consisted of two compartments in a thermostatically controlled environment. The upper compartment represented the oral cavity with the abutment, which was exposed to 20 mL of hot water. The temperature at each thermocouple was logged over a period of 10 minutes. An estimation of the "effective dose 50" (ED50) for the abutment (95% confidence interval) was done. It was found that, for 53 test series, the abutment temperature ranged from 52.80 °C to 71.72 °C. There was a positive correlation between the maximum temperature at the implant level and the temperature of the abutment. The 47 °C/1 min threshold was reached 31 times at the most cervical implant level and decreased in frequency farther away from the heat source (14, 6, 3, 1, and 1 times, respectively).The ED50 was estimated at 62.3 °C, indicating that for an abutment temperature of 62.3 °C, there was a 50% chance that 47 °C would be reached at the implant level for 1 minute. Therefore, it was concluded that abutment temperature was transmitted to the implant. Although results of *in vitro* studies should be interpreted with caution, clinicians should be aware of temperature changes along implants and the potential risks associated with them [182].

There may be temperature changes or gradients during surface treatments, as well as modifications. Geminiani et al. [183] investigated the temperature gradient (ΔT) generated by laser irradiation of an implant surface using a carbon dioxide (CO_2) and an Erbium:yttrium aluminium garnet (Er:YAG) laser. A dental implant was irradiated with CO_2 and Er:YAG lasers, with variable power settings. Temperature increase was measured at two locations on the implant surface: in the cervical area (ΔTc) and in the apical area (ΔTa). It was reported that (i) the CO_2 laser showed the following results: after 60 seconds of irradiation with continuous mode, ΔTc was 13.9 °C and ΔTa was 12.5 °C. The Er:YAG laser showed the following results: after 60 seconds of irradiation with continuous mode, the temperature rise ΔTc was 50.6 °C and ΔTa was 38.6 °C, (ii) the CO_2 laser with continuous mode generated a temperature increase of 10 °C after only 36 seconds, and (iii) the Er:YAG laser with continuous mode produced a more rapid temperature increase and took only 10 s to reach the critical threshold. It was, therefore, concluded that the irradiation of implant surfaces with CO_2 and Er:YAG lasers may produce a temperature increase above the critical threshold (10 °C) after 10 seconds of continuous irradiation [183].

6.13. Corrosion Behavior

It is generally believed that a material with excellent corrosion resistance should be evaluated to be good biocompatible with vital hard/soft tissues because the oxide film formed on surface substrates shows chemical or electrochemical stability, or both, which prevents further oxidation reaction and unwanted ion release. The corrosion behavior of variously surface-treated materials indicated that sandblasted surfaces showed the least corrosion resistance, while polished or pre-passivated surfaces in either HNO_3 or oxygenated saline solution exhibited better corrosion resistance in stainless steel and Co–Cr alloy [184].

The electrochemical behavior of TiO_2 deposited on 316L stainless steel was characterized in SBF. It was shown that (i) the titanium dioxide-coated 316L SS exhibited a higher corrosion resistance than uncoated 316L stainless steel and (ii) the titanium dioxide coated surface was porous, uniform, and acted as a barrier layer on the metallic substrate, and (iii) the porous titanium dioxide coating induces the formation of HA layer on the metal surface [185]. The passive oxide film formed on titanium and its natural growth in a phosphate buffered solution with and without an H_2O_2 addition were investigated by electrochemical impedance spectroscopy (EIS) and it was reported that (i) in the absence of H_2O_2, the impedance response indicated a stable thin oxide film on titanium; (ii) however, the addition of H_2O_2 to the solution led to a significant decrease in corrosion resistance of titanium and also to a thickening of the porous outer layer [186]. Titania-coated NiTi was subjected to EIS measurements in Hank's solution and it as reported that the corrosion resistance of titania-coated NiTi samples was increased by about two orders of magnitude compared with the substrate [187]. Anodized NiTi samples in a solution containing calcium and phosphate ions (solution Ca-P) were electrochemically characterized. It was reported that polarization tests in Hanks' solution showed significant increase in corrosion resistance due to anodization and further increase was obtained via hydrothermal treatment [188]. The corrosion resistance of titanium nitride (TiN)-coated and ion-nitrided Ti substrates for dental applications were investigated and the polarization resistance obtained from the EIS was ranked as follows: TiN-coated Ti>ion-nitrided Ti>untreated Ti [189]. Similar results were reported for TiN-coated nanotube-formed Ti–Ta–Zr alloy [190] and Hf containing ZrCN protective layers [191].

An amorphous Ta_2O_5 layer was prepared on a Ti surface using a simple hydrolysis-condensation process at room temperature and the corrosion resistance of the test specimens was evaluated from the potentiodynamic polarization curves and ion release measurements in simulated blood plasma. It was reported that the presence of an amorphous Ta_2O_5 layer on the Ti surface increased its corrosion resistance and biocompatibility [192]. Tantalum was coated on a NiTi substrate. Using X-ray photoelectron spectroscopy, it was found that a thin oxide film, with Ta_2O_5 in the outmost layer and tantalum suboxides in the inner layer, was formed on the tantalum coating as a result of natural passivation of Ta in the atmosphere. The Ni ion release from uncoated and coated samples was studied in the 0.9% NaCl solution and indicated that the Ta_2O_5 coating had a beneficial effect on the inhabitation of Ni ion release from the TiNi substrate [193].

Biodegradable Mg alloys are of great interest for osteosynthetic applications because they do not require surgical removal after they have served their purpose [194]. The surface-treated Mg alloy by microarc oxidation was investigated in terms of the degradation rate. It was reported that oxidation treatment appears to be very interesting for osteosynthetic implant applications, as it delays implant degradation immediately after implantation, enhances fracture stabilization, minimizes the burden on the postoperatively irritated surrounding tissue, and generates good bone/implant connections—all this is followed by accelerated degradation in the later stages of bone healing [195]. Bioglass-apatite coated Ti–6Al–4V was subjected to electrochemical corrosion tests in SBF. Electrochemical impedance spectroscopic tests revealed higher polarization resistance and lower capacitance values for the coated specimens, which is evidence of the stable nature of the formed coatings [196].

For decades, the design, development, and use of metallic biomaterials has focused on the corrosion resistance of these materials once implanted in the human body. Recently, degradable metallic biomaterials have been proposed for specific applications, including pediatric, orthopedic, and cardiovascular. Degradable metallic biomaterials are expected to disappear via corrosion after providing structural support for a certain period of time, which depends on the application site. Over the past decades, a wide-ranging and comprehensive set of *in vitro*, *in vivo*, and in some cases, *ex vivo* tests have been proposed and exhaustively investigated for conventional corrosion-resistant metallic biomaterials. Once implanted, this new class of biomaterials is expected to support the healing process of a diseased tissue or organ while degrading at a potentially adjustable degradation rate. The tests developed for corrosion-resistant metals cannot simply be transposed to degradable materials. The current challenge is how to assess the tolerance of surrounding tissues and organs to the presence of degradation products [197].

Studies on the corrosion behavior of HA coatings on various Ti alloys, including Ti–20Nb–10Zr–5Ta alloy [198], Ti–35Nb-(3–5)HF alloy [199], Ti–6Al–4V [200,201], and 316L stainless steel [201–203] indicate that the polarization resistance (R_p) of HA-coated surface was higher than that of uncoated substrates.

6.14. Effect of Sterilization

The effects of surface preparation and sterilization treatments of CpTi on *in vitro* osteoblast cell attachment were investigated. Surface characterization by XPS (X-ray photoelectron spectroscopy) and AES (Auger electron spectroscopy) and determination of wetting angles indicated that sterilization by exposure to ultraviolet light or gamma irradiation resulted in highly energetic, relatively contaminant-free CpTi surfaces, which supported high levels of osteoblast cell attachment. Steam autoclaving, however, resulted in relatively low energy surfaces with high levels of O-C-and N-containing contaminants. Other inorganic contaminants were also detected on the surface of selected samples. As a result, steam-autoclaved surfaces supported significantly lower levels of cell attachment. Two hours after initial attachment, osteoblast cells failed to spread and integrate on surface characteristics were bio-determined using contaminated and CpTi substrata first onto the surfaces sterilized by steam autoclaving. These results confirm previous studies regarding the contamination resulting from steam autoclaving and indicate that noncontaminating sterilization procedures should be employed for the sterilization of commercial metallic implant materials [204].

Biomaterials must be sterilized before implantation, but the effects of sterilization on their surface properties have been less well studied. The effects of cleaning and sterilization manufactured to present two different surface structures: pretreated titanium (PT, Ra – 0.4 μm) (i.e., surfaces that were not modified by sandblasting or acid etching, or the both); (SLA, Ra = 3.4 μm). Previously cultured cells and their ECM were removed from all bio-contaminated specimens by cleaning in a sonicator bath with a sequential acetone—isopropanol—ethanol—distilled water protocol. Cleaned specimens were sterilized with autoclave, gamma irradiation, oxygen plasma, or ultraviolet light. Small organic molecules present on contaminated Ti surfaces were removed with cleaning. It was found that (i) cleaning and sterilization affected hydrophobicity and roughness, (ii) these modified surface properties affected osteogenic differentiation of human MG63 osteoblast-like cells, (iii) specifically, autoclaved SLA surfaces lost the characteristic increase in osteoblast differentiation seen on starting SLA surfaces, which was correlated with altered surface wettability and roughness. These data indicated that recleaned and resterilized Ti implant surfaces can't be considered the same as the first surfaces in terms of surface properties and cell responses. It was, therefore, concluded that the re-use of Ti implants after resterilization may not result in the same tissue responses as found with never-before-implanted specimens [205].

6.15. Strontium Effect

Although studies have indicated systemic treatment with Sr as a potential route to increase bone quality and formation around osseointegrating implants, adverse effects are linked to such treatment [206–208]. Anderson et al. [209] demonstrated a surface modification method designed for sustained local release of Sr from implants. The four groups used were prepared by a magnetron co-sputtering process and selected on the basis of Sr release data. Mesenchymal stem cells (MSCs) were cultured on the different coatings to evaluate potential cytotoxic effects and the effect on cellular proliferation. It was reported that (i) no indication of toxicity was found, (ii) a rodent study demonstrated a significant increase in direct bone-to-implant contact and peri-implant bone volume for several of the groups four weeks after implantation, as compared to a CpTi (grade 4) reference group, (iii) median values of bone-to-implant contact and new bone formation was found to be 19% and 53%, respectively, for the best group compared to 0% for both parameters with respect to the CpTi reference, indicating that this method may have applications within the orthopedic and dental industry [209].

Development of biomedical titanium implants with high osteogenic ability for fast and good osseointegration under normal as well as osteoporotic conditions is being pursued. Strontium (Sr)-loaded nanotubular structures that allow controlled and long-term Sr release are expected to yield favorable osteogenic effects and properties [210]. The amount of Sr loaded is regulated by the length of hydrothermal treatment, 1 and 3 hours, in a $Sr(OH)_2$ solution. It was found that (i) long lasting and controllable Sr release was observed in NT-Sr samples with no cytotoxicity, and (ii) Sr incorporation enhances proliferation of rat MSCs on the nanotubular structure; Sr-incorporated nanotubes promote the spread of the MSCs into a polygonal osteoblastic shape [210].

6.16. Characterization of HA

HA coatings have proven effective in providing excellent short- and intermediate-term outcomes in terms of fixation, stability, function, and pain relief [211–214]. HA coatings enhance osteoblast attachment, proliferation, and differentiation [215].

While HA is generally considered to be an osteoconductive material, it has occasionally been shown to have osteoinductive properties, which have been attributed to the adsorption of bone morphogenetic proteins [216]. Osteoblastic activity is modulated by surface roughness and is enhanced when the R_a is between 1 and 7 μm [217–219]. In addition, surface roughness is an important factor affecting *in vivo* bone apposition and mechanical strength of the implant–bone interface [220]. Increasing surface roughness by grit-blasting or chemical etching has been associated with increased osseointegration in a variety of animal models [221–223]. Since HA coatings can alter surface roughness, it is important to determine the relative significance of the individual contributions of these factors [221,224]. One study concluded that surface roughness contributed more to increased bone apposition rates than HA coating [224]. However, another study found significantly increased bone apposition in HA-coated implants despite comparable surface roughness measures between coated and uncoated implants [225].

HA coatings on 316 L stainless steel were evaluated and it was reported that (i) the coating showed a high degree of crystallinity ~92%, a high porosity level of 20 vol.% and a moderate bonding strength of about 13 MPa, (ii) using the nanoindentation technique, the nano-hardness and modulus of elasticity were 6 and 92 GPa, respectively, (iii) the fracture toughness was ~0.6 MPa $m^{0.5}$, and (iv) from the nano-scratch experiments, the critical normal load at which localized microcracking led to delamination was measured to be ~400 mN [226]. Although HA is employed as a coating on a range of press-fit (cementless) orthopedic implants to enhance their osseointegration, the plasma spraying method for HA depositing often contains unwanted crystal phases that can lead to coating delamination.

HA particles were used as blasting media and the inclusion of HA abrasive agents can enhance the *in vitro* and *in vivo* performance of the modified surface [227]. It was reported that (i) when HA was used along with alumina, a stable surface that enhanced *in vitro* osteoblast attachment and viability was obtained, and (ii) implantation of the surface produced by blasting with alumina and HA in a rabbit model confirmed that this surface promoted the *in vivo* formation of early stage lamellar bone growth [227]. McLeod et al. conducted a systematic study on growth kinetics of biomimetically grown HA thin film in the SBF solution in terms of two important parameters: SBF immersion period and with and without periodic SBF replenishment [100]. It was reported that (i) a continuous, stable HA coating fully covered the titanium substrate after a growth period of 13 hours without SBF replenishment; (ii) thicker HA coatings of about 1 μm in thickness resulted after a growth period of 21 days, both with and without SBF replenishment; and (iii) the Ca/P ratio at the surface of the HA coating was significantly lower than that in its bulk [100].

The chemical stability of coated HA by the electron-beam method was investigated by measuring the calcium ion meter for obtaining the dissolution rate and it was reported that (i) the dissolution rate was strongly dependent on the Ca/P ratio of the layer, (ii) layers with a Ca/P ratio close to that of crystalline HA (Ca/P = 1.67) showed good stability in the physiological saline solution, and (iii) when the layer was crystallized by heat treatment in air at temperatures between 400 °C and 500 °C, the stability was enhanced further while maintaining good interfacial bonding strength with the substrate [228]. A similar study indicated that (i) the dissolution of plasma-sprayed HA coating in a physiologic saline solution decreased with the cystallinity, and (ii) preferential dissolution was observed on the amorphous phase [229].

Among a huge volume of reports, the majority of which indicate positive and beneficial influences of HA coatings, there are negative evaluations of HA coatings that bring to light remarkable adverse effects. Plasma-sprayed HA coating on Ti–6Al–4V was evaluated *in vivo* for its effect on the osteoconductivity and it was reported that (i) HA coating with denser microstructure and less thickness showed a higher bonding strength at the HA/Ti–6A1–4V interface; (ii) however, this denser HAC underwent adverse biological degradation in terms of a new bone healing index after 12 weeks of implantation, indicating that the HA coating with both high bonding strength and good osteoconductivity is difficult to achieve [230].The effects of HA-coated CpTi dental implants on nerve conduction were studied using isolated rat sciatic nerves [231]. HA-coated implants were brought into intimate contact with the nerves and evoked compound action potentials were recorded before and after contact with the implants. It was reported that although the intimate contact with HA-coated implants lead to a reduction in compound action potentials in nerves *in vitro*, neither this surface nor CpTi surface lead to irreversible neurotoxic effects [231].

HA is widely employed as coating on cementless hip stems. On 151 prostheses (implanted between June 1990 and December 1991) with an anatomic fully HA-coated Co–Cr stem, alumina bearing surfaces, and a threaded Ti–6Al–4V cup, implanted in 147 consecutive patients (57 males, 90 females, average age 58 years), a 12-year follow-up examination was conducted and reported that at 12 years the HA-coated stem showed an overall good outcome while the threaded non-HA-coated cup employed had a bad survival, which influenced the longevity of the prosthesis, concluding that HA is a viable and effective coating [232]. There are several clinical reports on HA effects. Between 1990 and 1994, 138 patients underwent primary total hip arthroplasty (THA) using a simple femoral component. Thirty-eight patients received a textured geometry, 50 were implanted with a HA coated stem, and 50 with a plasma sprayed stem. The average length of follow up was 8 years, 11 months (range: 6–10 years). It was reported that it is obvious that the coating enhancement of choice was HA [233]. To differentiate between the survival and success definitions of functional HA-coated implant prosthesis, a total of 248 implants (62 patients), 5–10 years in function, were evaluated. The implant distribution lengths were 8 mm (6.5%), 10 mm (29.4%), 13 mm (30.2%), and 15 mm (33.9%) and the diameters were 3.25 mm (60.1%) and 4 mm (39.9%). Probing depth (PD), gingival index (GI), height of keratinized mucosa (KM), and recession (REC) were key parameters for evaluation. Only implants that fulfilled the success rate criteria were considered successful. All other functional implants were assigned to the nonsuccessful group. All functional implant prostheses were defined as survival ones. Based on the above criteria, it was concluded that a distinguishable difference between the survival and success rate was observed, particularly in long-term observations, and implant length and diameter have an influence on the survival rate [234]. A clinical report on 146 primary total knee replacements, either fully or partially coated with HA of which 74 knees in 68 patients were available for clinical and radiological assessment at a mean of 11.2 years (10–15), was published and it was concluded that fixation with HA is a reliable option in primary total knee replacement [235]. Capilla et al. [236] conducted a clinical follow-up on 127 cylindrical implants placed in 21 patients after 5 years of function: 75 implants were coated with titanium plasma spray and 52 implants were coated with HA. It was reported that (i) no significant differences were found between the two implant systems according to the periodontal parameters studied; (ii) however, 5-year success rates were 86.7% for Ti plasma sprayed implants and 94.3% for HA-coatedimplants and (iii) long-term success rates were outstanding for HA-coated implants and acceptable for Ti plasma sprayed implants after 5 years of function [236].

Bioactive glass coating by the vitreous enamelling technique and HA coating by the air microplasma spray technique were performed. The behavior of HA and recently developed bioactive glass-coated implants (62 implants) was compared in osseous tissue following implantation in 31 patients. It was reported that (i) HA and bioactive glass coating materials were nontoxic and biocompatible and (ii) bioactive glass-coated implants were as equally successful as HA in achieving osseointegration and supporting final restorations. It was concluded that the newly developed bioactive glass is a good alternative coating material for dental implants [237]. A clinical study was conducted on 269 HA ceramic-coated hip arthroplasties in patients under the age of 50 with annual review using the Harris Hip Score (HHS); assessments were over a maximum of 19 years. Early patients (46) had implants with ceramic/plastic bearings. Later patients (223) all had ceramic on ceramic bearings [238]. It was reported that (i) HHS showed 90.3% scoring over 90 or 100; lower scores mostly relate to other joint and medical problems, (ii) osteolysis and debris disease have only been seen rarely in hips with ceramic on polythene bearings, (iii) fractured alumina components have been encountered (six heads and three acetabular liners, 2.1%), (iv) ceramic/ceramic hips have otherwise remained successful, (v) wear in polythene liners developed in 21 patients followed up more than 15 years (45.7%), and (vi) other complications include one post-operative death and 14 dislocations (5.2%). Based on these clinical findings, it was concluded that HA-coated arthroplasty in patients under the age of 50 does well, and HA bonding provides lasting implant/bone stability [238].

6.17. Characterization of Other Bio-Ceramics

In this section, Ti oxides, TiN, and other complex compounds will be discussed as bio-ceramic materials. The effect of low pressure radio frequency (rf) plasma treatment on TiO_2surface states has been studied using X-ray photoelectron spectroscopy and it was reported that a rapid decrease in the ratio of carbon to titanium (C/Ti) at the TiO_2 surface was observed after plasma treatment and more than 90% of carbon atoms were removed from the surface. This led to the conclusion that the plasma treatment of TiO_2 has advantages over surface carbon cleaning, increasing O^- and Ti^{3+} surface states, hence improving the activity of TiO_2 for different environmental, energy, and biological applications [239].

Titania (TiO_2) can be potentiostatically anodized on CpTi in sulfuric acid (0.5M H_2SO_4) [240] or in phosphoric acid (1.4M H_3PO_4) [240,241]. A corrosion resistance comparison between these TiO_2 films was conducted in the phosphate saline buffer solution, PSB (pH 7.4) at 25 °C, and it was reported that anodic oxide prepared in H_3PO_4 exhibited higher polarization resistance [241]. A bioactive fluoride-modified implant (Osseospeed) and a bioinert anodically oxidized implant (TiUnite) were implanted in the tibiae of New Zealand white rabbits [242,243]. Two weeks after implant placement, the removal torque values were measured according to time. Using the time–torque curve resulting from the measurements, the maximum values were determined, and the angular momentum were calculated. It was reported that (i) the anodically oxidized implant had significantly higher peak removal torque and angular momentum values than the fluoride-modified implant and (ii) the bioactive fluoride-modified surface may show no superiority to the bioinert anodized surface in early bone response [243]. Similarly, it was reported that anodized Ti miniscrews had improved surface characteristics compared with machined surface miniscrews [244].

Among three crystalline structures (brookite, rutile, and anatase), anatase-type titania has been commonly produced [245–247] by the mid-frequency AC magnetron sputtering technique. The anatase phase of TiO_2 has been shown to have very good biocompability. It was reported that, after studying the mechanisms of the Ti to TiO and the TiO to anatase phase transitions, the anodizing and annealing treatments of Ti were evaluated in a best way to produce anatase-type titania [248]. Meanwhile, Valilić et al. reported that, by the plasma electrolytic oxidation of titanium in sodium metasilicate at 200 mA/cm^2, a mixture of partly crystallized and mainly composed of anatase and rutile titania was produced [249]. Tsai et al. reported that the composite $Ti(Zn)O_2$ coating with a lower content of Zn (7.6 ± 1.3 at.%) not only improved antibacterial activity against human *S. aureus*, but also maintained the biocompatibility to bone cells of murine osteoblasts (MC3T3-E1) [250].

TiN films have been applied for medical cutting tools to improve their mechanical properties such as surface hardness and wear resistance, and also to provide biocompatibility to the surgical tools. The TiN film was deposited by the bipolar-pulsed DC discharge method in the gas mixture of $TiCl_4$, N_2, H_2, and Ar. It was reported that (i), after corrosion tests, the Hank's solution, the estimated corrosion rates of uncoated stainless, was 1300 nA/cm^2, while that of TiN-coated stainless steel was only 66 nA/cm^2; (ii) the TiN film also shows a good biocompatibility in the standard cytotoxicity test (ISO10993-5) [251]. It was reported that the rf inductively coupled plasma technique formed new hard phases of TN, including α-Ti(N), δ-TiN, and ε-Ti_2N in the treated layer with microhardness of 2650 HV [252]. Furthermore, Subramanian et al. [253] assessed the performance of three titanium nitride coatings (TiN, TiON, and TiAlN) on CpTi substrates for biomedical applications in terms of their surface properties, electrochemical corrosion in SBF and cytotoxicity. It was reported that (i) on control samples (uncoated CpTi), platelets were seen as aggregates, whereas on nitrided CpTi, platelets were seen as singles, without any significant spreading and (ii) after the cytocompatibility studies, coated CpTi showed good cytocompatbility with the cell lines used [253]. Double nitride coatings of TiN and ZrN nanotubular structures on Ti–35Ta–*x*Hf (3wt% > *x* > 15 wt%) ternary alloys for bio-implant applications were investigated [254] and it was reported that (i) highly ordered, high aspect ratio, and nanotubular morphology surface oxide layers can be formed on the ternary titanium alloys by anodization, (ii) the TiN and ZrN coatings formed on the nanotubular surfaces were uniform and stable, and (iii) the top of the nanotube layers was uniformly covered with the ZrN film compared to the TiN film when the Ti–35Ta–*x*Hf alloys had the high Hf content [254].

Anodized Zr in a 1 mol/L phosphoric acid solution at a fixed potential between 3 and 30 V was characterized by means of several surface techniques. It was reported that (i) the incorporation of P from the electrolyte to the surface oxide during the anodizing process changed the surface chemistry and (ii) after 30 days of immersion in the SBF solution, Ca-P rich compounds were present on anodized zirconium [255]. Although metallic implants are widely used in orthopedic surgery, metal ion release in surrounding tissues may play a major role in therapeutic failure. Two types of biological glasses (BVA and BVH) were investigated as coatings of metal implants. It was reported that (i) the BVA glass is bioactive, that is it developed a direct chemical bond between prosthesis and bone by the formation of a calcium phosphate layer at its surface, and (ii) the BVH glass was not bioactive and was used as a cement to isolate the metal implant from the biological environment, but the coating disaggregates with implantation time and glass grains migrate through the bony lacuna network [256].

There are several works on SiO_2 containing coating materials including chemically synthesized $CaO–ZrO_2–SiO_2$ plasma sprayed onto a Ti–6Al–4V alloy substrate [257], Ti/dicalcium silicate composite coatings with different ratios (weight ratios as Ca_2SiO_4: Ti=3:7, 5:5, 7:3), plasma sprayed on the Ti–6Al–4V substrate [258] and $CaSiO_3$ (Wollastonite) plasma sprayed on different substrates [259]. There are interesting findings: (i) bioactivity evaluation in the Tris–HCl buffer indicated that the degradation mass loss of $CaO–ZrO_2–SiO_2$ was much lower than that of the Wollastonite coating and close to that of the HA coating [257]; (ii) the dissolution of dicalcium silicate in the composite coatings in simulated physiological environment resulted in the decrease of flexural strength and flexural modulus of the coatings in the simulated physiological environment; (iii) the higher the titanium content in the composite coatings, the more stable the composite coatings in the physiological environment [258]; and (iv) increasing the substrate temperature is a feasible method to improve the mechanical properties and to decrease the dissolution rate of Wollastonite coatings [259].

Although Co–Cr Mo alloys have been used since the 1940s in the production of orthopedic implants due to their excellent corrosion resistance, problems such as the release of metal ions into tissues and crevice corrosion associated with casting defects, inclusions, and others are encountered with these materials; crevice corrosion increases the tendency to fatigue failure [260], since the applied stress can be intensified at the tip of crevice. To improve the biocompatibility of the Co–Cr–Mo alloy, a layer of glass was used to bind α-alumina particles to a surgical Co–Cr alloy since the α-alumina cannot be sprayed without porosity and without phase transformation during deposition. The data obtained indicated that (i) a morphological study of the coating proved that the binding layer of glass is totally continuous and there was no contact between the metal and external fluids, and (ii) the flexural strength and the large amount of alumina on the surface indicated a promising future for this coating in orthopedic applications [260].

Due to the clinical fact that in THA, UHMWPE wear debris generated at the articular surface has been recognized as a long-term cause of loosening and failure of artificial hip joints due to osteolysis, the plasma-based ion implantation has been used to improve wear resistance of the metal femoral head. The Co–Cr-based alloy substrate was subjected to nitrogen ion implantation and improved corrosion resistance was noticed [261]. A similar beneficial effect of nitrization on the Co–Cr-based alloy was reported [262].

6.18. Surface Texturing and Topology

Topology and surface chemistry have a profound effect on the way in which cells interact with an implant, which in turn impacts clinical use and performance. Birch et al. [263] examined an electrochemical polishing approach in H_2SO_4/methanol that could be applied to the widely used orthopedic/dentistry implant material (Ti–6Al–4V) to produce structured surfaces. The surface roughness, as characterized by R_a, was found to be dependent on the time of electropolishing. The surface chemistry, however, was dependent on the applied electrochemical potential. It was found that the chemical composition of the surface layer was modified during the electrochemical process, and at high potentials (9.0 V), a pure TiO_2 layer of at least 10 nm was created on top of the bulk alloy. Characterization of these surfaces with rat cells from the osteoblast lineage provided further evidence of contact guidance by microscale topography with morphology analysis correlating with surface roughness (R_a 300–550 nm). Formation of a bone-like matrix after long-term culture on these surfaces was not strongly dependent upon R_a values but followed the voltage parameter. It was suggested, based on these results, that the surfaces created by treatment at higher voltages (9.0 V) produced a nanoscale layer of pure TiO_2 on the Ti–6Al–4V surface that influenced cellular differentiation, culminating in osteogenesis [263]. The effects of submicron topography and microtopography on the phenomena of bone bonding and interfacial stability of endosseous implants were investigated [264], by placing custom-made titanium alloy implants of varying surface topographical complexity in rat femora, for 6, 9 or 12 days. The five surfaces were polished, machined, dual acid etched, and two forms of grit blasted and acid etched; each surface type was further modified with the deposition of nanocrystals of calcium phosphate to make a total of 10 material groups ($n = 10$ for each time point; total 300 implants). At sacrifice, the bone/implant interface was subjected to a mechanical disruption test. It was found that even the smoothest surfaces, when modified with sub-micron scale crystals, could be bonebonding. However, as locomotor loading through bone to the implant increased with time of healing, such interfaces failed while others, with submicron features superimposed on surfaces of increasing microtopographical complexity, remained intact under loading. It was, hence, demonstrated that micron or coarsemicron, topography is a requirement for longer term interfacial stability [264].

Wennerberg et al. [265] analyzed the possible effects of titanium surface topography on bone integration, collecting data from a PubMed search that identified 1184 publications of assumed relevance; of those, 1064 had to be disregarded because they did not accurately present *in vivo* data on bone response to surface topography. The remaining 120 papers were read and analyzed, after the removal of an additional 20 papers that mainly dealt with CaP-coated and Zr implants; 100 papers remained and formed the basis for their paper. The bone response to differently configured surfaces was mainly evaluated by histomorphometry (bone-to-implant contact), removal torque, and pushout/pullout tests. The obtained analytical results were as follows: (i) a huge number of the experimental investigations have demonstrated that the bone response was influenced by the implant surface topography; smooth ($S_a < 0.5$ μm) and minimally rough (S_a 0.5–1 μm) surfaces showed less strong bone responses than rougher surfaces and (ii) moderately rough (S_a > 1–2 μm) surfaces showed stronger bone responses than rough (S_a > 2 μm) in some studies. It was concluded that (i) surface topography influences bone response at the micrometer level, (ii) some indications exist that surface topography influences bone response at the nanometer level, (iii) the majority of published papers present an inadequate surface characterization, (iv) measurement and evaluation techniques need to be standardized, and (v) not only height descriptive parameters but also spatial and hybrid ones should be used [265].

Carimo et al. [266] topographically characterized a titanium alloy subjected to different surface treatments using roughness evaluation, scanning electron microscopy (SEM), and atomic force microscopy (AFM).

For each group, six disks of a titanium alloy had their surfaces modified by four treatments. All surfaces were blasted with Al_2O_3, cleaned, and the specimens were divided into four groups: G1, immersion in a standardized acid solution (SAS) (control group); G2, immersion in acetone, followed by immersion in SAS; G3, immersion in acetone, followed by immersion in SAS, followed by immersion in nitric acid; G4, immersion in acetone, followed by immersion in SAS, followed by immersion in sulfuric acid. It was reported that (i) regarding the roughness parameters, no significant differences were found, (ii) a similar roughness pattern was created for all the groups, and (iii) the images and topographic profiles indicated that all the groups showed high levels of roughness [266]. Ricci et al. [267] evaluated the characteristics and the topography of a new implant surface. Titanium disks were manufactured using master alloy powder (Ti–6Al–4V) with a particle size of 25–45 μm as the basic material. Images in three different dimensional ranges of decreasing dimensions: 30 (dimensional class A), 10 (dimensional class B), and 5 μm^2 (dimensional class C) were acquired. For each dimensional range, five (dimensional classes A and B) to ten (dimensional classes C) different images, belonging both to the center and to the edge of the slide, were collected. In dimensional class A, the implant surface showed an average roughness value (R_a) of 0.6 μm, whereas the root mean square roughness (R_{rms}) value was 0.78 μm. In the dimensional class B, the value of R_a was 133.4 μm and the value of R_{rms} was 161.7 μm. Finally, at a smaller level as in dimensional class C, the value of R_a was 68.5 μm and R_{rms} was 81.05 μm. Moreover, the peak to peak value was 369.5 μm and the average height value was 187.3 μm. The surface which results from the direct laser fabrication process has an ideal nano-roughness to enhance protein adsorption and to facilitate precursor osteoblast adhesion. In conclusion, direct laser surface formation seems to be a promising technique for producing dental implants from titanium alloys [267].

Pecora et al. [268] evaluated a tapered dental implant with a 2-mm wide collar that was laser micromachined in the lower 1.5 mm in order to preferentially encourage bone and connective tissue attachment while inhibiting epithelial down-growth. Data are reported at measurement periods from 1 to 37 months postoperative for 20 pairs of implants in 15 patients. The implants are placed adjacent to machined collar control implants of the same design. Measurement values are reported for bleeding index, plaque index, probing depth, and crestal bone loss. It was reported that (i) no statistical differences were measured for either bleeding or plaque index, (ii) at all measurement periods there were significant differences in the probing depths and the crestal bone loss differences were significant after 7 months, and (iii) at 37 months the mean probing depth was 2.30 mm and the mean crestal bone loss was 0.59 mm for LL versus 3.60 and 1.94 mm, respectively, for control implant. Furthermore, there was a nonstatistically significant suggestion that the LL crestal bone retention superiority was greater in the maxilla than in the mandible [268]. Laser engineering may create hemispherical porosities on titanium surfaces obtaining regular and predetermined rough titanium surfaces. Cei et al. [269] studied the viability and the proliferation of primary osteoblast-like cells to growth factors on titanium surfaces with a different roughness *in vitro*. The osteoblast-like cells were allowed to attach on four different titanium surfaces: sandblasted titanium disks, 5-, 10-, and 20-μm regular laser-engineered micropore titanium disks. A well with no disk was used as control. Cell morphology was evaluated with SEM. Viability was measured with the MTT (3[4, 5 dimethylthiazol 2yl]2, 5 diphenyltetrazolium bromide) assay. The proliferation rate of attached cells was evaluated with Cell Counting Kit-8 48 hours after the platelet-released supernatant (PRS) application. It was reported that (i) all surfaces showed osteoblast-like cells attachment on SEM, (ii) osteoblast-like cells appeared more numerous on 20-μm surfaces, and (iii) the laser-engineered surfaces showed higher osteoblast-like cells viability than the sandblasted Ti surfaces. In terms of proliferation, viability increase was noted for all groups after the PRS application. It was, therefore, concluded that the laser-engineered porous titanium surfaces promoted viability and proliferation of osteoblast-like cells [269]. The effect of micro/nanotextured titanium implant on osseointegration in ovariectomized (OVX) sheep was investigated [270]. The hierarchical micro/nanotextured surface of titanium implant was fabricated by acid in 0.5% (w/v) HF and anodized in HF acid electrolytes with a DC power of 20V, and the machined surface implants with no treatment served as a control group. The implants were placed in mandibles of OVX sheep. Twelve weeks after implantation, resonance frequency analysis (RFA), microcomputed tomography, histomorphometry, and biomechanical tests were applied to detect the osseointegration of the two groups. It was found that HF etching and anodized hierarchical micro/nanotextured surface titanium implant was placed in mandibles of ovariectomized sheep for 12 weeks, and it showed improved osseointegration by RFA, microcomputed tomography (micro-CT) evaluation, histomorphometry, and biomechanical test. Accordingly, it was concluded that implant modification by HF acid etching and anodization to form a hierarchical micro/nanotextured surface improved titanium implant osseointegration in OVX sheep 12 weeks after implantation [270].

The surface roughness of a medical implant is of great importance since the surface is in direct contact with the host tissue (e.g., bone and fibrous tissue). The response of cells to roughness (rugophilia) is different depending on the cell type. However, the influence of roughness on cell behavior has only rarely been systematically studied. Kunzler et al. [271] have developed a surface-modification process to produce roughness gradients that cover a wide range of roughness values on one substratum. Such gradients allow for systematic investigations of roughness on cell behavior. Gradients were fabricated using a two-step roughening and smoothening process, involving sandblasting and a subsequent chemical polishing step. The strategy is exactly what Oshida [272,273] proposed. In order to produce a set of identical surfaces, Kunzler et al. applied a replica technique [271]. Cell experiments were carried out with rat calvarial osteoblasts (RCO) and HGF. RCOs showed a significantly increased proliferation rate with increasing surface roughness. The footprint of osteoblasts varied in size at different positions on the gradient, remaining small on the rough end of the gradient and increasing considerably as the roughness decreased. HGF showed the opposite proliferation behavior: proliferation decreasing with increasing roughness. The fibroblast morphology was found to be similar to that seen for osteoblasts [271].

A porous structure comprises pores and pore throats with a complex 3D network structure, and many investigators have described the relationship between average pore size and the amount of bone ingrowth. However, the influence of network structure or pore throats for tissue ingrowth has rarely been discussed. Four types of bioactive porous titanium implants with different pore sizes and porosities (6 mm in diameter and 15 mm long) were analyzed using specific algorithms for 3D analysis of interconnectivity based on a micro focus X-ray computed tomography system. The *in vivo* histomorphometric analysis was performed using the very same implants implanted into the femoral condyles of male rabbits for 6 and 12 weeks. This matching study revealed that more poorly differentiated pores tended to have narrow pore throats, especially in their shorter routes to the outside. In addition, for assessment of the entire implant, Otsuki et al. proposed new two indices that represent the degree of bone and tissue ingrowth into an implant by considering the effect of narrow pore throats. Data obtained suggest that this sort of novel analysis can be useful for evaluating bone and tissue ingrowth into porous biomaterials [274].

A porous structure can be fabricated by various ways such as sintering, coating, or foams. In particular, metallic foams have the advantage of being more porous than the traditional coatings. Their high porosity provides more space for bone ingrowth and mechanical interlocking and presents more surface area for implant-bone contact. Wazen et al. [275] investigated *in vivo* bone ingrowth into Ti implants covered with a novel Ti foam coating. This foam contains 50% in volume of interconnected pores and a higher surface area compared to dense Ti. Both coated implants and dense Ti controls were placed transcortically in the rat tibia. The animals were sacrificed at 2 weeks after implantation, and the amount of bone in the implants was determined using backscattered electron imaging and X-ray microtomography. Already at this time interval, the pores within the Ti foam showed 97.7% bone filling, and the bone-implant contact area was significantly increased compared to dense Ti controls. It was concluded that the novel Ti foam is biocompatible, has the capacity to sustain bone formation, and can potentially improve osseointegration [275]. Porous bioactive titanium implants (porosity of 40%) were produced by a plasma-spray method and subsequent chemical and thermal treatments of immersion in a 5 M aqueous NaOH solution at 60 °C for 24 hours, immersion in distilled water at 40 °C for 48 hours, and heating to 600 °C for 1 hour. Compression strength and bending strength were 280 MPa (0.2% offset yield strength 85.2 MPa) and 101 MPa, respectively. For *in vivo* analysis, bioactive and nontreated porous titanium cylinders were implanted into 6 mm diameter holes in rabbit femoral condyles. The percentage of bone–implant contact (affinity index) of the bioactive implants (BGs) was significantly larger than for the nontreated implants (CGs) at all post-implantation times (13.5 versus 10.5, 16.7 versus 12.7, 17.7 versus 10.2, 19.1 versus 7.8 at 2, 4, 8 and 16 weeks, respectively). The percentage of bone area ingrowth showed a significant increase with the BGs, whereas with the CGs it appeared to decrease after 4 weeks (10.7 versus 9.9, 12.3 versus 13.1, 15.2 versus 9.8, 20.6 versus 8.7 at 2, 4, 8, and 16 weeks, respectively). Based on these results, it was suggested that porous bioactive titanium has sufficient mechanical properties and biocompatibility for clinical use under load-bearing conditions [276].

Surface structural modifications at the micrometer and nanometer scales have driven the improved success rates of dental and orthopedic implants by mimicking the hierarchical structure of bone. However, how initial osteoblast-lineage cells populating an implant surface respond to different hierarchical surface topographical cues remains to be elucidated, with bone marrow MSCs or immature osteoblasts as possible initial colonizers. After obtaining results (i) the sensitivity of osteoblasts to both surface microroughness and nanostructures led to a synergistic effect on maturation and local factor production, (ii) osteoblastic differentiation of MSCs was sensitive to Ti–6Al–4V surface microroughness with respect to production of differentiation markers, but no further enhancement was found when cultured on micro/nanostructured surfaces, and (iii) superposition of nanostructures to microroughened surfaces affected final MSC numbers and enhanced the production of VEGF but the magnitude of the response was lower than for HOB (human osteoblasts) cultures; Gittens et al. suggested that the differentiation state of osteoblast-lineage cells determines the recognition of surface nanostructures and subsequent cell response, which has implications for clinical evaluation of new implant surface nanomodifications [277]. Disks consisting of macroporous NiTi alloy (NiTi, Nitinol®, Actipore®) are used as implants in clinical surgery, for example, for the treatment of spinal dysfunctions. Their morphological properties were studied by SEM and by synchrotron radiation-based microtomography (SRμCT). Their composition was studied by X-ray diffraction (XRD), differential scanning calorimetry (DSC), and energy-dispersive X-ray spectroscopy (EDX). Their mechanical properties were studied with temperature-dependent dynamical mechanical analysis (DMA). Studies on their biocompatibility were performed by co-incubation of porous NiTi samples with isolated peripheral blood leukocyte fractions (polymorphonuclear neutrophil granulocytes, PMN; peripheral blood mononuclear leukocytes, PBMC) in comparison with control cultures without NiTi samples. The cell adherence to the NiTi surface was analyzed by fluorescence microscopy and SEM. The activation of adherent leukocytes was analyzed by measurement of the released cytokines using the enzyme-linked immunosorbent assay (ELISA). The cytokine response of PMN (analyzed by the release of IL-1ra and IL-8) was not significantly different between cell cultures with or without NiTi. There was a significant increase in the release of IL-1ra ($p < 0.001$), IL-6 ($p < 0.05$), and IL-8 ($p < 0.05$) from PBMC in the presence of NiTi samples. In contrast, the release of TNF-$\alpha$by PBMC was not significantly elevated in the presence of NiTi. IL-2 was released from PBMC only in the range of the lower detection limit in all cell cultures. The material, clearly macroporous with an interconnecting porosity, consisted of NiTi (martensite; monoclinic, and austenite; cubic) with small impurities of $NiTi_2$ and possibly NiC_x. The material was not superelastic upon manual compression and showed good biocompatibility [278].

Porous biomaterials are not limited to metallic materials but can also be found in ceramic and composite materials. Porous ceramics have demonstrated osteoconductive properties because of their biocompatibility and 3D macroporous structure, and these materials have recently been widely studied as bone replacement materials. The foam TiC/Ti composites discussed in this study possess good mechanical properties, balancing out metallic toughness with ceramic strength. Furthermore, because of the high porosity and pore connectivity of these TiC/Ti composites, they have the potential to be a new bone replacement material. The purpose of this study was to evaluate the osseointegration of foam TiC/Ti composites, to preliminarily discuss the TiC/Ti ossification mechanism, and to obtain reliable data on the use of foam TiC/Ti composites as bone replacement materials. The foam TiC/Ti composites were implanted into 40 Japanese white rabbits for 4, 8, 12, and 24 weeks. The foam TiC/Ti composites were compared to foam SiC. M-CT (micro-computed tomography) analysis, histological analysis, SEM observation, and energydispersive X-ray spectrometer (EDS) analysis were conducted to estimate the osseointegration of the materials. The histological observations and quantitative analysis exhibited significantly more ossification area (volume), trabeculae maturity, and calcium and phosphorus content in the foam TiC/Ti composites, compared to the foam SiC. The results from this study suggest that the foam TiC/Ti composites possessed good osseointegration capacity and have the potential to be a new bone replacement material [279]. A porous structural oxide film was formed on Ti–Nb alloys by anodic oxidation after cathodic pretreatment. The effects of titanium hydride compounds on the formation of an oxide film and the structural properties of a TiNb matrix were investigated by X-ray diffraction (XRD), SEM, transmission electron microscopy (TEM), and nano-indentation. The XRD spectra showed that composite films containing $TiH_{1.924}$ were formed by cathodic pretreatment and directly dissolved after anodic oxidation. Consequently, a thick and porous oxide surface was formed on a TiNb matrix, thereby increasing the bioactivity of TiNb. Nano-indentation showed that the elastic modulus of TiNb was reduced until it was close to that of bone tissue. These results showed that TiNb subjected to anodic oxidation after cathodic pretreatment had the potential to promote sufficient load sharing between the bone and the TiNb implant [280]. A method has recently been developed for producing fiber-reinforced composites (FRC) with porous surfaces, intended for use as load-bearing orthopedic implants. This study focuses on the evaluation of the bone-bonding behavior of FRC implants. Three types of cylindrical implants, that is FRC implants with a porous surface, solid polymethyl methacrylate (PMMA) implants and titanium (Ti) implants, were inserted in a transverse direction into the intercondular trabeculous bone area of distal femurs and proximal tibias of New Zealand White rabbits. Animals were sacrificed at 3, 6, and 12 weeks postoperation, and push-out tests were then carried out. At 12 weeks the shear force at the porous FRC–bone interface was significantly higher (283.3 ± 55.3N) than the shear force at interfaces of solid PMMA/bone (14.4 ± 11.0N) and Ti/bone (130.6 ± 22.2N). Histological observation revealed new bone growth into the porous surface structure of FRC implants. Solid PMMA and Ti implants were encapsulated mostly with fibrous connective tissue. FEA revealed that porous FRC implants had mechanical properties which could be tailored to smooth the shear stress distribution at the bone–implant interface and reduce the stress-shielding effect [281].

Surface texturing can be done by producing ultrafine grain microstructures. Bulk ultrafine-grained $Ni_{50.8}Ti_{49.2}$ alloy (UFG–NiTi) was successfully fabricated by the equal-channel angular pressing (ECAP) technique. To further improve its surface biocompatibility, surface modification techniques including sandblasting, acid etching, and alkali treatment were employed to produce either irregularly roughened surface or microporous surface or hierarchical porous surface with bioactivity. The effect of the above surface treatments on the surface roughness, wettability, corrosion behavior, ion release, apatite forming ability, and cytocompatibility of UFG–NiTi alloy was systematically investigated with the coarse-grained NiTi alloy as control. The pitting corrosion potential (E_{pit}) was increased from 393 mV (SCE) to 704 mV (SCE) with sandblasting and further increased to 1539 mV (SCE) with following acid etching in the HF/HNO_3 solution. All the above surface treatment increased the apatite forming ability of UFG-NiTi in varying degrees when soaked them in SBF. Meanwhile, both sandblasting and acid etching could promote the cytocompatibility for osteoblasts: sandblasting enhanced cell attachment and acid etching increased cell proliferation. The different corrosion behavior, apatite forming ability, and cellular response of UFG-NiTi after different surface modifications are attributed to the topography and wettability of the resulting surface oxide layer [282].

Similarly, bulk ultrafine-grained Ti (UFG Ti) was successfully fabricated by the ECAP technique to further improve its surface biocompatibility, and surface modification techniques including sandblasting, acid etching, and alkali treatment were employed to produce a hierarchical porous surface. The effect of the above surface treatments on the surface roughness, wettability, electrochemical corrosion behavior, apatite forming ability, and cellular behavior of UFG Ti was systematically investigated with the coarse-grained Ti as control. Results show that UFG-Ti with surface modification had no pitting corrosion and presented the low corrosion rate in SBF. The hierarchical porous surface yielded by surface modification enhanced the ability of UFG Ti to form a complete apatite layer when soaked in SBF and promoted osteoblast-like cells attachment and proliferation *in vitro*, which promises to have a significant impact on increasing bone-bonding ability and reducing healing time when implanted due to faster tissue integration [283].

Zr (zirconium) can also be treated to exhibit the UFG structure. This was obtained by severe plastic deformation (SPD), which resulted in a refinement of the grain size by several orders of magnitude. Compared to conventional Zr, higher hardness values were measured on UFG Zr. Polished surfaces having similar topographical features from both materials were prepared, as assessed by AFM. Surface hydrophobicity of Zr, evaluated by measuring water contact angles, was unaffected by grain size reduction. The *in vitro* biocompatibility was addressed on conventional and UFG Zr surfaces and, for comparative purposes, a polished Ti–6Al–4V alloy was also investigated. Cell attachment and spreading, actin and β-tubulin cytoskeleton reorganization, fibronectin secretion and cellular distribution as well as cell viability were evaluated by culturing human osteoblastic Saos-2 cells on the surfaces. The osteoblastic response to conventional Zr was found to be essentially identical to Ti–6Al–4V and was not affected by grain size reduction. In order to evaluate the ability of the surfaces to promote osteogenic maturation and bone matrix mineralisation, human mesenchymal cells from bone marrow were switched to the osteoblastic phenotype by incubation in osteogenic induction media. Compared to undifferentiated mesenchymal cells, alkaline phosphatase activity and formation of mineralisation nodules were enhanced to the same extent on both Zr surfaces and Ti–6Al–4V alloy after induction of osteoblastic differentiation. In summary, the improved mechanical properties, together with excellent *in vitro* biocompatibility, make UFG Zr a promising biomaterial for surgical implants [284].

6.19. Retrieved Implants

There are several reasons for implant failure, which should include contraindications, complications, and other unseen factors. As to contraindications, there are absolute contraindications and relative ones [285,286]. In a case of absolute contraindications, implants can't be placed in these situations. Such situations include (i) heart area: heart diseases affecting the valves (valvulopathy), recent infarcts, severe cardiac insufficiency, and cardiomyopathy; (ii) miscellaneous: active cancer, certain bone diseases (osteomalacia, Paget's disease, brittle bones syndrome, etc.), certain immunological diseases, immunosuppressant treatments, clinical AIDS, awaiting an organ transplant, certain mental diseases, strongly irradiated jaw bones (radiotherapy treatment), treatments of osteoporosis, or some cancers by bisphosphonates (as tablets: ACTONEL®, FOSAMAX®, DIDRONEL®, LYTOS®, SKELID® and so forth, and particularly as injections: ZOMETA®, AREDIA® etc.), even from treatment several years before; and (iii) age: children: not before the jaw bones have stopped growing (in general at 17–18 years old); on the other hand, advanced age does not pose problems if the patient's general condition is good. For relative contraindications, the indication to place implants should be evaluated on a case-by-case basis, with the greatest caution, and the following situations can include diabetes (particularly insulin-dependent), angina pectoris (angina), seropositivity (absolute contraindication for clinical AIDS), significant consumption of tobacco, certain mental diseases, radiotherapy to the neck or face (depending on the zone, quantity of radiation, and localization of the cancerous lesion etc.), certain auto-immunes diseases, drug and alcohol dependency, and pregnancy. Furthermore, there are relative local contraindications, for which the indication to place implants should be evaluated on a case-by-case basis, with caution, and the following situations should include an insufficient quantity of bone, certain diseases of the mucous membranes of the mouth, periodontal diseases (loosening of the teeth); it is necessary to clean up the gums and stabilize the disease first, severe grinding or clenching of the teeth, an unbalanced relationship between the upper and lower teeth, infections in the neighboring teeth (pockets, cysts, and granulomas), major sinusitis, and poor hygiene of the mouth and teeth.

The possible complications when an implant is inserted are classified into two groups: (i) the immediate complications, and (ii) late complications. As to (i) the immediate complications, there are (i) risk from the anesthetic (even though it is performed under local anesthesia in the vast majority of cases, the risk from an anesthetic is never zero. An allergy, although extremely rare, is always possible. However, this type of anesthesia is very widely used and the "at risk" subjects are often already known). (ii) Non-osseointegration of the implant (called "rejection," but wrongly): it becomes apparent in the weeks or months that follow insertion of the implant. The material used is pure titanium, whose physical and biological properties are very well known and which has been used for many years in orthopedic surgery (hip and knee prostheses, etc.). It is very well tolerated by the body and no rejection or allergic reactions have been reported so far. The bone cells have not colonized the surface of the implant and it is mobile as it is not "soldered" to the bone. So the implant will have to be removed. For this reason we generally wait 2–6 months before finally making the prosthesis on the implant. The causes are not always identified; however, tobacco and hygiene play a non negligible role. Overall this involves 5% of implants placed. A 100% success rate does not exist for implant treatments. However, if it is possible, an implant can be re-inserted in the same site some weeks or months later, and quite often, this second attempt is successful. (iii) Infection: postoperative infections are rare. An abscess sometimes occurs in the neighborhood, or (much more rarely) an infection of the soft tissues around the jaw bone (the infection is called cellulitis) or a sinus infection (sinusitis). For this reason antibiotic therapy is prescribed, since the conditions of asepsis must be as near as possible to absolute and we should avoid operating when the body is weakened (by another infection, poorly controlled diabetes, etc.). (iv) Hemorrhage: as with any buccal surgery, a hemorrhage or a hematoma may occur, but this is not serious in the vast majority of cases. And (v) lesions of the nerves: in the lower jaw (mandible) lies the nerve serving the lip and the chin which runs inside the bone (in the region of the premolars and the molars). For this reason a scan is also requested in order to locate it accurately, and sometimes, if the depth of bone is insufficient, implants should not be considered in this area. Very rarely the nerve can be touched, while the implant is being performed (due to a technical error, a poor understanding of the scan, the patient moving at the moment of drilling, etc.), or afterward by a compressive hematoma or edema. This results in a reduction in the sensitivity of the lip and chin (not paralysis). These disorders are generally reversible upon appropriate treatment. Exceptionally, there can also be a lesion of the lingual nerve which gives anesthesia of the tip of the tongue. For (ii) the late complications—several years after placement—can be due to mechanical factors, loosening of the implant (as a natural tooth may), lack of hygiene or a generally weak condition. This results in the loss of the implant (which no longer holds) or more rarely its fracture. Hence, very rigorous hygiene and regular checkups are very important [285–289].

As mentioned before, the failure of adental implant is often related to the failure of the implant to osseointegrate correctly with the bone. A dental implant is considered to be a failure if it is lost, mobile, or shows peri-implant (around the implant) bone loss of greater than 1.0 mm in the first year and greater than 0.2 mm a year after [288,289]. A total of 68 patients, 26 men and 42 women, aged 21–86 years, were treated with 204 endosseous implants (TPS®, ITI®, Bonefit, or Biolox) from 1985 to 1990. They were examined at their latest recall visit approximately 22.5 months after surgery, the range varying greatly between the implant systems used (from 4–60 months). Fourteen implants were lost during the observation period because of failures in osseointegration. There were no statistically significant differences in success rates between the implant systems during the observation period. The Periotest values, however, differed between the Bonefit and ITI implants in maxillae and mandibles, and between successful and failed TPS implants. In four of the failures, all ITI implants, the prosthetic restorations (fixed dentures and single crowns), had been lost. All other failures were treated by using the previous complete denture. Possible causes of failure included advanced age and poor general health of the patient, complications in the surgical procedures, and compromised oral hygiene [289].

Shibli et al. [290] evaluated the microbiota and surface of failed titanium dental implants from four manufacturers. Twelve mobile dental implants were retrieved from 10 smokers after 3 to 10 years of functional loading. Before implant removal, microbial samples were taken and evaluated using the polymerase chain reaction. After implant removal, analyses of the failed implant surfaces were performed using SEM and energy-dispersive spectrometer X-ray. Periodontal pathogens such as *Aggregactibacter actinomycetemcomitans, Campylobacter rectus, Eikenella corrodens, Fusobacterium nucleatum, Porphyromonas gingivalis, Prevotella intermedia, Tannerella forsythia,* and *Treponema denticola* were detected in all implants in different proportions. Surface analysis showed varying degrees of surface roughness between the samples and the presence of proteinaceous material, appearing mainly as dark stains. Foreign carbon, oxygen, sodium, calcium, aluminum, and silicon elements were also found. Although no material-related causes of implant failure were detected, several periodontal pathogens were identified independently of the surface topography or manufacturer [290].

Steflik et al. [291] analyzed the reports obtained from 200 implant cases retrieved from humans and submitted to the American Academy of Implant Dentistry Research Foundation, Medical College of Georgia implant retrieval center. The samples that were not decalcified were embedded in polymethylmethacrylate and examined with SEM and routine light, polarized, or Nomarski microscopy. Cases included both orthopedic and dental implants, as well as entire mandibles and portions of maxillae obtained at autopsy. A significant number of submitted implants had substantial amounts of adhered bone, which permitted evaluation of human bone remodeling to osseointegrated implants. These implants failed because of implant fracture. As was observed with animal studies, healthy bone supported these implants, with the bone containing an interdigitating canaliculi network that provided communication between interfacial osteocytes and osteocytes deeper within the remodeled osteonal and trabecular bone. Early dental implants containing a coating of beads showed a connective tissue interface, which corresponded to the bead surface of specific orthopedic implants that underwent some degree of micromovement. This is in contrast with the excellent response reported for successful contemporary beaded implants. Significant numbers of osseointegrated fractured HA-coated dental implants demonstrated the adequate serviceability of these implants before biomaterial fracture. In contrast, the HA coating was dissociated from retrieved orthopedic implants, leading to extensive cup loosening and case failure. This study, therefore, underscores the need for evaluation of failed human dental and orthopedic implants. Correlations can be drawn between human retrieval and experimental animal studies [291].

There should be precaution about the storage of implant materials, although titanium implants are sold in the market as storable medical devices. All the implants have a certain shelf life during which they maintain their sterility, but variations of the surface properties through this duration have not been subject to a comprehensive assessment. Lu et al. [292] investigated the effects of storage methods on time-related changes of titanium surface properties. Acid-etched titanium disks (Sa = 0.82 μm) were placed in a sealed container (tradition method) or submerged in the ddH_2O/NaCl solution (0.15 mol L^{-1})/$CaCl_2$ solution (0.15 mol L^{-1}), and new titanium disks were used as a control group. It was reported that (i) SEM and optical profiler showed that surface morphology and roughness did not change within different groups, but the XPS analysis confirmed that the surface chemistry altered by different storage protocols as the storage duration increased, (ii) the contact angle also varied with storage methods, (iii) the storage method also affected the protein adsorption capacity and cellular response on the titanium surface, and (iv) all titanium disks stored in the solution maintained their excellent bioactivity even after four weeks storage time, but titanium disks stored in a traditional manner decreased substantially in an age-dependent manner, suggesting that much effort is needed to improve the storage methods in order to maintain the bioactivity of a titanium dental implant [292].

During the operation for placing implants, the appropriate selection of instruments becomes a crucial factor. Louropoulou et al. [293] conducted a literature survey to systematically collect and evaluate existing evidence on the effects of different mechanical instruments on the surface characteristics of smooth and rough titanium surfaces. PubMed-MEDLINE, Cochrane-CENTRAL, and EMBASE databases were searched up to December 2010 to identify appropriate studies—3275 unique papers were identified. The eligible studies were controlled studies investigating titanium surface alterations following treatment with different mechanical instruments. A screening of the titles and abstracts resulted in 34 publications that met all of the eligibility criteria. Surface roughness was evaluated using SEM in most studies and using a profilometer in only 10 studies. The rough surfaces evaluated were titanium plasma sprayed and SBA surfaces only. Nonmetal instruments were found to cause minimal or no damage to both smooth and rough titanium surfaces. Metal instruments were found to cause major damage to smooth surfaces. Burs seemed to be the instruments of choice, if smoothening of a rough surface was required. It was, hence, concluded that (i) nonmetal instruments and rubber cups seem to be the instruments of choice for the treatment of smooth surfaces; (ii) similarly, for rough implant surfaces, nonmetal instruments and air abrasives are the instruments of choice, if surface integrity needs to be maintained; and (iii) metal instruments and burs are recommended only in cases requiring the smoothening of the surface roughness, indicating that the clinical impact of these findings requires clarification [293].

References

1. Bruinink, A. and Luginbuehl, R., 2012, Evaluation of biocompatibility using in vitro methods: interpretation and limitations, *Adv Biochem Eng Biotechnol* 126:117–152. doi: http://dx.doi.org/10.1007/10_2011_111.
2. Anusavice, A.J., 2003, Overview of materials for dental applications, In: A.J. Anusavice, ed., *Phillip's Science of Dental Materials,* 11th ed. Saunders, St. Louis, MO, pp. 3–19.
3. Moore, B.K. and Oshida, Y., 1995, Materials science and technology in dentistry, In: D.L. Wise, ed., *Encyclopedic Handbook of Biomaterilas and Bioengineering*, Marcel Dekker, Boston, MA, pp. 1325–1430.
4. ISO/FDIS:7405:2008, 2008, *Dentistry—Evaluation of Biocompatibility of Medical Devices Used in Dentistry*; BSI, London, UK.

5. Dearnley, P.A., 2005, A brief review of test methodologies for surface-engineered biomedical implant alloys, *Surf Coat Tech* 198:483–490. doi: http://dx.doi.org/10.1016/j.surfcoat.2004.10.067.
6. Smith, T., 2004, Biomedical testing, *JOM* 162:41–43.
7. Yokoyama, K., Kaneko, K., Miyamoto, Y., ASaoka, K., Sakai, J. and Nagumo, M., 2004, Fracture associated with hydrogen absorption of sustained tensile-loaded titanium in acid and neutral fluoride solutions, *J Biomed Mater Res A* 68:150–158. doi: http://dx.doi.org/10.1002/jbm.a.20067.
8. Manda, M.G., Psyllaki, P.P., Tsipas, D.N. and Koidis, P.T., 2009, Observations on an *in-vivo* failure of a titanium dental implant/abutment screw system: A case report, *J Biomed Mater Res B Appl Biomater* 89:264–273. doi: http://dx.doi.org/10.1002/jbm.b.31211.
9. Michailidis, N., Karabinas, G., Tsouknidas, A., Mailiaris, G., Tsipas, D. and Koidi, P., 2013, A FEM based endosteal implant simulation to determine the effect of peri-implant bone resorption on stress induced implant failure, *Biomed Mater Eng* 23:317–327. doi: http://dx.doi.org/10.3233/BME-130756.
10. Lauterbur, P.C., 1973, Image formation by induced local interactions: Example employing nuclear magnetic resonance, *Nature* 242:190–191. doi: http://dx.doi.org/10.1038/242190a0.
11. Shellock, F.G. and Crues, J.V., 1988, High field strength MR imaging and metallic biomedical implants: An ex vivo evaluation of deflection forces, *Am J Roentgenol* 151:389–392.
12. Shellock, F.G., Morisoli, S. and Kanal, E., 1993, MR procedures and biomedical implants, materials, and devices, update, *Radiology* 189:587–599.
13. Shellock, F.G., Mink, J.H., Curtin, S. and Friesman, M.J., 1992, MR imaging and metallic implants for anterior cruciate ligament reconstruction: Assessment of ferromagnetism and artifact, *J Magn Reson Imaging* 2:225–228. doi: http://dx.doi.org/10.1002/jmri.1880020217.
14. Shellock, F.G., 2002, Biomedical implants and devices: Assessment of magnetic field interactions with a 3.0 tesla MR system, *J Magn Reson Imaging* 16:721–732. doi: http://dx.doi.org/10.1002/jmri.10207.
15. Shellock, F.G., Fieno, D.S., Thompson, L.J., Talavage, T.M. and Berman, D.S., 2006, Cardiac pacemaker: In vitro assessment at 1.5 T, *Am Heart J* 151:436–443. doi: http://dx.doi.org/10.1016/j.ahj.2005.04.015.
16. Oshida, Y., Tuna, E.B., Aktören, O. and Gençay, K., 2010, Dental implant systems, *Int J Mol Sci* 11:1580–1678. doi: http://dx.doi.org/10.3390/ijms11041580.
17. www.stmri.com/ht_docs/safety-2.html; www.mri.tju.edu/Policies-contraindications.html
18. Lim, Y.J., Oshida, Y., Barco, T. and Andres, C.J., 2001, Surface characterizations of variously treated titanium materials, *Int J Oral Maxillofac Implants* 16:333–342.
19. Wei, Q.F., Huang, F.L., Hou, D.Y. and Wang, Y.Y., 2006, Surface functionalization of polymer nanofibers by sputter coating of titanium dioxide, *Appl Surf Sci* 252:7874–7877. doi: http://dx.doi.org/10.1016/j.apsusc.2005.09.074.
20. Tian, Y., Ding, S., Peng, H., Lu, S., Wang, G., Xia, L. and Wang, P., 2012, Osteoblast growth behavior on porous-structure titanium surface, *Appl Surf Sci* 261:25–30. doi: http://dx.doi.org/10.1016/j.apsusc.2012.07.035.
21. Lin, Z., Lee, G-H., Liu, C-M. and Lee, I-S., 2010, Controls in wettability of TiOx films for biomedical applications, *Surf Coat Tech* 205:S391-S397. doi: http://dx.doi.org/ 10.1016/j.surfcoat.2010.08.052.
22. Park, J.H., Schwartz, Z., Olivares-Navarrete, R., Boyan, B.D. and Tannenbaum, R., 2011, Enhancement of surface wettability via the modification of microtextured titanium implant surfaces with polyelectrolytes, Langmuir 27:5976–5985. doi: http://dx.doi.org/10.1021/la2000415.

23. Fleming, R.A. and Min Zou, M., 2012, Fabrication of stable superhydrophilic surfaces on titanium substrates, *J Adhes Sci Tech* 28:823–832. doi: http://dx.doi.org/10.1080/01694243.2012.697754.
24. Khosroshahi, M.E., Mahmoodi, M. and Tavakoli, J., 2007, Characterization of Ti6Al4V implant surface treated by Nd:YAG laser and emery paper for orthopedic applications, *Appl Surf Sci* 253:8772–8781. doi: http://dx.doi.org/10.1016/j.apsusc.2007.04.084.
25. Shtansky, D.V., Batenina, I.V., Yadroitsev, I.A., Ryashin, N.S., Kiryukhantsev-Korneev, P.V., Kudryashov, A.E., Sheveyko, A.N., Zhitnyak, I.Y., Gloushankova, N.A., Smurov, I.Y. and Levashov, E.A., 2012, A new combined approach to metal-ceramic implants with controllable surface topography, chemistry, blind porosity, and wettability, *Surf Coat Tech* 208:14–23. doi: http://dx.doi.org/10.1016/j.surfcoat.2012.07.008.
26. Vasilev, K., Poh, Z., Kant, K., Chan, J., Michelmore, A. and Losic, D., 2010, Tailoring the surface functionalities of titania nanotube arrays, *Biomaterials* 31:532–540. doi: http://dx.doi.org/10.1016/j.biomaterials.2009.09.074.
27. Barshilia, H.C., Chaudhary, A., Kumar P. and and Manikandanath, N.T., 2012, Wettability of Y_2O_3: A relative analysis of thermally oxidized, reactively sputtered and template assisted nanostructured coatings, *Nanomaterials* 2:65–78. doi: http://dx.doi.org/10.3390/nano2010065.
28. Park, J.H., Wasilewski, C.E., Almodovar, N., Olivares-Navarrete, R., Boyan, B.D., Tannenbaum, R. and Schwartz, Z., 2012, The responses to surface wettability gradients induced by chitosan nanofilms on microtextured titanium mediated by specific integrin receptors, *Biomaterials* 33:7386–7393. doi: http://dx.doi.org/10.1016/j.biomaterials.2012.06.066.
29. Park, J.H., Olivares-Navarrete, R., Wasilewski, C.E., Boyan, B.D., Tannenbaum, R. and Schwartz, Z., 2012, Use of polyelectrolyte thin films to modulate Osteoblast response to microstructured titanium surfaces, *Biomaterials* 33:5267–5277. doi: http://dx.doi.org/10.1016/j.biomaterials.2012.03.074.
30. Mekayarajjananonth, T. and Winkler, S., 1999, Contact angle measurement on dental implant biomaterials, *J Oral Implantol* 25:230–236. doi: http://dx.doi.org/10.1563/1548-1336(1999)025<0230:CAMODI>2.3.CO;2.
31. Paital, S.R,, He, W. and Dahotre, N.B., 2010, Laser pulse dependent micro textured calcium phosphate coatings for improved wettability and cell compatibility, *J Mater Sci Mater Med* 21:2187–2200. doi: http://dx.doi.org/10.1007/s10856-010-4085-6.
32. Park, J-W., Kim, Y-J. and Jang, J-H., 2010, Enhanced osteoblast response to hydrophilic strontium and/or phosphate ions-incorporated titanium oxide surfaces, *Clin Oral Implants Res* 21:398–408. doi: http://dx.doi.org/10.1111/j.1600-0501.2009.01863.x.
33. Tsuji, H., Satoh, H., Ikeda, S., Gotoh, Y. and Junzo Ishikawa, J., 1998, Contact angle lowering of polystyrene surface by silver-negative-ion implantation for improving biocompatibility and introduced atomic bond evaluation by XP, *Nucl Instrum Meth Phys Res B* 141:197–201. doi: http://dx.doi.org/10.1016/S0168-583X(98)00090-1.
34. Lin, Z., Lee, G-H., Liu, C-M. and In-Seop Lee, I-S., 2006, Controls in wettability of TiOx films for biomedical applications, *Surf Coat Tech* 205:S391–S397. doi: http://dx.doi.org/10.1016/j.surfcoat.2010.08.052.
35. Wu, K-R., Wang, J-J., Liu, W-C., Chen, Z-S. and Wu, J-K., 2006, Deposition of graded TiO_2 films featured both hydrophobic and photo-induced hydrophilic properties, *Appl Surf Sci* 252:5829–5838. doi: http://dx.doi.org/10.1016/j.apsusc.2005.08.016.
36. Panjwani, B. and Sujeet.K. Sinha, S.K., 2012, Tribology and hydrophobicity of a biocompatible GPTMS/PFPE coating on Ti6Al4V surfaces, *J Mech Behav Biomed Mater* 15:103–111. doi: http://dx.doi.org/10.1016/j.jmbbm.2012.06.016.

37. Ou, J., Liu, M., Li, W., Wang, F., Xue, M. and Li, C., 2012, Corrosion behavior of superhydrophobic surfaces of Ti alloys in NaCl solutions, *Appl Surf Sci* 258:4724–4728. doi: http://dx.doi.org/10.1016/j.apsusc.2012.01.066.
38. Duske, K., Koban, I., Kindel, E., Schröder, K., Nebe, B., Holtfreter, B., Jablonowski, L., Weltmann, K.D. and Kocher, T., 2012, Atmospheric plasma enhance wttability and cell spreading on dental implant metals, *J Cin Periodontol* 39:400–407. doi: http://dx.doi.org/10.1111/j.1600-051X.2012.01853.x.
39. Schliephake, H., Scharnweber, D., Dard, M., Sewing, A., Aref, A. and Roessler, S., 2005, Functionalization of dental implant surfaces using adhesion molecules, *J Biomed Mater Res B Appl Biomater* 73:88–96. doi: http://dx.doi.org/10.1002/jbm.b.30183.
40. Tsyganov, I., Maitz, M.F. and Wieser, E., 2004, Blood compatibility of titanium-based coatings prepared by metal plasma immersion ion implantation and deposition, *Appl Surf Sci* 235:156–163. doi: http://dx.doi.org/10.1016/j.apsusc.2004.05.134.
41. Chen, J.L., Li, Q.L., Chen, J.Y., Chen, C. and Huang, N., 2009, Improving blood-compatibility of titanium by coating collagen–heparin multilayers, *Appl Surf Sci* 255:6894–6900. doi: http://dx.doi.org/10.1016/j.apsusc.2009.03.011.
42. Xue, X., Wang, J., Zhu, Y., Tu, Q. and Huang, N., 2010, Biocompatibility of pure titanium modified by human endothelial cell-derived extracellular matrix, *Appl Surf Sci* 256:3866–3873. doi: http://dx.doi.org/10.1016/j.apsusc.2010.01.042.
43. Huang, C-F., Cheng, H-C., Liu, C-M., Chen, C-C. and Ou, K-L., 2009, Microstructure and phase transition of biocompatible titanium oxide film on titanium by plasma discharging, *J Alloys Compounds* 476:683–688. doi: http://dx.doi.org/10.1016/j.jallcom.2008.09.122.
44. Wang, M., Wang, Y., Chen, Y. and Gu, H., 2013, Improving endothelialization on 316L stainless steel through wettability controllable coating by sol–gel technology, *Appl Surf Sci* 268:73–78.doi: http://dx.doi.org/10.1016/j.apsusc.2012.11.159.
45. Milleret, V., Tugulu, S., Schlottig, F. and Hall, H., 2011, Alkali treatment of microrough titanium surfaces affects macrophage/monocyte adhesion, platelet activation and architecture of blood clot formation, *Eur Cell Mater* 21:430–444.
46. Lai, H-C., Zhuang, L-F., Zhang, Z-Y., Wieland, M. and Liu, X., 2009, Bone apposition around two different sandblasted, large-grit and acid-etched implant surfaces at sites with coronal circumferential defects: an experimental study in dogs, *Clin Oral Implants Res* 20:247–253. doi: http://dx.doi.org/10.1111/j.1600-0501.2008.01651.x.
47. Mustafa, K., Wroblewski, J., Hultenby, K., Lopez, B.S. and Kristina Arvidson, K., 2000, Effects of titanium surfaces blasted with TiO_2 particles on the initial attachment of cells derived from human mandibular bone—A scanning electron microscopic and histomorphometric analysis, *Clin Oral Implants Res* 11:116–128. doi: http://dx.doi.org/10.1034/j.1600-0501.2000.110204.x.
48. Hao, Y.Q., Li, S.J., Hao, Y.L., Zhao, Y.K. and Ai, H.J., 2013, Effect of nanotube diameters on bioactivity of a multifunctional titanium alloy, *Appl Surf Sci* 268:44–51. doi: http://dx.doi.org/10.1016/j.apsusc.2012.11.142.
49. Pae, A., Kim, S-S., Kim, H-S. and Woo, Y-H., 2011, Osteoblast-like cell attachment and proliferation on turned, blasted, and anodized titanium surfaces, *Int J Oral Maxillofac Implants* 26:475–481.
50. Chen, C-S., Tsao, Y-L., Wang, D-J., Ou, S-F., Cheng, H-Y., Chiang, Y-C. and Ou, K-L., 2013, Research on cell behavior related to anodized and hydrothermally treated titanium surface, *Appl Surf Sci* 271:1–6. doi: http://dx.doi.org/10.1016/j.apsusc.2012.11.169.
51. Yang, W-E. and Huang, H-H., 2010, Improving the biocompatibility of titanium surface through formation of a TiO_2 nano-mesh layer, *Thin Solid Films* 518:7545–7550. doi: http://dx.doi.org/10.1016/j.tsf.2010.05.045.

52. Guo, J., Padilla, R.J., Ambrose, W., De Kok, I.J. and Cooper, L.F., 2007, The effect of hydrofluoric acid treatment of TiO_2 grit blasted titanium implants on adherent osteoblast gene expression in vitro and in vivo, *Biomaterials* 28:5418–5425. doi: http://dx.doi.org/10.1016/j.biomaterials.2007.08.032.
53. Galli, C., Piemontese, M., Ravanetti, F., Lumetti, S., Passeri, G., Gandolfini, M. and Macaluso, G.M., 2012, Effect of surface treatment on cell responses to grades 4 and 5 titanium for orthodontic mini-implants, *Am J Orthod Dentofacial Orthop* 141:705–714. doi: http://dx.doi.org/10.1016/j.ajodo.2011.12.022.
54. Wang, X., Wang, G., Liang, J., Cheng, J., Ma, W. and Zhao, Y., 2009, Staphylococcus aureus adhesion to different implant surface coatings: An in vitro study, *Surf Coat Tech* 203:3454–3458. doi: http://dx.doi.org/10.1016/j.surfcoat.2009.05.009.
55. Chiang, C-Y., Chiou, S-H., Yang, W-E., Hsu, M-L., Yung, M-C., Tsai, M-L., Chen, L-K. and Huang, H-H., 2009, Formation of TiO_2 nano-network on titanium surface increases the human cell growth, *Dent Mater* 25:1022–1029. doi: http://dx.doi.org/10.1016/j.dental.2009.03.001.
56. Zhang, F., Huang,Y., Li, X. and Zhao, S., 2011, Surface modification and its effect on attachment, spreading, and proliferation of human gingival fibroblasts, *Int J Oral Maxillofac Implants* 26:1183–1192. doi: http://dx.doi.org/10.1002/jbm.b.32784.
57. Neoh, K.G., Hu, X., Zheng, D. and Kang, E.T., 2012, Balancing osteoblast functions and bacterial adhesion on functionalized titanium surfaces, *Biomaterials* 33:2813–2822. doi: http://dx.doi.org/10.1016/j.biomaterials.2012.01.018.
58. Zhang, S., Xianting, Z., Yongsheng, W., Kui, C. and Wenjian, W., 2006, Adhesion strength of sol–gel derived fluoridated hydroxyapatite coatings, *Surf Coat Tech* 200:6350–6354. doi: http://dx.doi.org/10.1016/j.surfcoat.2005.11.033.
59. Landuyt, P.V., Streydio, J-M. and Delanny, F., 1998, Comparison of surface treatment methods for promoting the adhesion of glass on titanium, *J Mater Sci* 33:4991–4999. doi: http://dx.doi.org/10.1023/A:1004407007593.
60. Park, Y-J., Shin, K-H. and Song, H-J., 2007, Effects of anodizing conditions on bond strength of anodically oxidized film to titanium substrate, *Appl Surf Sci* 253:6013–6018. doi: http://dx.doi.org/10.1016/j.apsusc.2006.12.112.
61. Qu, H. and Wei, M., 2008, Improvement of bonding strength between biomimetic apatite coating and substrate, *J Biomed Mater Res B Appl Biomater* 84:436–443. doi: http://dx.doi.org/10.1002/jbm.b.30889.
62. Wang, Y.M., Guo, L.X., Ouyang, J.H., Zhou, Y. and Jia, D.C., 2009, Interface adhesion properties of functional coatings on titanium alloy formed by microarc oxidation method, *Appl Surf Sci* 255:6875–6880. doi: http://dx.doi.org/10.1016/j.apsusc.2009.03.007.
63. Fernández-Pradas, J.M., García-Cuenca, M.V., Clèries, L., Sardin, G. and Morenza, J.L., 2002, Influence of the interface layer on the adhesion of pulsed laser deposited hydroxyapatite coatings on titanium alloy, *Appl Surf Sci* 195:31–37. doi: http://dx.doi.org/10.1016/S0169-4332(02)00002-8.
64. Bull, S.J. and Berasetegui, E.G., 2006, An overview of the potential of quantitative coating adhesion measurement by scratch testing, *Tribol Int* 39:99–114. doi: http://dx.doi.org/10.1016/j.triboint.2005.04.013.
65. Lahiri, D. and Agarwal, A., 2012, Scratch based technique quantifies adhesion strength at micro and nanoscales, *Adv Mater Process* 170:22–27.
66. Kieswetter, K., Schwartz, Z., Dean, D.D. and Boyan, B.D., 1996, The role of implant surface characteristics in the healing of bone, *Crit Rev Oral Biol Med* 7:329–345.
67. Albrektsson T. and Johansson, C., 2001, Osteoinduction, osteoconduction and osseointegration, *Eur Spine J* 10:S96–S101. doi: http://dx.doi.org/10.1007/s005860100282.

68. Kakuta, S., Miyaoka, K., Fujimori, S., Lee, W.S., Miyazaki, T. and Nagumo, M., 2000, Proliferation and differentiation of bone marrow cells on titanium plates treated with a wire-type electrical discharge machine, *J Oral Implantol* 26:156–162. doi: http://dx.doi.org/10.1563/1548-1336(2000)026<0156:PADOBM>2.3.CO;2.
69. Albrektsson, T., Eriksson, A.R., Friberg, B., Lekholm, U., Lindahl L., Nevins, M., Oikarinen, V., Roos, J., Sennerby, L. and Astrand, P., 1993, Histologic investigations on 33 retrieved nobelpharma implants, *Clin Mater* 12:1–9. doi: http://dx.doi.org/10.1016/0267-6605(93)90021-X.
70. Boyan, B.D., Hummert, T.W., Dean, D.D. and Z. Schwartz, Z., 1996, Role of material surfaces in regulating bone and cartilage cell response, *Biomaterials* 17:137–146. doi: http://dx.doi.org/10.1016/0142-9612(96)85758-9.
71. Chae, G-J., Jung, U-W., Jung, S-M., Lee, I-S., Cho, K-S., Kim, C-K. and Choi, S-H., 2008, Healing of surgically created circumferential gap around nano-coating surface dental implants in dogs, *Surf Interface Anal*, 40:184–187. doi: http://dx.doi.org/10.1002/sia.2745.
72. Johansson, C.B., Cosentino, F., Tundo, S. Milella, E., Ramires, P.A. and Wennerberg, A., 2003, Biological behavior of sol–gel coated dental implants, *J Mater Sci Mater Med* 14:539–545. doi: http://dx.doi.org/10.1023/A:1023412131314.
73. Harimoto, K., Yoshida, Y., Yoshihara, K., Nagaoka, N., Matsumoto, T. and Tagawa, Y., 2012, Osteoblast compatibility of materials depends on serum protein absorbability in osteogenesis, *Dent Mater J* 31:674–680. doi: http://dx.doi.org/10.4012/dmj.2012-075.
74. Zagury, R., Harari, N.D., Conz, M.B., Soares, G.de A. and Vidigal, G.M.Jr., 2007, Histomorphometric analyses of bone interface with titanium–aluminum–vanadium and hydroxyapatite-coated implants by biomimetic process, *Implant Dent* 16:290–296. doi: http://dx.doi.org/10.1097/ID.0b013e3180e9d9ed.
75. Zechner, W., Tangl, S., Fürst, G., Tepper, G., Thams, U., Mailath, G. and Georg Watzek, G., 2003, Osseous healing characteristics of three different implant types—A histologic and histomorphometric study in mini-pigs, *Clin Oral Implants Res* 14:150–157. doi: http://dx.doi.org/10.1034/j.1600-0501.2003.140203.x.
76. Grandfield, K., Palmquist, A., Gonçalves, S., Taylor, A., Taylor, M., Emanuelsson, L., Thomsen, P. and Engqvist, H. J., 2011, Free form fabricated features on CoCr implants with and without hydroxyapatite coating in vivo: a comparative study of bone contact and bone growth induction, *J Mater Sci Mater Med* 22:899–906. doi: http://dx.doi.org/10.1007/s10856-011-4253-3.
77. Junker, R., Manders, P.J.D., Wolke, J., Borisov, Y. and Jansen, J.A., 2010, Bone reaction adjacent to microplasma-sprayed CaP-coated oral implants subjected to occlusal load, an experimental study in the dog. Part I: short-term results, *Clin Oral Implants Res* 21:1251–1263. doi: http://dx.doi.org/10.1111/j.1600-0501.2010.01940.x.
78. Schiegnitz, E., Palarie, V., Nacu, V., Al-Nawas, B. and Kämmerer, P.W., 2012, Vertical osteoconductive characteristics of titanium implants with calcium-phosphate-coated surfaces—A pilot study in rabbits, *Clin Implant Dent Related Res.* doi: http://dx.doi.org/10.1111/j.17-8-8208.2012.00469.x.
79. Chen, H-T., Chung, C-J., Yang, T-C., Tang, C-H. and He, J-L., 2012, Microscopic observations of osteoblast growth on microarc oxidized β titanium, *Appl Surf Sci* 266:73–80. doi: http://dx.doi.org/10.1016/j.apsusc.2012.11.087.
80. Chung, C-J., Su, R-T., Chu, H-J., Chen, H-T., Tsou, H-K. and He, J-L., 2013, Plasma electrolytic oxidation of titanium and improvement in osseointegration, *J Biomed Mater Res B Appl Biomater* 101:1023–1030. doi: http://dx.doi.org/10.1002/jbm.b.32912.
81. Ballo, A.M., Bjöörn, D., Åstrand, M., Palmquist, A., Lausmaa, J. and Peter Thomsen, P., 2013, Bone response to physical-vapour-deposited titanium dioxide coatings on titanium

implants, *Clin Oral Implants Res* 24:1009–1017. doi: http://dx.doi.org/10.1111/j.1600-0501.2012.02509.x.

82. Chung, S.H., Kim, H-K., Shon, W-J. and Park, Y-S., 2013, Peri-implant bone formations around (Ti,Zr)O_2-coated zirconia implants with different surface roughness, *J Clin Periodon* 40:404–411. doi: http://dx.doi.org/10.1111/jcpe.12073.
83. Plecko, M., Sievert, C., Andermatt, D., Frigg, R., Kronen, P., Klein, K., Stübinger, S., Nuss, K., Bürki, A., Ferguson, S., Stoeckle, U. and von Rechenberg, B., 2012, Osseointegration and biocompatibility of different metal implants—A comparative experimental investigation in sheep, *BMC Musculoskeletal Disorders* 13:32–44. doi: http://dx.doi.org/10.1186/1471-2474-13-32.
84. Scarano, A., Piattelli, M., Vrespa, G., Petrone, G., Iezzi, G. and Piattelli, A., 2003, Bone healing around titanium and titanium nitride-coated dental implants with three surfaces: an experimental study in rats, *Clin Implant Dent Related Res* 5:103–111. doi: http://dx.doi.org/10.1111/j.1708-8208.2003.tb00191.x.
85. Freeman, C.O. and Brook, I.M., 2006, Bone response to a titanium aluminium nitride coating on metallic implants, *J Mater Sci Mater Med* 17:465–470. doi: http://dx.doi.org/10.1007/s10856-006-8474-9.
86. Choi, C-R., Yu, H-S., Kim, C-H., Lee, J-H., Oh, C-H., Kim, H-W. and Lee, H-H., 2010, Bone cell responses of titanium blasted with bioactive glass particles, *J Biomater Appl* 25:25: 99–117. doi: http://dx.doi.org/0.1177/0885328209337345.
87. Hacking, S.A., Harvey, E.J., Tanzer, M., Krygier, J.J. and Bobyn, J.D., 2003, Acid-etched microtexture for enhancement of bone growth into porous-coated implants, *J Bone Joint Surg Br* 85:1182–1189.
88. Herrero-Climent, M., Lázaro, P., Rios, J.V., Lluch, S., Marqués, M., Guillem-Martí, J. and Gil, F.J., 2013, Influence of acid-etching after grit-blasted on osseointegration of titanium dental implants: in vitro and in vivo studies, *J Mater Sci Mater Med* 24:2047–2055. doi: http://dx.doi.org/10.1007/s10856-013-4935-0.
89. Oshida, Y., 2007, *Bioscience and Bioengineering of Titanium Materials*, Elseveier, London, UK, pp. 236–237.
90. Wall, I., Donos, N., Carlqvist, K., Jones, F. and Peter Brett, P., 2009, Modified titanium surfaces promote accelerated osteogenic differentiation of mesenchymal stromal cells in vitro, *J Bone* 45:17–26. doi: http://dx.doi.org/10.1016/j.bone.2009.03.662.
91. Jeong, R., Marin, C., Granato, R., Suzuki, M., Gil, J.N., Granjeiro, J.M. and Paulo G. Coelho. P.G., 2010, Early bone healing around implant surfaces treated with variations in the resorbable blasting media method. A study in rabbits, *Med Oral Patol Oral Cir Bucal* 15:119–125. doi: http://dx.doi.org/10.4317/medoral.15.e119.
92. Park, J.W., Jang, I.S. and Suh, J.Y., 2008, Bone response to endosseous titanium implants surface- modified by blasting and chemical treatment: A histomorphometric study in the rabbit femur, *J Biomed Mater Res B* 84:400–407. doi: http://dx.doi.org/10.1002/jbm.b.30884.
93. An, S-H., Matsumoto, T., Miyajima, H., Sasaki, J., Narayanan, M. and Kyo-Han Kim, K-H., 2012, Surface characterization of alkali- and heat-treated Ti with or without prior acid etching, *Appl Surf Sci* 258:4377–4382. doi: http://dx.doi.org/10.1016/j.apsusc.2011.12.119.
94. Stadlinger, B., Pilling, E., Huhle, M., Mai, R., Bierbaum, S., Bernhardt, R., Scharnweber, D., Kuhlisch, E., Hempel, U. and Eckelt, U., 2007, Influence of extracellular matrix coatings on implant stability and osseointegration: An animal study, *J Biomed Mater Res B Appl Biomater* 83:222–231. doi: http://dx.doi.org/10.1002/jbm.b.30787.
95. Alcheikh, A., Pavon-Djavid, G., Helary, G., Petite, H., Migonney, V. and F. Anagnostou, F., 2013, PolyNaSS grafting on titanium surfaces enhances osteoblast differentiation and

inhibits Staphylococcus aureus adhesion, *J Mater Sci Mater Med* 24:1745–1754. doi: http://dx.doi.org/10.1007/s10856-013-4932-3.

96. Ferraris, S., Spriano, S., Pan, G., Venturello, A., Bianchi, C.L., Chiesa, R., Faga, M.G., Maina, G. and Vernè, E., 2011, Surface modification of Ti–6Al–4V alloy for biomineralization and specific biological response: Part I, inorganic modification, *J Mater Sci Mater Med* 22:533–545. doi: http://dx.doi.org/10.1007/s10856-011-4246-2.
97. Pham, M.H., Landin, M.A., Tiainen, H., Reseland, J.E., Ellingsen, J.E. and Haugen, H.J., 2013, The effect of hydrofluoric acid treatment of titanium and titanium dioxide surface on primary human osteoblasts, *Clin Oral Implants Res.* doi: http://dx.doi.org/10.1111/clr.12150.
98. Park, J-W., 2012, Osseointegration of two different phosphate ion-containing titanium oxide surfaces in rabbit cancellous bone, *Clin Oral Imaplnats Res* 100:145–151. doi: http://dx.doi.org/10.1111/j.1600-0501.2011.02406.x.
99. Sul, Y-T., 2010, Electrochemical growth behavior, surface properties, and enhanced in vivo bone response of TiO_2 nanotubes on microstructured surfaces of blasted, screw-shaped titanium implants, *Int I Nanomedicine* 5:87–100.
100. McLeod, K., Kumar, S., Dutta, N.K., Smart, R.S.C., Voelcker, N.H. and Anderson, G.I., 2010, X-ray photoelectron spectroscopy study of the growth kinetics of biomimetically grown hydroxyapatite thin-film coatings, *Appl Surf Sci* 256:7178–7185. doi: http://dx.doi.org/10.1016/j.apsusc.2010.05.047.
101. Vidigal, G.M.Jr., Groisman, M., de Sena, L.Á. and de Almeida Soares, G., 2009, Surface characterization of dental implants coated with hydroxyapatite by plasma spray and biomimetic process, *Implant Dent* 18:353–361. doi: http://dx.doi.org/10.1097/ID.0b013e3181ac9a3d.
102. Biemond, L., Hannink, G., Verdonschot, N. and Buma, P., 2012, Assessment of bone ingrowth potential of e-beam produced surface topographies with a biomimetic coating, *J Bone Joint Surg Br* 94-B:2529.
103. Kim, M.H., Lee, S-Y., Kim, M-J., Kim, S-K., Heo, S-J. and Koak, J.Y., 2011, Effect of biomimetic deposition on anodized titanium surfaces, *J Dent Res* 90:711–716. doi: http://dx.doi.org/10.1177/0022034511400074.
104. Bumgardner, J.D., Chesnutt, B.M., Yuan, Y., Yang, Y., Appleford, M., Oh, S., McLaughlin, R., Elder, S.H. and Ong, J.L., 2007, The integration of chitosan-coated titanium in bone: An in vivo study in rabbits, *Implant Dent* 16:66–79. doi: http://dx.doi.org/10.1097/ID.0b013e3180312011.
105. Kim, S.E., Song, S-H., Yun, Y.P., Choi, B-J., Kwon, I.K., Bae, M.S., Moon, H-J. and Kwon, Y-D., 2011, The effect of immobilization of heparin and bone morphogenic protein-2 (BMP-2) to titanium surfaces on inflammation and osteoblast function, *Biomaterials* 32:366–373. doi: http://dx.doi.org/10.1016/j.biomaterials.2010.09.008.
106. Miron, R.J., Oates, C.J., Molenberg, A., Dard, M., Hamilton, D.W., 2010, The effect of enamel matrix proteins on the spreading, proliferation and differentiation of osteoblasts cultured on titanium surfaces, *Biomaterials* 31:449–460. doi: http://dx.doi.org/10.1016/j.biomaterials.2009.09.075.
107. Schliephake, H., Bötel, C., Förster, A., Schwenzer, B., Reichert, J. and Scharnweber, D., 2012, Effect of oligonucleotide mediated immobilization of bone morphogenic proteins on titanium surfaces, *Biomaterials* 33:1315–1322. doi: http://dx.doi.org/10.1016/j.biomaterials.2011.10.027.
108. Yang, Z. and Zhang, C., 2009, Adsorption/desorption behavior of protein on nanosized hydroxyapatite coatings: A quartz crystal microbalance study, *Appl Surf Sci* 255:4569–4574. doi: http://dx.doi.org/10.1016/j.apsusc.2008.11.078.
109. Assmann, A., Delfs, C., Munakata, H., Schiffer, F., Horstkötter, K., Huynh, K., Barth, M., Stoldt, V.R., Kamiya, H., Boeken, U., Lichtenberg, A. and Akhyari, P., 2013, Acceleration

of autologous in vivo recellularization of decellularized aortic conduits by fibronectin surface coating, *Biomaterials* 34:6015–6026. doi: http://dx.doi.org/10.1016/j.biomaterials.2013.04.037.
110. Poh, C.K., Shi, Z., Lim, T.Y., Neoh, K.G. and Wang, W., 2010, The effect of VEGF functionalization of titanium on endothelial cells in vitro, *Biomaterials* 31:1578–1585. doi: http://dx.doi.org/10.1016/j.biomaterials.2009.11.042.
111. Santander, S., Alcane, C., Lyahyai, J., Pěrez, M.A., Rodellar, C., Doblarě M. and Ochoa, I., 2012, In vitro osteoinduction of human mesenchymal stem cells in biomimetic surface modified titanium alloy implants, *Dent Mater J* 31:843–850. doi: http://dx.doi.org/10.4012/dmj.2012-015.
112. Sanpo, N., Ang, S.M., Cheang, P. and K. A. Khor, K.A., 2009, Antibacterial property of cold sprayed chitosan-Cu/Al coating, *J Therm Spray Technol* 18:600–608. doi: http://dx.doi.org/10.1007/s11666-009-9391-5.
113. Zheng, D., Neoh, K.G., Shi, Z. and Kang, E-T., 2013, Assessment of stability of surface anchors for antibacterial coatings and immobilized growth factors on titanium, *J Colloid Interf Sci* 406:238–246. doi: http://dx.doi.org/10.1016/j/jcis.2013.05.060.
114. Ando, Y., Miyamoto, H., Noda, I., Miyaji, F., Shimazaki, T., Yonekura, Y., Miyazaki, M., Mawatari, M. and Hotokebuchi, T., 2010, Effect of bacterial media on the evaluation of the antibacterial activity of a biomaterial containing inorganic antibacterial reagents or antibiotics, *Biocontrol Sci* 15:15–19.
115. Chang, Y-Y., Huang, H-L., Chen, Y-C., Weng, J-C. and Lai, C-H., 2012, Characterization and antibacterial performance of ZrNO–Ag coatings, *Surf Coat Technol* 231:224–228. doi: http://dx.doi.org/10.1016/j.surfcoat.2012.05.084.
116. Kang, M-K., Moon, S-K., Kim, K-M. and Kim, K-N., 2011, Antibacterial effect and cytocompatibility of nano-structured TiO_2 film containing Cl, *Dent Mater J* 30:790–798. doi: http://dx.doi.org/10.4012/dmj.2011-021.
117. Sanaa, M.F., El-Rab, G., Fadl-allah, S.A. and Montser, A.A., 2012, Improvement in antibacterial properties of Ti by electrodeposition of biomimetic Ca–P apatite coat on anodized titania, *Appl Surf Sci* 261:1–7. doi: http://dx.doi.org/10.1016/j.apsusc.2012.05.139.
118. Yoon, H., Joshi, B., Na, S-H. and Yoon, S.S., 2012, Antibacterial activity and photocatalysis of electrosprayed titania films physical and analytical electrochemistry, electrocatalysis, and photoelectrochemistry, *J Electrochem Soc* 159:H823–H827. doi: http://dx.doi.org/10.1149/2.002211jes.
119. Duerig, T., Pelton, A, and Stöckel, D., 1999, An overview of nitinol medical appliations, *Mater Sci Eng (A)* 273/275:149–160. doi: http://dx.doi.org/10.1016/S0921-5093(99)00294-4.
120. Thompson, A., 2000, An overview of nickel-titanium alloys used in dentistry, *Inter Endo J* 33:297–310. doi: http://dx.doi.org/10.1046/j.1365-2591.2000.00339.x.
121. Feninat, F.E., Laroche, G., Fiset, M. and Mantovani, D., 2002, Shape memory materials for biomedical applications, *Adv Eng Mater* 4:91–104. doi: http://dx.doi.org/10.1002/1527-2648(200203)4:3<91::AID-ADEM91>3.0.CO;2-B.
122. Shabalovskaya, S.A., 2002, Surface, corrosion and biocompatibility aspects of Nitinol as an implant material, *Biomed Mater Eng* 12:69–109.
123. Wever, D.J., Veldhuizen, A.G., Vriesv, J., Busscher, H.J. Uges, D.R.A. and van Horn, J.R., 1998, Electrochemical and surface characterization of a nickel-titanium alloy, *Biomaterials* 19:761–769. doi: http://dx.doi.org/10.1016/S0142-9612(97)00210-X.
124. Putters, J.L., Kaulesar, S.D., De Zeeuw, G.R. and Besselink, P.A., 1992, Comparative cell culture effects of shape memory metal (Nitinol), nickel and titanium: A biocompatibility estimation, *Eur Surg Res* 24:378–379.

125. Shabalovskaya, S.A., Anderegg, J. and Van Humbeeck, J., 2008, Critical overview of Nitinol surfaces and their modifications for medical applications, *Acta Biomater* 4:447–467. doi: http://dx.doi.org/10.1016/j.actbio.2008.01.013.
126. Starosvetsky, D. and Gotman, I., 2001, Corrosion behavior of titanium nitride coated Ni-Ti shape memory surgical alloy, *Biomaterials* 22:18531859. doi: http://dx.doi.org/10.1016/S0142-9612(00)00368-9
127. Villermaux, F., Tabrizian, M., Yahia, L.H., Meunier, M. and Piron, D.L., 1997, Excimer laser treatment of NiTi shape memory alloy biomaterials, *Appl Surf Sci* 109/110:62–66. doi: http://dx.doi.org/10.1016/S0169-4332(96)00619-8
128. Nose, M., Deguchi, Y., Mae, T., Honbo, E, Nagae, T. and Nogi, K., 2004, Influence of puttering conditions on the structure and properties of Ti–Si–N thin films prepared by r.f.-active sputtering, *Surf Coat Technol* 176:261–265.
129. Steegmueller, R., Wagner, C., Fleckenstein, T. and Schuessler, A., 2002, Gold Coating of Nitinol devices for medical Applications, *Mater Sci Forum* 394/395:161–164. doi: http://dx.doi.org/10.4028/www.scientific.net/MSF.394-395.161
130. Cheng, Y., Cai, W., Li, H.T. and Y. F. Zheng, Y.F., 2006, Surface modification of NiTi alloy with tantalum to improve its biocompatibility and radiopacity, *J Mater Sci* 41:4961–4964. doi: http://dx.doi.org/10.1007/s10853-006-0096-6
131. Oshida, Y., 2007, *Bioscience and Bioengineering of Titanium Materials*, Elsevier, London, UK, pp. 61–64.
132. Ju, X. and Dong, H., 2006, Plasma surface modification of NiTi shape memory alloy, *Surf Coat Technol* 201:1542–1547. doi: http://dx.doi.org/10.1016/j.surfcoat.2006.02.022
133. Zhao, T., Li, Y., Zhao, X., Chen, H. and Zhang, T., 2012, Ni ion release, osteoblast–material interactions, and hemocompatibility of hafnium-implanted NiTi alloy, *J Biomed Mater Res B Appl Biomater* 100:646–659. doi: http://dx.doi.org/ 10.1002/jbm.b.31989
134. de Camargo, E.N., Lobo, A.O., da Silva, M.M., Ueda, M., Garcia, E.E., Pichon, L., Reuther, H. and Otubo, J., 2011, Determination of Ni release in NiTi SMA with surface modification by nitrogen plasma immersion ion implantation, *J Mater Eng Perform* 20:798–801.
135. Satoh, K., Ohtsu, N., Sato, S. and Wagatsuma, K., 2013, Surface modification of Ti-6Al-4 V alloy using an oxygen glow-discharge plasma to suppress the elution of toxic elements into physiological environment, *Surf Coat Technol* 232:298–302. doi: http://dx.doi.org/10.1016/j.surfcoat.2013.05.018
136. Gordin, D.M., Gloriant, T., Chane-Pane, V., Busardo, D., Mitran, V., Höche, D., Vasilescu, C., Drob, S.I. and Cimpean, A., 2012, Surface characterization and biocompatibility of titanium alloys implanted with nitrogen by Hardion+ technology, *J Mater Sci Mater Med* 23:2953–2966. doi: http://dx.doi.org/ 10.1007/s10856-012-4750-z
137. Kung, K-C., Lee, T-M. and Lui, T-S., 2010, Bioactivity and corrosion properties of novel coatings containing strontium by microarc oxidation, *J Alloys Compounds* 508:384–390. doi: http://dx.doi.org/10.1016/j.jallcom.2010.08.057
138. Huang, H-H., Wu, C-P., Sun, Y-S. and Lee, T-H., 2013, Improvements in the corrosion resistance and biocompatibility of biomedical Ti–6Al–7Nb alloy using an electrochemical anodization treatment, *Thin Solid Films* 528:157–162. doi: http://dx.doi.org/10.1016/j.tsf.2012.08.063
139. Grant, D.M., Lo, W.J., Parker, K.G. and Parker, T.L., 1996, Biocompatible and mechanical properties of low temperature deposited quaternary (Ti, Al, V) N coatings on Ti6Al4V titanium alloy substrates, *J Mater Sci Mater Med* 7:579–584. doi: http://dx.doi.org/10.1007/BF00122181

140. Luo, R., Liu, Z., Yan, F., Kong, Y. and Zhang, Y., 2013,The biocompatibility of hydroxyapatite film deposition on microarc oxidation Ti6Al4V alloy, *Appl Surf Sci* 266:57–61. doi: http://dx.doi.org/10.1016/j.apsusc.2012.11.074
141. Xue, W., B. Krishna, V., Bandyopadhyay, A. and Bose, S., 2007, Processing and biocompatibility evaluation of laser processed porous titanium, *Acta Biomater* 3:1007–1018. doi: http://dx.doi.org/10.1016/j.actbio.2007.05.009
142. Jin, S., Zhang, Y., Wang, Q., Zhang, D. and Zhang, S., 2013, Influence of TiN coating on the biocompatibility of medical NiTi alloy, *Colloids Surf Biointerf*ace 101:343–349. doi: http://dx.doi.org/10.1016/j.colsurfb.2012.06.029
143. Hahn, B-D., Lee, J-M., Park, D-S., Choi, J-J., Ryu, J., Yoon, W-H., Choi, J-H., Lee, B-K., Kim, J-W., Kim, H-E. and Kim, S-G., 2011, Enhanced bioactivity and biocompatibility of nanostructured hydroxyapatite coating by hydrothermal annealing, *Thin Solid Films* 519:8085–8090. doi: http://dx.doi.org/10.1016/j.tsf.2011.07.008
144. Dong, Z., Li, Y. and Zou, Q., 2009, Degradation and biocompatibility of porous nanohydroxyapatite/polyurethane composite scaffold for bone tissue engineering, *Appl Surf Sci* 255:6087–6091. doi: http://dx.doi.org/10.1016/j.apsusc.2009.01.083
145. Casaletto, M.P., Ingo, G.M., Kaciulis, S., Mattogno, G., Pandolfi, L. and Scavia, G., 2001, Surface studies of in vitro biocompatibility of titanium oxide coatings, *Appl Surf Sci* 172:167–177. doi: http://dx.doi.org/10.1016/S0169-4332(00)00844-8
146. Jung, S-C., Lee, K. and Kim, B-H., 2012, Biocompatibility of plasma polymerized sandblasted large grit and acid titanium surface, *Thin Solid Films* 521:150–154. doi: http://dx.doi.org/10.1016/j.tsf.2011.12.089
147. Kaklamani, G., Mehrban, N., Chen, J., Bowen, J., Dong, H., Grover, L. and A Stamboulis, A., 2010, Effect of plasma surface modification on the biocompatibility of UHMWPE, *Biomed Mater* 5: 054102. doi: http://dx.doi.org/ 10.1088/1748-6041/5/5/054102
148. Shim, C.D., Won, D.H., Cho, H.W. and Kim, B.I., 2007, Comparative biocompatibility of pure Ti and Ti alloy with and without surface treatment, *J Jpn Inst Met Mater* 71:113–119. doi: http://dx.doi.org/10.2320/jinstmet.71.113
149. Lavos-Valereto, I.C., Wolynec, S., Deboni, M.C.Z. and B. König Jr, B., 2001, In vitro and in vivo biocompatibility testing of Ti–6Al–7Nb alloy with and without plasma-sprayed hydroxyapatite coating, *J Biomed Mater Res* 58:727–733. doi: http://dx.doi.org/10.1002/jbm.1072
150. Lee, E-J., Kim, H-W. and Kim, H-E., 2005, Biocompatibility of Fluor-Hydroxyapatite Bioceramics, *J Am Ceram Soc* 88:130–1311. doi: http://dx.doi.org/10.1111/j.1551-2916.2004.00172.x
151. Li, Y., Lee, I-S., Cui, F-Z. and Choi, S-H., 2008, The biocompatibility of nanostructured calcium phosphate coated on microarc oxidized titanium, *Biomaterials* 29:2025–2032. doi: http://dx.doi.org/10.1016/j.biomaterials.2008.01.009
152. Bruni, S., Martinesi, M., Stio, M., Treves, C., Bacci, T. and Borgioli, F., 2005, Effects of surface treatment of Ti–6Al–4V titanium alloy on biocompatibility in cultured human umbilical vein endothelial cells, *Acta Biomater* 1:223–234. doi: http://dx.doi.org/10.1016/j.actbio.2004.11.001
153. Zhao, J., Cai, X.M., Tang, H.Q., Liu, T., Gu, H.Q. and Cui, R.Z., 2008, Bactericidal and biocompatible properties of TiN/Ag multilayered films by ion beam assisted deposition, *J Mater Sci Mater Med* 20: 101–105. doi: http://dx.doi.org/10.1007/s10856-008-3491-5
154. Liu, H.Y., Wang, X.J., Wang, L.P., Lei, F.Y., Wang, X.F. and Ai, H.J., 2008, Effect of fluoride-ion implantation on the biocompatibility of titanium for dental applications, *Appl Surf Sci* 254:6305–6312. doi: http://dx.doi.org/10.1016/j.apsusc.2008.03.075

155. Wei, D. and Zhou, Y., 2009, Characteristic and biocompatibility of the TiO_2-based coatings containing amorphous calcium phosphate before and after heat treatment, *Appl Surf Sci* 255:6232–6239. doi: http://dx.doi.org/10.1016/j.apsusc.2009.04.019
156. Oshida, Y., Munoz, C.A., Winkler, M.M., Hashem, A. and Ito, M., 1993, Fractal dimension analysis of aluminum oxide particle for sandblasting dental use, *J Bio-Med Mater Eng* 3:117–126.
157. Rüger, M., Gensior, T.J., Herren, C., von Walter, M., Ocklenburg, C., Marx, R. and Erli, H-J., 2010, The removal of Al_2O_3 particles from grit-blasted titanium implant surfaces: Effects on biocompatibility, osseointegration and interface strength in vivo, *Acta Biomater* 6:2852–2861. doi: http://dx.doi.org/10.1016/j.actbio.2010.01.009
158. Lima, R.S. and Marple, B.R., 2003, High weibull modulus HVOF titania coatings, *J Therm Spray Technol* 12:240–249. doi: http://dx.doi.org/10.1361/105996303770348230
159. Masmoudi, M., Assoul, M., Wery, M., Abdelhedi, R., Halouani, F.E. and Monteil, G., 2006, Friction and wear behaviour of cp Ti and Ti6Al4V following nitric acid passivation, *Appl Surf Sci* 253:2237–2243. doi: http://dx.doi.org/10.1016/j.apsusc.2006.04.047
160. Bhatt, H. and Goswami, T., 2008, Implant wear mechanisms—basic approach, *Biomed Mater* 3:042001. doi: http://dx.doi.org/10.1088/1748-6041/3/4/042001
161. Spriano, S., Vernè, E., Faga, M.G., Bugliosi, S. and Maina, G., 2005, Surface treatment on an implant cobalt alloy for high biocompatibility and wear resistance, *Wear* 259:919–925. doi: http://dx.doi.org/10.1016/j.wear.2005.02.011
162. Raoufi, M., Mirdamadi, S., Mahboubi, F., Ahangarani, S., Mahdipoor, M,S. and Elmkhah. H., 2012, Effect of active screen plasma nitriding pretreatment on wear behavior of TiN coating deposited by PACVD technique, *Appl Surf Sci* 258:7820–7825. doi: http://dx.doi.org/10.1016/j.apsusc.2012.04.041
163. Wang, Y., Lei, T., Guo, L. and Jiang, B., 2006, Fretting wear behaviour of microarc oxidation coatings formed on titanium alloy against steel in unlubrication and oil lubrication, *Appl Surf Sci* 252:8113–8120. doi: http://dx.doi.org/10.1016/j.apsusc.2005.10.032
164. Surowska, B., Bieniaś, J., Walczak, M., Sangwal, K. and Stoch, A., 2004, Microstructure and mechanical properties of ceramic coatings on Ti and Ti-based alloy, *Appl Surf Sci* 238:288–294. doi: http://dx.doi.org/10.1016/j.apsusc.2004.05.219
165. Spector, M., Ries, M.D., Bourne, R.B., Sauer, W.S., Long, M. and Gordon Hunter, G., 2001,Wear performance of ultra-high molecular weight polyethylene on oxidized zirconium total knee femoral components, *J Bone Joint Surg Am* 83:S80-S86.
166. Santos, C.B., Haubold, L., H. Holeczek, H., Becker, M. and Metzner, M., 2010, Wear–corrosion resistance of DLC/CoCrMo system for medical implants with different surface finishing, *Tribol Letters* 37:251–259. doi: http://dx.doi.org/10.1007/s11249-009-9501-z
167. Wang, C.T., Gao, N., Gee, M.G., Wood, R.J.K. and Langdon, T.G., 2013,Tribology testing of ultrafine-grained Ti processed by high-pressure torsion with subsequent coating, *J Mater Sci* 48: 4742–4748. doi: http://dx.doi.org/ 10.1007/s10853.012.7110-y
168. Johansson, E., Klintberg, L., Akdogan, G. and Axén, N., 2004, Microstructure and Sliding Wear of Nitrided Ti–13Nb–13Zr and Nitrided CP–Ti, *Tribol Letters* 16:65–72. doi: http://dx.doi.org/10.1023/B:TRIL.0000009716.69086.5d
169. Ji, H., Xia, L., Ma, X. and Sun, Y., 2000, Tribological performance of Ti-6Al-4V plasma-based ion implanted with nitrogen, *Wear* 246:40–45. doi: http://dx.doi.org/10.1016/S0043-1648(00)00444-0
170. Díaz, C., Lutz, J., Mändl, S., García, J.A., Martínez, R. and R. J. Rodríguez, R.J., 2009, Improved bio-tribology of biomedical alloys by ion implantation techniques, *Nucl Instrum Meth Phy Res* 267:1630–1633. doi: http://dx.doi.org/10.1016/j.nimb.2009.01.118

171. Bazzoni, A., Mischler, S. and Espallargas, N., 2013, Tribocorrosion of Pulsed Plasma-Nitrided CoCrMo Implant Alloy, *Tribol Letters* 49:157–167. doi: http://dx.doi.org/10.1007/s11249-012-0047-0
172. Huang, S.Y., Huang, J.J., Kang, T., Diao, D.F. and Y. Z. Duan, Y.Z., 2013, Coating NiTi archwires with diamond-like carbon films: Reducing fluoride-induced corrosion and improving frictional properties, *J Mater Sci Mater Med* 24:2287–2292. doi: http://dx.doi.org/10.1007/s10856-013-4988-0
173. Oshida, Y. and Daly, J., 1990, Fatigue damage evaluation of shot-peened high strength aluminum alloy, In: S.A. Meguid ed., *Surface Engineering*, Elsevier Applied Science, London, UK, pp. 404–416. doi: http://dx.doi.org/10.1007/978-94-009-0773-7_42
174. Gil, F.J., Planell, J.A., Padrós, A. and Aparicio, C., 2007, The effect of shot blasting and heat treatment on the fatigue behavior of titanium for dental implant applications, *Dent Mater* 23:486–491. doi: http://dx.doi.org/10.1016/j.dental.2006.03.003
175. Apachitei, I., Leoni, A., Riemslag, A.C., Fratila-Apachitei, L.E. and Duszczyk, J., 2011, Enhanced fatigue performance of porous coated Ti6Al4V biomedical alloy, *Appl Surf Sci* 257:6941–6944. doi: http://dx.doi.org/10.1016/j.apsusc.2011.03.038
176. Hiromoto, S., Tomozawa, M. and Maruyama, N., 2013, Fatigue property of a bioabsorbable magnesium alloy with a hydroxyapatite coating formed by a chemical solution deposition, *J Mech Behav Biomed Mater* 25:1–10. doi: http://dx.doi.org/10.1016/j.jmbbm.2013.04.021
177. He, Y., Zhang, J., Yao, W., Li D. and Teng, X., 2009, Effect of temperature on residual stress and mechanical properties of Ti films prepared by both ion implantation and ion beam assisted deposition, *Appl Surf Sci* 255:4484–4490. doi: http://dx.doi.org/10.1016/j.apsusc.2008.11.053
178. Jiang, W., Wang, W.D., Shi, X.H., Chen, H.Z., Zou, W., Guo, Z., Luo, J.M., Gu, Z.W. and Zhang, X.D., 2008, The effects of hydroxyapatite coatings on stress distribution near the dental implant–bone interface, *Appl Surf Sci* 255:273–275. doi: http://dx.doi.org/10.1016/j.apsusc.2008.06.165
179. Stráský, J., Janeček, M., Harcuba, P., Bukovina, M. and Lothar Wagner, L., 2011, The effect of microstructure on fatigue performance of Ti–6Al–4V alloy after EDM surface treatment for application in orthopedics, *J Mech Behav Biomed Mater* 4:1955–1962. doi: http://dx.doi.org/10.1016/j.jmbbm.2011.06.012
180. Pazos, L., Corengia, P. and Svoboda, H., 2010, Effect of surface treatments on the fatigue life of titanium for biomedical applications, *J Mech Behav Biomed Mater* 3:416–424. doi: http://dx.doi.org/10.1016/j.jmbbm.2010.03.006
181. Zhang, X.C., Xu, B.S., Wang, H.D. and Wu, Y.X., 2008, Effect of graded interlayer on the mode I edge delamination by residual stresses in multilayer coating-based systems, *Appl Surf Sci* 254:1881–1889. doi: http://dx.doi.org/10.1016/j.apsusc.2007.07.108
182. Patel, Z. and Greta A.V.M. Geerts, G.A.V.M., 2011, Temperature changes along a dental implant, *Int J Prosthodont* 24:58–63.
183. Geminiani, A., Caton, J.G. and Romanos, G.E., 2011, Temperature increase during CO2 and Er:YAG irradiation on implant surfaces, *Implant Dent* 20:379–382.
184. Revie, R.W. and Norbert D. Greene, N.D., 1969, Corrosion behaviour of surgical implant materials: II. Effects of surface preparation, *Corr Sci* 9:763–770. doi: http://dx.doi.org/10.1016/S0010-938X(69)80081-8
185. Nagarajan, S. and Rajendran, N., 2009, Surface characterisation and electrochemical behaviour of porous titanium dioxide coated 316L stainless steel for orthopedic applications, *Appl Surf Sci* 255:3927–3932. doi: http://dx.doi.org/10.1016/j.apsusc.2008.10.058
186. Pan, J., Thierry, D. and Leygraf, C., 1996, Electrochemical impedance spectroscopy study of the passive oxide film on titanium for implant application, *Electrochim Acta* 41:1143–1153. doi: http://dx.doi.org/10.1016/0013-4686(95)00465-3

187. Chiu, K.Y., Wong, M.H., Cheng, F.T. and Man, H.C., 2007, Characterization and corrosion studies of titania-coated NiTi prepared by sol–gel technique and steam crystallization, *Appl Surf Sci* 253:6762–6768. doi: http://dx.doi.org/10.1016/j.apsusc.2007.01.121
188. Wong, M.H., Cheng, F.T. and Man, H.C., 2007, Characteristics, apatite-forming ability and corrosion resistance of NiTi surface modified by AC anodization, *Appl Surf Sci* 253:7527–7534. doi: http://dx.doi.org/10.1016/j.apsusc.2007.03.055
189. Huang, H-H., Hsu, C-H., Pan, S-J., He, J-L., Chen, C-C. and Tien-Ling Lee, T-L., 2005, Corrosion and cell adhesion behavior of TiN-coated and ion-nitrided titanium for dental applications, *Appl Surf Sci* 244:252–256. doi: http://dx.doi.org/10.1016/j.apsusc.2004.10.144
190. Kim, W-G. and Choe, H-C., 2012, Effects of TiN coating on the corrosion of nanostructured Ti–30Ta–xZr alloys for dental implants, *Appl Surf Sci* 258:1929–1934. doi: http://dx.doi.org/10.1016/j.apsusc.2011.06.151
191. Cotrut, C-M., Braic, V., Balaceanu, M., Titorencu, I., Braic, M. and Parau, A.C., 2013, Corrosion resistance, mechanical properties and biocompatibility of Hf-containing ZrCN coatings, *Thin Solid Films* 538:48–55. doi: http://dx.doi.org/10.1016/j.tsf.2012.12.100
192. Sun, Y-S., Chang, J-H. and Huang, H-H., 2013, Corrosion resistance and biocompatibility of titanium surface coated with amorphous tantalum pentoxide, *Thin Solid Films* 528:130–135. doi: http://dx.doi.org/10.1016/j.tsf.2012.06.088
193. Cheng, Y., Cai, W., Zheng, Y.F., Li, H.T. and Zhao, L.C., 2005, Surface characterization and immersion tests of TiNi alloy coated with Ta, *Surf Coat Technol* 190:428–433. doi: http://dx.doi.org/10.1016/j.surfcoat.2004.03.051
194. Xin, Y., Hu, T. and Chu, P.K., 2010, Influence of test solutions on in vitro studies of biomedical magnesium alloys corrosion, passivation, and anodic films, J Electrochem Soc 157:C238–C243.
195. Fischerauer, S.F., Kraus, T., Wu, X., Tangl, S., Sorantin, E., Hänzi, A.C., Löffler, J.F., Uggowitzer, P.J. and Weinberg, A.M, 2013, In vivo degradation performance of microarc-oxidized magnesium implants: A micro-CT study in rats, *Acta Biomater* 9:5411–5420. doi: http://dx.doi.org/10.1016/j.actbio.2012.09.017
196. Balamurugan, A., Balossier, G., Michel, J. and Ferreira, J.M.F., 2009, Electrochemical and structural evaluation of functionally graded bioglass-apatite composites electrophoretically deposited onto Ti6Al4V alloy, *Electrochimica Acta* 54:1192–1198. doi: http://dx.doi.org/10.1016/j.electacta.2008.08.055
197. Purnama, A., Hermawan, H., Couet, J. and Mantovani, D., 2010, Assessing the biocompatibility of degradable metallic materials: State-of-the-art and focus on the potential of genetic regulation, *Acta Biomater* 6:1800–1807. doi: http://dx.doi.org/10.1016/j.actbio.2010.02.027
198. Popa, M., Vasilescu, E., Drob, P., Popa, M.V., Moreno, J.M.C., Vasilescu, C. and Drob, S.I., 2012, Deposition, characterization, and corrosion resistance of nanocrystalline bioactive hydroxyapatite ceramic coating on new Ti-20Nb-10Zr-5Ta Alloy, *J Am Ceram Soc* 95:3807–3814. doi: http://dx.doi.org/10.1111/jace.12029
199. Kim, J-U., Jeong, Y-H. and Choe, H-C., 2012, Measurement of oxide thin film dissolution rate on the HA-coated Ti alloy by scanning electron microscopy and impedance spectroscopy, *Surf Interface Anal* 44:1468–1472. doi: http://dx.doi.org/10.1002/sia.4977
200. Kwok, C.T., Wong, P.K., Cheng, F.T. and Man, H.C., 2009, Characterization and corrosion behavior of hydroxyapatite coatings on Ti6Al4V fabricated by electrophoretic deposition, *Appl Surf Sci* 255:6736–6744. doi: http://dx.doi.org/10.1016/j.apsusc.2009.02.086
201. Aksakal, B., Gavgali, M. and Dikici, B., 2010, The effect of coating thickness on corrosion resistance of hydroxyapatite coated Ti6Al4V and 316L SS implants, *J Mater Eng Perform* 19:894–899. doi: http://dx.doi.org/10.1007/s11665-009-9559-7

202. Singh, T.P., Singh, H. and Singh, H., 2012, Characterization, corrosion resistance, and cell response of high-velocity flame-sprayed HA and HA/TiO_2 coatings on 316L SS, *J Therm Spray Technol* 21:917–927. doi: http://dx.doi.org/10.1007/s11666-012-9782-x
203. Kannan, S., Balamurugan, A. and Rajeswari, S., 2005, Electrochemical characterization of hydroxyapatite coatings on HNO_3 passivated 316L SS for implant applications, *Electrochim Acta* 50:2065–2072. doi: http://dx.doi.org/10.1016/j.electacta.2004.09.015
204. Keller, J.C., Wick, D.Z.G., Draughn, R.A. and Wightman, J.P., 1995, The effects of sterilization treatments on adhesion of bone cells to titanium, *J Adhes* 54:145–153. doi: http://dx.doi.org/10.1080/00218469508014387
205. Park, J.H., Olivares-Navarrete, R., Baier, R.E., Meyer, A.E., Tannenbaum, R., Boyan, B.D. and Schwartz, Z., 2012, Effect of cleaning and sterilization on titanium implant surface properties and cellular response, *Acta Biomater* 8:1966–1975. doi: http://dx.doi.org/10.1016/j.actbio.2011.11.026
206. Marie P.J., Felsenberg, D. and Brandi, M.I., 2011, How strontium ranelate, via opposite effect on bone resorption and formation, prevents osteoporosis, *Osteoporos Int* 22:1659–1667. doi: http://dx.doi.org/10.1007/s00198-010-1369-0
207. Peng, S., Zhou G., Luk K.D., Cheung, K.M.C., Li, Z., Lam, W.M., Zhou, Z. and Lu, W.W., 2009, Strontium promotes osteogenic differentiation of mesenchymal stem cells through the Ras/MAPK singnaling pathay, *Cell Physiol Biochem* 23:165–174. doi: http://dx.doi.org/10.1159/000204105
208. Maimoun, L., Brennan, T.C., Badoud, I., Dubois-Ferriere, V., Rizzoli, R. and Ammann, P., 2010, Strntium ranelate improves implant osseointegration, *Bone* 46:1436–1441. doi: http://dx.doi.org/10.1016/j.bone.2010.01.379
209. Andersen, O.Z., Offermanns, V., Sillassen, M., Almtoft, K.P., Andersen, I.H., Sørensen, S., Jeppesen, C.S., Kraft, D.C.E., Bøttiger, J., Rasse, M., Kloss, F. and Foss, M., 2013, Accelerated bone ingrowth by local delivery of strontium from surface functionalized titanium implants, *Biomaterials* 34:5883–5890. doi: http://dx.doi.org/10.1016/j.biomaterials.2013.04.031
210. Zhao, L., Wang, H., Huo, K., Zhang, X., Wang, W., Zhang, Y., Wu, Z. and Paul K. Chu, P.K., 2013, The osteogenic activity of strontium loaded titania nanotube arrays on titanium substrates, *Biomaterials* 34:19–29. doi: http://dx.doi.org/10.1016/j.biomaterials.2012.09.041
211. D'Antonio, J.A., Capello, W.N., Crothers, O,D., Jaffe, W.L. and Manley, M.T., 1992, Early clinical experience with hydroxyapatite-coated femoral implants, J Bone Joint Surg Am 74:995–1008.
212. D'Antonio, J.A., Capello, W.N. and Manley, M.T., 1996, Remodeling of bone around hydroxyapatite-coated femoral stems, *J Bone Joint Surg Am* 78:1226–1234.
213. D'Lima, D.D., Walker, R.H. and Colwell, C.W. Jr., 1999, Omnifit-HA stem in total hip arthroplasty. A 2- to 5-year followup, *Clin Orthop Relat Res* 363:163–169.
214. Geesink, R.G. and Hoefnagels, N.H., 1995, Six-year results of hydroxyapatite-coated total hip replacement, *J Bone Joint Surg Br* 77:534–547.
215. Beck, G.R. Jr., 2003, Inorganic phosphate as a signaling molecule in osteoblast differentiation, *J Cell Biochem* 90:234–243. doi: http://dx.doi.org/10.1002/jcb.10622
216. Reddi, A.H., 2000, Morphogenesis and tissue engineering of bone and cartilage: inductive signals, stem cells, and biomimetic biomaterials, *Tissue Eng* 6:351–359. doi: http://dx.doi.org/10.1089/107632700418074
217. Michaels, C.M., Keller, J.C., Stanford, C.M. and Solursh, M., 1989, In vitro cell attachment of osteoblast-like cells to titanium, *J Dental Res* 68:276–282.
218. Curtis, A. and Clark, P., 1990, The effects of topographical and mechanical properties of materials on cell behavior, *CRC Crit Rev Biocompatibil* 5:343–362.

219. Oshida, Y, 2007, *Bioscience and Bioengineering of Titanium Materials*, Elseveir, London, UK, pp. 180–182.
220. Oshida, Y, 2007, *Bioscience and Bioengineering of Titanium Materials*, Elseveir, London, UK, pp. 142–145.
221. D'Lima, D.D., Lemperle, S.M., Chen, P.C., Holmes, R.E. and Colwell, C.W. Jr., 1998, Bone response to implant surface morphology, *J Arthroplasty* 13:928–934. doi: http://dx.doi.org/10.1016/S0883-5403(98)90201-7
222. Feighan, J.E., Goldberg, V.M., Davy, D., Parr, J.A. and Stevenson, S., 1995, The influence of surface-blasting on the incorporation of titanium-alloy implants in a rabbit intramedullary model, *J Bone Joint Surg Am* 77:1380–1395.
223. Wennerberg, A., Albrektsson, T., Johansson, C. and Andersson, B., 1996, Experimental study of turned and grit-blasted screw-shaped implants with special emphasis on effects of blasting material and surface topography, *Biomaterials* 17:15–22. doi: http://dx.doi.org/10.1016/0142-9612(96)80750-2
224. Hacking, S.A., Tanzer, M., Harvey, E.J., Krygier, J.J. and Bobyn, J.D., 2002, Relative contributions of chemistry and topography to the osseointegration of hydroxyapatite coatings, *Clin Orthop Relat Res* 405:24–38. doi: http://dx.doi.org/10.1097/00003086-200212000-00004
225. Daugaard, H., Elmengaard, B., Bechtold, J.E., Jensen, T. and Soballe, ., 2010, The effect on bone growth enhancement of implant coatings with hydroxyapatite and collagen deposited electrochemically and by plasma spray, *J Biomed Mater Res* A 92:913–921.
226. Dey, A., Mukhopadhyay, A.K., Gangadharan, S., Sinha, M.K. and Debabrata Basu, D., 2009, Characterization of Microplasma Sprayed Hydroxyapatite Coating, *J Therm Spray Technol* 18:578–592. doi: http://dx.doi.org/10.1007/s11666-009-9386-2
227. O'Hare, P., Meenan, B.J., Burke, G.A., Byrne, G., Dowling, D. and Hunt, J.A., 2010, Biological responses to hydroxyapatite surfaces deposited via a co-incident microblasting technique, *Biomaterials* 31:515–522. doi: http://dx.doi.org/10.1016/j.biomaterials.2009.09.067
228. Kim, D-H., Kong, Y-M., Lee, S-H., Lee, I-S., Kim, H-E., Heo, S-J. and Koak, J-Y., 2003, Composition and crystallization of hydroxyapatite coating layer formed by electron beam deposition, *J Am Ceram Soc* 86:186–188. doi: http://dx.doi.org/10.1111/j.1151-2916.2003.tb03301.x
229. Sun, L., Berndt, C.C., Khor, K.A., Cheang, H.N. and Gross, K.A., 2002, Surface characteristics and dissolution behavior of plasma-sprayed hydroxyapatite coating, *J Biomed Mater Res* 62:228–236. doi: http://dx.doi.org/10.1002/jbm.10315
230. Wang, B.C., Chang, E., Yang, C.Y., Tu, D. and Tsai, C.H., 1993, Characteristics and osteoconductivity of three different plasma-sprayed hydroxyapatite coatings, *Surf Coat Technol* 58:107–117. doi: http://dx.doi.org/10.1016/0257-8972(93)90181-M
231. Çehreli, M.C., Onur, M.A. and Şahin, S., 2003, Effects of hydroxyapatite-coated and commercially pure titanium oral implant surfaces on compound nerve action potentials—A study on the rat sciatic nerve, *Clin Oral Implants Res* 14:269–272. doi: http://dx.doi.org/10.1034/j.1600-0501.2003.140303.x
232. Traina, F., Bordini, B., De Clerico, M. and Aldo Toni, A., 2008, Twelve years follow up experience with hydroxapatite coated hip arthroplasty with ceramic bearing surfaces, *J Bone Joint Surg* 90-B:188–194.
233. Schaper, L., 2004, The effect of surface coating on a single stem design: A 6 to 10 years study, *J Bone Joint Surg* 86-B:402–406.
234. Artzi, Z., Carmeli, G. and Kozlovsky, A., 2006, A distinguishable observation between survival and success rate outcome of hydroxyapatite-coated implants in 5–10 years in function, *Clin Oral Implants Res* 17:85–93. doi: http://dx.doi.org/10.1111/j.1600-0501.2005.01178.x

235. Epinette, J-A. and Manley, M.T., 2007, Hydroxyapatite-coated total knee replacement, *J Bone Joint Surg* 89-B:34–38. doi: http://dx.doi.org/10.1302/0301-620X.89B1.17864
236. Capilla , M.V., Olid , M.N.R., Gaya , M.V.O., Botella, C.R. and Romera, C.Z., 2007, Cylindrical dental implants with hydroxyapatite- and titanium plasma, spray–coated surfaces: 5-year, *J Oral Implantol* 33:59–68. doi: http://dx.doi.org/10.1563/1548-1336(2007)33[59:CDIWHA]2.0.CO;2
237. Mistry, S., Kundu, D., Datta, S. and Basu, D., 2011, Comparison of bioactive glass coated and hydroxyapatite coated titanium dental implants in the human jaw bone, *Austral Dent J* 56:68–75. doi: http://dx.doi.org/10.1111/j.1834-7819.2010.01305.x
238. Buchanan, J., 2012, Review of patients at or under the age of fifty having total hip replacement using hydroxyapatite ceramic coated hip implants: a clinical and radiological evaluation with up to nineteen year follow-up, *J Bone Joint Surg Br* 94-B:24–29.
239. Jun, J., Shin, J-H. and Dhayal, M., 2006, Surface state of TiO_2 treated with low ion energy plasma, *Appl Surf Sci* 252:3871–3877. doi: http://dx.doi.org/10.1016/j.apsusc.2005.06.004
240. Fadl-allah, S.A. and Mohsen, Q., 2010, Characterization of native and anodic oxide films formed on commercial pure titanium using electrochemical properties and morphology techniques, *Appl Surf Sci* 256:5849–5855. doi: http://dx.doi.org/10.1016/j.apsusc.2010.03.058
241. Chen, Z.X., Takao, Y., Wang, W.X., Matsubara, T. and L M Ren, L.M., 2009, Surface characteristics and in vitro biocompatibility of titanium anodized in a phosphoric acid solution at different voltages, *Biomed Mater* 4: doi: http://dx.doi.org/10.1088/1748-6041/4/6/065003
242. Choi, J-Y., Lee, H-J., Jang, J-U. and Yeo, I-S., 2012, Comparison between bioactive fluoride modified and bioinert anodically oxidized implant surfaces in early bone response using rabbit tibia model, *Implant Dent* 21:124–128. doi: http://dx.doi.org/10.1097/ID.0b013e318249f283
243. Kwon, T-K., Lee, H-J., Min, S-K. and Yeo, I-S., 2012, Evaluation of early bone response to fluoride-modified and anodically oxidized titanium implants through continuous removal torque analysis, *Implant Dent* 21:427–432. doi: http://dx.doi.org/10.1097/ID.0b013e31826917f6
244. Choi, S-H., Cha, J-Y., Joo, U-H. and Hwang, C-J., 2012, Surface changes of anodic oxidized orthodontic titanium miniscrew, *The Angle Orthodon* 82:522–528. doi: http://dx.doi.org/10.2319/071311-448.1
245. Chung, Y-L., Gan, D-S., Ou, K-L. and Chiou, S-Y., 2011, Formation of anatase and TiO from Ti Thin Film after anodic treatment and thermal annealing corrosion, passivation, and anodic films, *J Electrochem Soc* 158:C319–C324. doi: http://dx.doi.org/10.1149/1.3615999
246. Hou, Y-Q., Zhuang, D-M., Zhang, G., Zhao, M. and Wu, M-S., 2003, Influence of annealing temperature on the properties of titanium oxide thin film, *Appl Surf Sci* 218:98–106. doi: http://dx.doi.org/10.1016/S0169-4332(03)00569-5
247. Drnovšek, N., Rade, K., Milačič, R., Štrancar, J. and Novak, S., 2012, The properties of bioactive TiO_2 coatings on Ti-based implants, *Surf Coat Technol* 209:177–183. doi: http://dx.doi.org/10.1016/j.surfcoat.2012.08.037
248. Chung, Y-L., Gan, D-S. and Ou, K-L., 2012, The Ti to TiO and TiO to anatase transformations induced by anodizing and annealing treatments of Ti thin filmcorrosion, passivation, and anodic films, *J Electrochem Soc* 159:C133-C136. doi: http://dx.doi.org/10.1149/2.097203jes
249. Stojadinović, S., Vasilić, R., Petković, M., Kasalica, B., Belča, I., Žekić, A. and Zeković, I., 2013, Characterization of the plasma electrolytic oxidation of titanium in sodium metasilicate, *Appl Surf Sci* 265:226–233. doi: http://dx.doi.org/10.1016/j.apsusc.2012.10.183

250. Tsai, M-T., Chang, Y-Y., Huang, H-L., Hsu, J-T., Chen, Y-C. and Aaron Yu-Jen Wu, A.Y-J., 2013, Characterization and antibacterial performance of bioactive Ti–Zn–O coatings deposited on titanium implants, *Thin Solid Films* 528:143–150. doi: http://dx.doi.org/10.1016/j.tsf.2012.05.093
251. Park, J., Kim, D-J., Kim, Y-K., Lee, K-H., Lee, H. and Ahn, S., 2003, Improvement of the biocompatibility and mechanical properties of surgical tools with TiN coating by PACVD, *Thin Solid Films* 435:102–107. doi: http://dx.doi.org/10.1016/S0040-6090(03)00412-7
252. El-Hossary, F.M., Negm, N.Z., Khalil, S.M. and Raaif, M., 2005, Effect of continuous and cyclic Rf plasma processing time on titanium surface, *Appl Surf Sci* 239:142–153. doi: http://dx.doi.org/10.1016/j.apsusc.2004.05.256
253. Subramanian, B., Muraleedharan, C.V., Ananthakumar, R. and Jayachandran, M., 2011, A comparative study of titanium nitride (TiN), titanium oxy nitride (TiON) and titanium aluminum nitride (TiAlN), as surface coatings for bio implants, *Surf Coat Technol* 205:5014–5020. doi: http://dx.doi.org/10.1016/j.surfcoat.2011.05.004
254. Moon, B-K., Choe, H-C. and Brantley, W.A., 2012, Surface characteristics of TiN/ZrN coated nanotubular structure on the Ti–35Ta–xHf alloy for bio-implant applications, *Appl Surf Sci* 258:2088–2092. doi: http://dx.doi.org/10.1016/j.apsusc.2011.04.050
255. Sanchez, A.G., Schreiner, W., Duffó, G. and S. Ceré, S., 2011, Surface characterization of anodized zirconium for biomedical applications, *Appl Surf Sci* 257:6397–6405. doi: http://dx.doi.org/10.1016/j.apsusc.2011.02.005
256. Barbotteau, Y., Irigaray, J.L. and Jallot, e., 2003, Physicochemical characterization of biological glass coatings, *Surf Interface Anal* 35:450–458. doi: http://dx.doi.org/10.1002/sia.1559
257. Xie, Y., Zheng, X., Ding, C., Zhai, JW., Chang, L. and Ji, H., 2009, Preparation and characterization of CaO–ZrO_2–SiO_2 coating for potential application in biomedicine, *J Therm Spray Technol* 18:678–685. doi: http://dx.doi.org/10.1007/s11666-009-9394-2
258. Xie, Y., Zheng, X., Liu, X. and Ding, C., 2007, Durability of titanium/dicalcium silicate composite coatings in simulated body fluid, *J Therm Spray Technol* 16:588–592. doi: http://dx.doi.org/10.1007/s11666-007-9071-2
259. Wang, W., Liang, J., Guo, X., Xuan, F. and Hong, H., 2012, Mechanical properties and dissolution behavior of plasma sprayed wollastonite coatings deposited at different substrate temperatures, *J Therm Spray Technol* 21:496–504. doi: http://dx.doi.org/10.1007/s11666-011-9699-9
260. Cavalheiro, J., Ribeiro, C. and Branco, R., 1991, Morphological study of an alumina-glass coating, *Surf Coat Technol* 45:209–213. doi: http://dx.doi.org/10.1016/0257-8972(91)90225-L
261. Ikeda, D., Ogawa, M., Hara, Y., Nishimura, Y., Odusanya, O., Azuma, K., Matsuda, S., Yatsuzuka, M. and Murakami, A., 2002, Effect of nitrogen plasma-based ion implantation on joint prosthetic material, *Surf Coat Technol* 156:301–305. doi: http://dx.doi.org/10.1016/S0257-8972(02)00094-4
262. Yamanaka, K., Mori, M. and Chiba, A., 2013, Nanoarchitectured Co–Cr–Mo orthopedic implant alloys: Nitrogen-enhanced nanostructural evolution and its effect on phase stability, *Acta Biomater* 9:6259–6267. doi: http://dx.doi.org/10.1016/j.actbio.2012.12.013
263. Birch, M.A., Johnson-Lynn, S., Nouraei, S., Wu, Q-B., Ngalim, S., Lu, W-J., Watchorn, C., Yang, T-Y., McCaskie, A.W. and Ro, S., 2012, Effect of electrochemical structuring of Ti6Al4V on osteoblast behaviour in vitro, *Biomed. Mater.* 7:doi: http://dx.doi.org/10.1088/1748-6041/7/3/035016
264. Davies, J.E., Ajami, E., Moineddin, R. and Mendes, V.C., 2013, The roles of different scale ranges of surface implant topography on the stability of the bone/implant interface, *Biomaterials* 34:3535–3546. doi: http://dx.doi.org/10.1016/j.biomaterials.2013.01.024

265. Wennerberg, A. and Albrektsson, T., 2009, Effects of titanium surface topography on bone integration: A systematic review, *Clin Oral Implants Res* 20:172–184. doi: http://dx.doi.org/10.1111/j.1600-0501.2009.01775.x
266. Carimo, M.C., Leila, A., Deliberador, T.M., Zielak, J.C., Correr, G.M., Giovanini, A.F. and Gonzaga, C.C., 2012, Microstructural and topographical characterization of different surface treatments of a surgical titanium alloy for dental implants; *Implant Dent* 21:207–212. doi: http://dx.doi.org/10.1097/ID.0b013e3182566e19
267. Ricci, M., Mangano, F., Tercio, T., Tonelli, P., Barone, A., Raspanti, M. and U. Covani, U., 2012, Nanometrical evaluation of direct laser implant surface, *Surf Interface Anal* 44:1582–1586. doi: http://dx.doi.org/10.1002/sia.5087
268. Pecora, G.E., Ceccarelli, R., Bonelli, M., Alexander, H. and Ricci, J.L., 2009, Clinical evaluation of laser microtexturing for soft tissue and bone attachment to dental implants, *Implant Dent* 18:57–66. doi: http://dx.doi.org/10.1097/ID.0b013e31818c5a6d
269. Cei, S., Legitimo, A., Barachini, S., Consolini, R., Sammartino, G., Mattii, L., Gabriele, M. and Graziani, F., 2011, Effect of laser micromachining of titanium on viability and responsiveness of osteoblast-like cell, *Implant Dent* 20:285–291. doi: http://dx.doi.org/10.1097/ID.0b013e31821bfa9f
270. Xiao, J., Zhou, H., Zhao, L., Sun, Y., Guan, S., Liu, B. and L. Kong, L., 2011, The effect of hierarchical micro/nanosurface titanium implant on osseointegration in ovariectomized sheep, *Osteoporosis Int* 22:1907–1913. doi: http://dx.doi.org/10.1007/s00198-010-1413-0
271. Kunzler, T.P., Drobek, T., Schuler, M. and Spencer, N.D., 2007, Systematic study of osteoblast and fibroblast response to roughness by means of surface-morphology gradients, *Biomaterials* 28:2175–2182. doi: http://dx.doi.org/10.1016/j.biomaterials.2007.01.019
272. Oshida, Y., 2007, *Bioscience and Bioengineering of Titanium Materials*, Elseveier, London, UK, pp. 406–411.
273. Oshida, Y. and Tuna, E.B., 2009, Science and technology integrated titanium dental implant systems, In: B.Basu, D.S. Katti, A. Kumar ed., *Advanced Biomaterials*, Wiley & Sons, Hoboken, NJ, pp. 165–167.
274. Otsuki, B., Takemoto, M., Fujibayashi, S., Neo, M., Kokubo, T. and Nakamura, T., 2006, Pore throat size and connectivity determine bone and tissue ingrowth into porous implants: Three-dimensional micro-CT based structural analyses of porous bioactive titanium implants, *Biomaterials* 27:5892–5900. doi: http://dx.doi.org/10.1016/j.biomaterials.2006.08.013
275. Wazen, R.M., Lefebvre, L-P., Baril, E. and Nanci, A., 2010, Initial evaluation of bone ingrowth into a novel porous titanium coating, *J Biomed Mater Res* B 94B:64–71.
276. Takemoto, M., Fujibayashi, S., Neo, M., Suzuki, J., Kokubo, T. and Nakamura, T., 2005, Mechanical properties and osteoconductivity of porous bioactive titanium, *Biomaterials* 26:6014–6023. doi: http://dx.doi.org/10.1016/j.biomaterials.2005.03.019
277. Gittens, R.A., Olivares-Navarrete, R., McLachlan, T., Cai, Y., Hyzy, S.L., Schneider, J.M., Schwartz, Z., Sandhage, K.H. and Boyan, B.D., 2012, Differential responses of osteoblast lineage cells to nanotopographically-modified, microroughened titanium–aluminum–vanadium alloy surfaces, *Biomaterials* 33:8986–8994. doi: http://dx.doi.org/10.1016/j.biomaterials.2012.08.059
278. Prymak, O., Bogdanski, D., Köller, M., Esenwein, S.A., Muhr, G., Beckmann, F., Donath, T., Assad, M. and Epple, M., 2005, Morphological characterization and in vitro biocompatibility of a porous nickel–titanium alloy, *Biomaterials* 26:5801–5807. doi: http://dx.doi.org/10.1016/j.biomaterials.2005.02.029
279. Jingyu, W., Lin, W., Yong, G., Jinsong, Z. and Cuicui, Z., 2013, Experimental study on the osseointegration of foam TiC/Ti composites. *Biomed Mater* 8. doi: http://dx.doi.org/10.1088/1748-6041/8/4/045001

280. Kuo, P.C-H., Chou, H-H., Lin, Y-H., Peng, P-W., Ou, K-L. and Lee, W-R., 2012, Effects of surface functionalization on the nanostructure and biomechanical properties of binary titanium–niobium alloys electrochemical synthesis and engineering, *J Electrochem Soc* 159:E103–E107. doi: http://dx.doi.org/10.1149/2.094204jes
281. Mattila, R.H., Laurila, P., Rekola, J., Gunn, J., Lassila, L.V.J., Mäntylä, T., Aho, A.J. and Vallittu, P.K., 2009, Bone attachment to glass-fibre-reinforced composite implant with porous surface, *Acta Biomater* 5:1639–1646. doi: http://dx.doi.org/10.1016/j.actbio.2009.01.020
282. Zheng, C.Y., Nie, F.L., Zheng, Y.F., Cheng, Y., Wei, S.C. and Valiev, R.Z., 2011, Enhanced in vitro biocompatibility of ultrafine-grained biomedical NiTi alloy with microporous surface, *Appl Surf Sci* 257:9086–9093. doi: http://dx.doi.org/10.1016/j.apsusc.2011.05.105
283. Zheng, C.Y., Nie, F.L., Zheng, Y.F., Cheng, Y., Wei, S.C. and Valiev, R.Z., 2011, Enhanced in vitro biocompatibility of ultrafine-grained titanium with hierarchical porous surface, *Appl Surf Sci* 257:5634–5640. doi: http://dx.doi.org/10.1016/j.apsusc.2011.05.105
284. Saldaña, L., Méndez-Vilas, A., Jiang, L., Multigner, M., González-Carrasco, J.L., Pérez-Prado, M.T., González-Martín, M.L., Munuera, L. and Vilaboa, N., 2007, In vitro biocompatibility of an ultrafine grained zirconium, *Biomaterials* 28:4343–4354. doi: http://dx.doi.org/10.1016/j.biomaterials.2007.06.015
285. Hwang, D. and Wang, H.L., 2006, Medical contraindications to implant therapy: part I: absolute contraindictaions, *Implant Dent* 15:353–360. doi: http://dx.doi.org/10.1097/01.id.0000247855.75691.03
286. Hwang, D and Wang, H.L., 2007, Medical contraindications to implant therapy: part II: relative contraindictaions, *Implant Dent* 16:13–23. doi: http://dx.doi.org/10.1097/01.id.0000247855.75691.03
287. De Bruyn, H. and Collaert, B., 1994, The effect of smoking on early implant failure, *Clin Oral Implant Res* 5:260–264. doi: http://dx.doi.org/10.1034/j.1600-0501.1994.050410.x
288. Moy, P.K., Medina, D., Shetty, V. and Aghaloo, T.L., 2005, Dental implant failure rates and associated risk factors, *Int Oral Maxillofac Implants* 20:56–577.
289. Salonen, M.A.M., Oikarinen, K., Virtanen, K. and Pernu, H., 1993, Failures in the Osseointegration of Endosseous Implants, *J Oral Maxillofac Implants* 8:92–97.
290. Shibli, J.A., Vitussi, T.R.C., Garcia, R.V., Zenóbio, E.G., Ota-Tsuzuki, C., Cassoni, A., Piattelli, A. and d'Avila, S., 2007, Implant surface analysis and microbiologic evaluation of failed implants retrieved from smokers, *J Oral Implantol* 33:232–238. doi: http://dx.doi.org/10.1563/1548-1336(2007)33[232:ISAAME]2.0.CO;2
291. Steflik, D.E., Corpe, R.S., Young, T., Parr, G., Tucker, M., Sims, M., Tinley, J., Sisk, A. and McDaniel, M., 2001, Light microscopic and scanning electron microscopic retrieval analyses of implanted biomaterials retrieved from humans and experimental animals, *J Oral Implantol* 27:5–15. doi: http://dx.doi.org/10.1563/1548-1336(2001)027<0005:LMASEM>2.3.CO;2
292. Lu, H., Zhou, L., Wan, L., Li, S., Rong, M. and Guo, Z., 2012, Effects of storage methods on time-related changes of titanium surface properties and cellular response, *Biomed Mater* 7. doi: http://dx.doi.org/10.1088/1748-6041/7/5/055002
293. Louropoulou, A., Slot, D.E. and Van der Weijden, F.A., 2012, Titanium surface alterations following the use of different mechanical instruments: A systematic review, *Clin Oral Implants Res* 23:643–658. doi: http://dx.doi.org/10.1111/j.1600-0501.2011.02208.x

Chapter 7

New Materials, New Structures, and New Technologies

Material design, development, and new manufacturing R&D are developing very rapidly. Some of the new materials are under animal evaluation and others are already under clinical trials. New production technologies such as 3D bio-printing can be applied directly in dental and medical fields. For the purpose of matching new materials and technologies, new concepts for building new structures have been advanced, such as gradient functional material through controlling porosity during powder sintering. In this chapter, new items which are not yet established well in the dental/medical area are introduced.

7.1. Introduction

Development of materials for manufacturing of the biomedical implants in medicine—biomaterials (metals and alloys, polymers, ceramics, and hybrids and composites) is directly determined by characteristics and nature of the tissue, organs, and systems that are being replaced or supplemented [1]. The application of biomaterials requires the knowledge of their complex nature and different variables in regard to biocompatibility, corrosion behavior, mechanical characteristics, stability and durability in an aggressive environment, wear mechanisms and wear rates during exploitation, and many others [2]. Additive manufacturing technologies, rapid manufacturing, rapid prototyping, 3D printing, and nanotechnology are general terms that describe a variety of methods used to directly fabricate physical objects (three-dimensional models and end-use products) from electronic CAD (computer-aided design) data. Today's additive technologies offer advantages in many applications compared to classical subtractive fabrication methods such as milling or turning [1]. Biologic coatings have been incorporated into orthopedic implants in order to modulate the surrounding biological environment. While many of these coatings are still in the preclinical testing stage,

DOI 10.5643/9781606506288/ch7

bioengineers, material scientists, and surgeons continue to explore surface coatings as a means of improving the clinical outcome of patients undergoing orthopedic surgery [3]. In this chapter, we will introduce newly developed biomaterials, as well as new structures, texturing methods and technologies that are currently in use in the medical and dental fields or possess potential application.

7.2. New Materials

If any material, which has been developed in the engineering field, is considered to apply as a biomaterial, a test should be conducted as to whether or not it contains any element exhibiting toxicity. For example, V-element in the Ti–6Al–4V alloy is considered as a potentially toxic element. Even so, there were various clinical evidences indicating that this alloy has been used in orthopedic implants and posterior area dental implants. Since the V-toxicity issue has been receiving medical attention, the V-free Ti-based alloy needed to be developed. As a result, there is now Ti–6Al–7Nb (which is replaceable to Ti–6Al–4V due to equivalent mechanical properties). In addition, some newly developed materials will be reviewed here.

7.2.1. Bone Materials

Biological studies indicate that numerous materials present in living tissues owe their success to an optimal combination of properties and adaptive structures, rather than to extreme properties *per se*. Through studying natural tissues and by biomimesis, new polymer and composite materials may be designed to emulate the structural and functional responses of bone. These materials must ensure biochemical affinity with host tissue through judicious mixing of specific chemical cues. Also, they must mimic the response under load exhibited by natural bone through complex organization of material phases, that is, embedding of collagen fibers in the extracellular substance. Fiber and particulate reinforced polymers are increasingly significant in the development of new biomedical materials, since they can be engineered more accurately than monolithic structures. Meanwhile, design of nanocomposites with specific morphological and chemical signals is emerging as a powerful approach to the mimesis of extracellular matrix (ECM) of natural bone. In both cases, the manipulation of the main materials features at the micro- and nano-metric scale offers an intriguing strategy for improvement of biological and mechanical response [4].

Inorganic polymer nanocomposites are of significant interest for emerging materials due to their improved properties and unique combination of properties. Methacrylic acid (MA), a functionalization agent that can chemically link TiO_2 nanomaterials (n-TiO_2) and polymer matrix, was used to modify the surface of n-TiO_2 using a Ti−carboxylic coordination bond. Then, the double bond in MA was copolymerized with methyl methacrylate (MMA) to form an n-TiO_2−PMMA nanocomposite. The resulting n-TiO_2−PMMA nanocomposite materials were characterized by using thermal analysis, electron microscopy, and elemental analysis [5]. The dynamic mechanical properties (Young's and shear moduli) were measured using an ultrasonic pulse technique. It was found that (i) the glass transition temperature, thermal degradation temperature, and dynamic elastic moduli of the nanocomposites were shown to increase with an increase in the weight percentage of nanofibers in the composite, and (ii) the resulting nanocomposites exhibited improved elastic properties and have potential application indental composites and bone cements [5].

Hydroxyapatite (HA)/alginate nanocomposite fibrous scaffolds were fabricated via electrospinning and a novel *in situ* synthesis of HA that mimics mineralized collagen fibrils in bone tissue. Poorly crystalline HA nanocrystals were induced to nucleate and grow at the [$-COO^-$]–Ca^{2+}–[$-COO^-$] linkage sites on electrospun alginate nanofibers impregnated with PO_4^{3-} ions [6]. This novel process resulted in a uniform deposition of HA nanocrystals on the nanofibers, overcoming the severe agglomeration of HA nanoparticles processed by the conventional mechanical blending/electrospinning method. Preliminary *in vitro* cell study showed that rat calvarial osteoblasts attached more stably on the surface of the HA/alginate scaffolds than on the pure alginate scaffold. It was reported that (i), in general, the osteoblasts were stretched and elongated into a spindle-shape on the HA/alginate scaffolds, whereas the cells had a round-shaped morphology on the alginate scaffold, and (ii) the unique nanofibrous topography combined with the hybridization of HA and alginate can be advantageous in bone tissue regenerative medicine applications [6].

Continuously increasing life expectancy results in a rising number of bone diseases and fractures. Replacements from natural sources are not only limited in their availability, they also have some serious disadvantages such as possible immunological reactions or transmission of diseases. New synthetic biodegradable materials based on photopolymers could be an alternative solution. Schuster et al. [7] developed an acrylate-based monomer formulation, consisting of a biodegradable basis monomer which is derived from gelatin, different reactive diluents, an appropriate photoinitiator and filler materials. For the three-dimensional shaping process stereolithography is the method of choice because of its capability to produce cellular structures with high resolutions [7].

Searching for a flexible yet rigid like a human bone, and immediately capable of bearing loads, a new kind of implant, made of titanium foam, resembles the inside of a bone in terms of its structural configuration [8]. Not only does this make it less stiff than conventional massive implants, it also promotes ingrowth into surrounding bones. The force of stress stimulates the growth of the matrix. The foam-like structure of the substance resembles the spongiosa found inside the bone. The titanium foam is the result of a powder metallurgy-based molding process that has already proven its value in the industrial production of ceramic filters for aluminum casting. Open-cell polyurethane (PU) foams are saturated with a solution consisting of a binding medium and a fine titanium powder. The powder cleaves to the cellular structures of the foams. The PU and binding agents are then vaporized. What remains is a semblance of the foam structures. The mechanical properties of titanium foams made this way closely approach those of the human bone. Bone-like rigidity allows for stress forces to be transmitted; with the new formation of bone cells, it also fosters healing of the implant. Consequently, stress can and should be applied to the implant immediately after insertion [8,9].

A steel foam using a combination of powder and cast metal that has a similar elasticity to bone was developed [10]. The metal foam is lighter than solid aluminum and can also be made of 100% steel, suggesting that the foam could be used for biomedical implants and helps avoid the bone rejection that can result from more rigid implant materials, such as titanium. The rough surface of the foam would also foster bone growth into the implant, improving the strength of implant. If the modulus of elasticity (MOE) of the implant is too much bigger than the bone, the implant will take over the load bearing and the surrounding bone will start to die. While titanium has an MOE of approximately 100 GPa, the new composite foam has a value of MOE between 10 and 30 GPa, the same as bone [10], as seen in Figure 4.1 in this book.

7.2.2. Porous Materials

Porous tantalum trabecular metal has recently been incorporated in titanium dental implants as a new form of implant surface enhancement. However, there is little information on the applications of this material in implant dentistry. Porous tantalum metal is used to improve the contact between the osseous structure and dental implants and therefore presumably facilitate osseointegration. The success of porous tantalum metal in orthopedic implants led to the incorporation of porous tantalum metal in the design of root-form endosseous titanium implants. The porous tantalum three-dimensional enhancement of titanium dental implant surface allows for combining bone ongrowth together with bone ingrowth, or osseoincorporation, indicating that there seems to be several possible advantages of this implant design [11].

Over the past few decades there has been great interest in the use of orthopedic and dental implants that integrate into tissue by promoting bone ingrowth or bone adhesion, thereby eliminating the need for cement fixation. However, strategies to create bioactive implant surfaces to direct cellular activity and mineralization leading to osseointegration are lacking. Sargeant et al. [12] prepared a hybrid bone implant material consisting of Ti–6Al–4V foam, whose 52% porosity is filled with a peptide amphiphile (PA) nanofiber matrix. These PA nanofibers can be highly bioactive by molecular design and are used here as a strategy to transform an inert titanium foam into a potentially bioactive implant. Using scanning electron microscopy (SEM) and confocal microscopy, it was shown that PA molecules self-assemble into a nanofiber matrix within the pores of the metallic foam, fully occupying the foam's interconnected porosity [12]. Furthermore, the method allows the encapsulation of cells within the bioactive matrix, and under appropriate conditions the nanofibers can nucleate mineralization of calcium phosphate phases with a Ca:P ratio that corresponds to that of HA. An *in vivo* experiment was performed using a bone plug model in the diaphysis of the hind femurs of a Sprague Dawley rat and examined by histology to evaluate the performance of these hybrid systems after 4 weeks of implantation. The *de novo* bone formation was noticed around and inside the implant, vascularization around the implant, as well as the absence of a cytotoxic response. It was concluded that the PA–Ti hybrid strategy could be potentially tailored to initiate mineralization and direct a cellular response from the host tissue into porous implants to form new bone and thereby improve fixation, osseointegration, and long-term stability of implants [12].

Porous NiTi shape memory alloys provide enhanced osseointegration by facilitating tissue ingrowth and transport of body fluid to the implant. To retain the excellent thermomechanical properties of bulk NiTi and to improve its biocompatibility, Man et al. [13] fabricated a porous surface layer on bulk NiTi samples using laser surface engineering techniques. A powder mixture of NiTi and TiH_2 was laser surface alloyed on the NiTi. The macrostructure and microstructure of the modified surface layer were studied. It was reported that (i) a porous layer of a few hundred micrometers thick was formed, composed of NiTi, Ti_2Ni, $TiNi_3$, and TiN, (ii) the pores in the layer exhibited an interconnected morphology in 3D, and (iii) the Ni content was reduced from 49.2at.% in the substrate to 12.5 at.% near the surface of the modified layer [13]. Comparative microanalysis and histological studies of porous titanium and NiTi implants fabricated by selective laser sintering are conducted [14]. Sintered Ti and NiTi nanoporous structures are developed with grain sizes ranging from dozens to several hundreds nanometer and their formation is discussed. Dependence of the surface morphology of the implant on laser processing parameters (laser power, scanning velocity and beam diameter) is observed by analyzing the fractal-type nanostructure and its self-organization from the nano- to the macro-passing through the microlevel. It was shown that functional characteristics of the synthesized medical implants depend on the pores size distribution and their relative location as well as on the nanostructural morphology of the sintered surface [14].

The 3D fiber deposition is a technique that allows the development of metallic scaffolds with accurately controlled pore size, porosity, and interconnecting pore size. Li et al. [15] analyzed the *in vivo* performance of titanium alloy scaffolds, fabricated using 3D fiber deposition. The titanium alloy scaffolds with different structural properties, such as pore size, porosity, and interconnecting pore size were implanted on the decorticated transverse processes of the posterior lumbar spine of 10 goats. To monitor the bone formation over time, fluorochrome markers were administered at 3, 6, and 9 weeks and the animals were sacrificed at 12 weeks after implantation. Bone formation in the scaffolds was investigated by histology and histomorphometry of nondecalcified sections using traditional light- and epifluorescent microscopy. It was reported that the *in vivo* results showed an increase of porosity and pore size, and thus increase of permeability of titanium alloy implants positively influenced their osteoconductive properties [15].

Wei et al. [16] reported the anodic formation of highly ordered nanoporous Ta_2O_5 layers that exhibit a self-ordered alignment of pores uniformly over the anodized surface. These layers are grown by anodization of tantalum in a nonaqueous electrolyte consisting of an optimized glycerol/ethylene glycol mixture with the addition of NH_4F. To reach an optimized nanoporous structure, it was mentioned that several factors—fluoride concentration and content of supporting electrolyte $(NH_4)_2SO_4$—need to be controlled. Once optimized, the nanopore diameter can be adjusted using the applied voltage in the range of 7–18 nm, and layers with a thickness of more than 10 μm can be grown. As a result, a pore aspect ratio of 1,000 can be reached [16].

7.2.3. Nanomaterials

There are several studies on different types of material nanotube, including carbon nanotube, titania or zirconia nanotubes, Ti metal nanotubes, and composite nanotubes.

Carbon nanotubes (CNTs) are promising to be the next generation of viable tools for biomedical applications [17]. Further advances in such bioapplications may depend on improved understanding of physical and chemical properties as well as control over their biocompatibility. Dong et al. [17] conducted a systematic study to show how acid oxidation treatment changes CNTs physical and chemical properties and leads to improved CNTs biocompatibility. It was reported that systematically characterized CNTs were subsequently tested for their biocompatibility in relation to human epithelial cells or enzymes. Such selected examples are building pertinent relationships between CNTs biocompatibility and their intrinsic properties by showing that acid oxidation treatment lowers CNTs toxicity providing feasible platforms to be used for biomedical applications or the next generation of biosensors [17].

Chitosan-multiwalled carbon nanotubes/HAnanocomposites were synthesized by a novel *in situ* precipitation method [18]. The electrostatic adsorption between multiwalled carbon nanotubes and chitosan was investigated and explained by Fourier transform infrared spectroscopy analysis. Morphology studies showed that uniform distribution of HA particles and multiwalled carbon nanotubes in the polymer matrix was observed. In chitosan-multiwalled carbon nanotubes/HAnanocomposites, the diameters of multiwalled carbon nanotubes were about 10 nm. The elastic modulus and compressive strength increased sharply from 509.9 to 1089.1 MPa and from 33.2 to 105.5 MPa with an increase of multiwalled carbon/chitosan weight ratios from 0 to 5%, respectively. Finally, the cell biocompatibility of the composites was tested *in vitro*, which showed that they have good biocompatibility. These results suggest that the chitosan-multiwalled carbon nanotubes/HA nanocomposites are promising biomaterials for bone tissue engineering [18]. Mazare et al. [19] fabricated controlled-diameter TiO_2 nanotubes using electrochemical anodizing of two different substrates (Ti and Ti–6Al–7Nb) in an aqueous electrolyte. As-formed TiO_2 nanotubes are amorphous and by subjecting to thermal treatments, the structure becomes crystalline. It was found that the annealed samples have a more hydrophilic character than as-formed as well as a better stability in bioliquids, suggesting that such behavior of annealed samples is connected with a better biocompatibility expressed in terms of cell morphology and gene expression of bone-specific markers obtained from the Reverse Transcription Polymerase Chain Reaction (RT-PCR) [19]. To utilize carbon nanotubes (CNTs) in various commercial and scientific applications, the graphene sheets that comprise CNT surfaces are often modified to tailor properties, such as dispersion. Wepasnick et al. [20] reviewed the techniques used to explore the chemical and structural characteristics of CNTs modified by covalent surface modification strategies that involve the direct incorporation of specific elements and inorganic or organic functional groups into the graphene sidewalls, using not only the popular techniques such as transmission electron micrograph (TEM), XPS (X-ray photoelectron spectroscopy), IR, and Raman spectroscopy but also more specialized techniques such as chemical derivatization, Boehm titrations, EELS (electron energy-loss spectroscopy), NEXAFS (near edge X-ray absorption fine structure spectroscopy) , TPD (temperature programmed desorption), and TGA (thermogravimetric analysis) [20].

The carbon nanofiber film was formed on bulk pure titanium via hybrid surface mechanical attrition treatment (SMAT). The microstructure of the sample was investigated by SEM, TEM, and RAMAN characterization. It was reported that (i) the carbon nanofiber films are extremely long and uniform, exhibiting a high degree of uniformity of size of about 20 nm, and (ii) the SMAT Ti played the role of catalyst and substrate during synthesizing process [21].

Size-controlled synthesis of pure rutile-phase TiO_2 nanorods was prepared by a hydrothermal method using different organic acids as modifiers, and metatitanic acid and concentrated sulfuric acid as raw materials [22]. It was reported that (i) the steric effect occurred by the organic modifiers and nonpolarity of organic acids were beneficial to the formation of small-sized rutile TiO_2 nanorods and (ii) the strongly coordinative interaction between the carboxyl (or hydroxyl) group of the modifier and the surface of TiO_2 nanoparticles effectively inhibited the crystal growth [22]. Titanium dioxide (TiO_2) nanotubes can accelerate the adhesion and differentiation of osteoblasts, yet little is known how this nano-modified implant surface affects osseointegration at molecular level *in vivo*. Wang et al. [23] investigated the effects of TiO_2 nanotubes with different diameters (30 nm, 70 nm and 100 nm) on biological attachment mechanism of implants to bone *in vivo* by studying the gene expression and bone formation around the implants. The histological features and fluorochrome labeling changes of bone around implants on the nondecalcified sections (at 3, 5, and 8 weeks after implantation) were investigated by using traditional light- and fluorescent microscopy, and the gene expression of alkaline phosphatase (ALP), osterix (Osx), collagen-I (Col-I) and tartrate-resistant acid phosphatase (TRAP) was examined by using real-time PCR at 1, 2, 3, 4, and 5 weeks after implantation. It was reported that, comparing with machined titanium implants, (i) a significant increase in bone–implant contact (BIC) and gene expression levels was found in the bone attached to implants with TiO_2 nanotubes, especially with 70 nm diameter nanotubes, and (ii) at the same time, the sequential fluorescent labeling images illustrated dynamic bone deposition, concluding that TiO_2 nanotubes can modulate bone formation events at the bone–implant interface as to reach favorable molecular response and osseointegration, in addition, the diameters of nanotubes can be precisely controlled in order to obtain better bone formation [23].

Hassan et al. [24] formed TiO_2 nanotubes (TiNTs) by the electrochemical anodization of titanium in 2-propanol/water containing 0.14 MNH4F as the supporting electrolyte. The effects of the water content, time of anodization, and potential on the growth behavior of TiNT were studied. At the optimum solvent composition of 16 vol% water/84 vol% 2-propanol, the reaction was kinetically controlled. The TiNTs obtained under optimum conditions had heights of up to 1800 nm and inner diameters of about 90 nm. Increasing the potential beyond 20 V did not improve the quality of the nanotubes because of the introduction of disordering. The scanning electron microscopy and X-ray diffraction analysis revealed a preferred growth direction of the TiNTs relative to the substrate surface. It was also found that a thin barrier layer existed at the nanotubes/metal interface, which was also confirmed by ellipsometry, and this barrier layer was enriched with the rutile phase, whereas the nanotubes were enriched with the anatase phase [24]. Anodization of valve metals and alloys is a powerful tool to control nanoscale architecture for many metal oxides. Except for aluminum, the most explored system is self-organized oxide formed on titanium, namely self-organized TiO_2 nanotubes, because of the unique combination of geometry with the semiconductive nature of titania that is applicable in photocatalysis, light harvesting systems, electrochromic devices, batteries, matrices, templates, filtration membranes, and biocompatible materials [25]. There are several different methods to fabricate TiO_2 nanostructures. TiO_2 nanorods have been fabricated from the simple chemical bath deposition method [26]. Three-dimensional architecture of TiO_2 hollow spheres were fabricated by the hydrothermal process [27].

Highly ordered zirconium dioxide (ZrO_2: zirconia) nanotubes were prepared with porous anodic alumina as the template by the liquid phase deposition technique [28]. The obtained ZrO_2 nanotubes were characterized by TEM and X-ray diffraction (XRD). A new biocompatible nano-platform for the immobilization of hemoglobin (Hb) was developed by coating a chitosan (CHI) solution, in which the ZrO_2 nanotubes, 1-butyl-3-methylimidazolium tetrafluoroborate ionic liquid—(BMIM)BF_4— and Hb were dispersed, onto a glassy carbon electrode surface. Direct electrochemistry of the immobilized Hb on the electrode surface was then investigated. It was reported that (i) remarkable improvements on the direct electrochemistry of Hb were achieved, and (ii) the potential application of the Hb immobilized electrode (Hb/ZrO_2/[BMIM] BF_4/CHI/GCE) in biosensing was demonstrated by the catalytic electrochemical reduction of nitrite ion (NO_2^-) in an aqueous solution [28].

The nanotubular surface of Ti-binary and Ti-ternary alloys for biomaterials has been investigated using various methods of surface characterization. Binary Ti–*x*Nb (x = 10, 20, 30, and 40 wt.%) and ternary Ti–30Ta–*x*Nb (x = 3, 7, and 15 wt.%) alloys were prepared by using the high-purity sponges: Ti, Ta, and Zr spheres. The nanotube on the alloy surface was formed in 1.0 M $H_3PO_4$with small additions of NaF (0.5 and 0.8 wt.%), using a potentiostat. For cell proliferation, an MC3T3-E1 mouse osteoblast was used. It was reported that (i) the binary Ti–*x*Zr alloys had a lamellar and a needle-like structure, whereas, ternary Ti–30Ta–*x*Zr alloys had equiaxed grains with a lamellar martensitic α' structure, (ii) the thickness of the needle-like laths of the α-phase increased as the Zr content increased, (iii) the nanotubes formed on the α and β phases showed a different size and shape appearance with Zr content, and (iv) as the Zr content increased from 3 to 40 wt.%, the diameter of the nanotubes in Ti–*x*Zr and Ti–30Ta–*x*Zr alloy decreased from 200 nm to 50 nm. It was concluded that the nanotubular Ti–30Ta–15Zr alloy surface with a diameter of 50 nm provided a good osseointegration: cell proliferation, migration, and differentiation [29]. The nanotubes of Ti–50Zr alloy were formed in glycol with 15 vol.% H_2O and 0.2 M NH_4F by a two-step anodization process [30].

Hsu et al. [31] fabricated nanocomposites from a polyester-type water-borne PU containing different amounts (17.4–174 ppm) of gold (Au) nanoparticles (~5 nm) to study their biostability and biocompatibility. The nanocomposites were characterized by transmission electron microscopy and X-ray photoelectron spectroscopy, and their oxidative stability and free radical scavenging ability were tested. The inflammatory response was evaluated by monocyte activation *in vitro* and rat subcutaneous implantation *in vivo*. It was found that (i) the nanocomposites containing 43.5–65 ppm of Au had the least monocyte activation and tissue reactions, (ii) PU and the nanocomposites were rather resistant to oxidative degradation *in vitro* and biodegradation *in vivo*, and (iii) the nanocomposites exhibited greater free radical scavenging abilities than the original PU. Based on these findings, it was concluded that the significantly enhanced biocompatibility of the PU–Au nanocomposites with 43.5–65 ppm of gold over the original PU appeared to be a result of the extensively modified surface morphology and greater free radical scavenging ability, instead of due to the difference in biostability [31].

Nanoparticles are normally considered to be of a size no greater than 100 nm, and the exploitation of their unique attributes to combat infection has increased markedly over the past decade. The potential of nanoparticles to control the formation of biofilms within the oral cavity, as a function of their biomedical, anti–adhesive, and delivery capabilities, is now coming under close scrutiny [31]. Possible uses as constituents of prosthetic device coatings, as topically applied agents, and within dental materials are being explored. Allaker [32] reviewed the latest insights into the application of nanoparticles in the control of oral infections, including their use in photodynamic therapy, in particular, the use of nanoparticulate silver, copper, zinc, silicon, and their oxides was considered in relation to their effects on bacterial populations. The recent interest in the applications of nanoparticulate polymers and calcium phosphates and particular attention to the toxicity issues surrounding the potential impact of nanoparticles on oral and other tissues was addressed [32]. A simple preparation method for biocompatible nanoparticles in high concentration (0.5 wt%) by self-assembly of chitosan and carboxymethyl cellulose hydrolysates was developed [33]. Chitosan and carboxymethyl cellulose were hydrolyzed beforehand with chitosanase and cellulase respectively to make fragments having lower molecular weights. Nanoparticles were spontaneously formed only by mixing the two hydrolysate solutions. It was reported that (i) the particle size distribution was relatively narrow, about 200 nm in mean size, (ii) the mean particle size decreased from 226 nm to 165 nm with decreasing molecular weight of chitosan hydrolysate from 9.5 to 6.8 kDa, (iii) the mixing ratio of chitosan and carboxymethyl cellulose hydrolysates also affected particle size, and (iv) the chitosan-carboxymethyl cellulose nanoparticles were stably suspended over 1 week even under low pH (pH 3.0), high ionic strength (NaCl 1M), or low temperature (4 °C) conditions [33].

The fabrication of a smart magnetically controllable bio-based polymeric nanocomposite has immense potential in the biomedical field. Das et al. [34] prepared magneto-thermoresponsive sunflower oil modified hyperbranched polyurethane (HBPU)/Fe_3O_4 nanocomposites with different wt.% of magnetic nanoparticles (Fe_3O_4) by an *in situ* polymerization technique. It was reported that (i) good interfacial interactions between HBPU and well-dispersed superparamagnetic Fe_3O_4, with an average diameter of 7.65 nm was found, (ii) the incorporation of Fe_3O_4 in HBPU significantly improved the thermomechanical properties along with the shape-memory behavior, antibacterial activity, biocompatibility as well as biodegradability in comparison to the pristine system. It was also reported that, the *in vivo* biocompatibility and nonimmunological behavior, as tested in Wistar rats after subcutaneous implantation, showed promising signs for the nanocomposites to be used as antibacterial biomaterial for biomedical device and implant applications [34].

Titanium plates and apatite blocks are commonly used for restoring large osseous defects in dental and orthopedic surgery. Matsumoto et al. [35] fabricated a composite material that has mechanical properties similar to biocortical bone and high bioaffinity by compounding HA with the base material zirconia (ZrO_2), which possesses high mechanical properties and low toxicity toward living organisms. After mixing the raw material powders at several different ZrO_2/HA mixing ratios, the material was compressed in a metal mold (8 mm in diameter) at 5 MPa. Subsequently, it was sintered for 5 h at 1500 °C to obtain the ZrO_2/HA composite. The mechanical property and biocompatibility of materials were investigated. Furthermore, osteoconductivity of materials was investigated by animal studies. A composite material with a minute porous structure was successfully created using ZrO_2/HA powders, having different particle sizes, as the starting material. The material also showed high protein adsorption and a favorable cellular affinity. When the mixing ratio of ZrO_2/HA was 70/30, the strength was equal to cortical bone. Furthermore, it was reported that, (i) the *in vivo* experiments confirmed its high osteoconductivity, (ii) the composite material had strength similar to biocortical bones with high cell and tissue affinities by compounding ZrO_2 and HA, and (iii) the ZrO_2/HA composite material having a micro porous structure would be a promising bone restorative material [35].

7.2.4. Functionally Gradient Materials

Material is composed of multilayer, with each layer having unique characteristics, yet adjacent layers having some similarity is called functionally gradient (or gradient function) material (FGM) [36]. Although such functions can include various properties, it is limited to mechanical, physical, or thermal properties since other properties, such as chemical or electrochemical, is more likely important to the surface layer, and not related to bulky or semi-bulky behavior. For example, if HA is needed to spray-coat onto CpTi, this FGM concept can be applied. Instead of applying HA powder directly onto CpTi surface, a multilayer of HA/HA–Al_2O_3/Al_2O_3–TiO_2/TiO_2/CpTi can be prepared to enhance the bonding strength in between [36].

Functionally gradient and micro-channeled Al_2O_3–(*t*-ZrO_2)/HA composites were fabricated using the multi-pass extrusion process depending on the sintering temperature [37]. The continuous pores were homogeneously formed in the second-passed samples and their size was about 180 μm in diameter. The functionally gradient Al_2O_3–(*t*-ZrO_2)/HAp composites consisted of three layers, that is, HA/HA–Al_2O_3–ZrO_2/Al_2O_3–ZrO_2. It was also reported that the relative density and bending strength increased as the sintering temperature increased and in the sample sintered at 1400 °C, their maximum values were about 62.2% and 107.8 MPa, respectively [37].

Functionally gradient material (FGM) had been developed as a potential implant material to replace titanium for its improved capability of initial osseointegration. The idea behind FGM dental implant is that its properties can be tailored in accordance with the biomechanical needs at different regions adapting to its hosting bony tissues, therefore creating an improved overall integration and stability in the entire restoration. However, there have been very few reports available so far on predicting bone remodeling induced by FGM dental implants. Lin et al. [38] evaluated bone remodeling when replacing the titanium with a HA/collagen (HAP/Col) FGM model. A finite element model was constructed in the buccal–lingual section of a dental implant–bone structure generated from *in vivo* CT scan images. The remodeling simulation was performed over a 4-year healing period. Comparisons were made between the titanium implant and various FGM implants of this model. As a conclusion, it was mentioned that the FGM implants showed an improved bone remodeling outcome [38].

7.3. New Structures

Materials are not necessarily always solid forms, rather they can have very rough surfaces or various degrees of porosity at only surface zone or entire whole body structure. Some materials can have different properties from inner core to outer case zone. The others can have different functions which can gradually changing from core to case. This newly developed structure concept for material design will be introduced.

7.3.1. Nanostructures

To put the nano-scale (10^{-9} m or 10^{-3} μm) in context, the comparative size of a nanometer is the same as that of a marble to the size of the earth [39]. Nanomaterials are of interest from a fundamental point of view because with new materials, come new properties, which result in new opportunities for technological and commercial development, and applications of nanoparticles have been proposed in areas as a diverse as microelectronics, coatings and paints, and biotechnology. From these applications, nanopharmaceutiacals, nanosensors, nanoswithces, and nanodelivery systems have been developed. Two principal factors cause the properties of nanomaterials to differ significantly from other materials: the increase in the relative surface area and quantum effects. For example, a particle of 30 nm has 5% of its atoms on its surface, at 10 nm 20%, and at 3 nm 50% [40]. With the advent of nanotechnology, an opportunity exists for the engineering of new dental implant materials. Metallic dental implants have been successfully used for decades, but they have shortcomings related to osseointegration and mechanical properties that do not match those of bone. Without the development of an entirely new class of materials, faster osseointegration of currently available dental implants can be accomplished by various surface modifications. To date, there is no consensus regarding the preferred method(s) of implant surface modification, and further development will be required before the ideal implant surface can be created. Current approaches can generally be categorized into three areas: ceramic coatings, surface functionalization, and patterning on the micro- to nanoscale. The distinctions among these are imprecise, as some or all of these approaches can be combined to improve *in vivo* implant performance. These surface improvements have resulted in durable implants with a high percentage of success and long-term function. Nanotechnology has provided another set of opportunities for the manipulation of implant surfaces in its capacity to mimic the surface topography formed by ECM components of natural tissue. The possibilities introduced by nanotechnology now permit the tailoring of implant chemistry and structure with an unprecedented degree of control. For the first time, tools are available that can be used to manipulate the physicochemical environment and monitor key cellular events at the molecular level. These new tools and capabilities will result in faster bone formation, reduced healing time, and rapid recovery to function [41].

For implantable materials [39], the nano-structuring technology can be used in the following areas; tissue repair and replacement; implant coatings; tissue regeneration scaffolds; structural implant materials; bone repair; bioresorbable materials; smart materials; assessment and treatment devices; sensory aids; and retinal and cochlear implants. Bone is a natural nanostructured (i.e., a material with constituent features less than 100 nm in at least one dimension) composite composed of organic compounds (mainly collagen) reinforced with inorganic ones (HA: hydroxyapatite). It is this natural nanostructure that nanotechnology aims to emulate for orthopedic and dental applications. The smaller the particle is, the larger the surface area is in volume, as mentioned before. Nano-bone [42] uses this principle. The nanocrystallites show a loose microstructure, with nanopores situated between the crystallites. This material structure will be completed by pores in the micrometer area. By following this process, a rough surface area is formed on the boundary later between the biomaterial and cell, which is very important for fast cell growth. Porosity values of around 60% can be found in both the nano- and the micro-meter pores. All pores are interconnecting (i.e., by being in contact with the patient's blood, bodily substances merge into pores). Because the cells are too big for the small pores, blood plasma containing all the important proteins is retained in the interstices. The surface of the pores (and also of the nanopores) is modified in such a way that it literally "hang on" to the proteins. This is to be carried out by silica molecule. The compound silica is most important. Special features of bone graft materials should possess; osteoinductive; fully synthetic; net sintered; highly porous; nanostructured; absorbs natural body-produced proteins into the nanopores; degradation by osteoclasts; very good processability; and no ionic solution products [39].

Cryomilled nanocrystalline CpTi powders were spark plasma sintered using different process parameters (heating rate, temperature, pressure, and dwell time) to study densification, microstructure, and mechanical behavior [43]. It was reported that (i) the measured high ductility was accompanied by a moderate strength (yield strength: 770 MPa, ultimate tensile strength: 840 MPa with ~27% elongation to failure), and (ii) the combinations of microstructure and mechanical response were attributed to the multistep processing at different temperature ranges as well as to the presence of interstitial solutes [43].

Peng et al. [44], using an electrical discharge machining (EDM), fabricated porous recast layer on a titanium surface. Subsequently, an α-phase and a γ-TiH-(γ-hydride)-phase were formed on the recast layer by electrical-discharging. Nano-(δ+γ) hydrides play important roles in the formation of nanostructural oxide layers. Electrical-discharging not only generates a nanostructural recast layer but also converts the alloy surface into a nanostructured oxide surface, which increases the alloy biocompatibility. A γ-hydride microstructure was also formed on the recast layer following electrical-discharging. It was reported that (i) the microstructure had a tetragonal structure with lattice constant a = 0.421 nm (or 4.21 Å), (ii) in the recast layer, a transition, $\alpha \rightarrow (\alpha+\delta) \rightarrow (\delta+\gamma) \rightarrow \gamma$, occurred during electrical discharging, and (iii) the recast layer that contains nanophases was dissolved during electrical discharging; by this process, electrical-discharging for a short duration yields nanoporous TiO_2, concluding that electric discharging for a short duration leads to the production of nanostructures as well as bioactive titanium [44].

Nanostructuring technology has been proven to create unique biological properties in various biomaterials. Ogawa et al. [45] reported about the discovered phenomenon of titanium nanonodular self-assembly that occurs during physical vapor depositions

(PVD) of titanium onto specifically conditioned micro-textured titanium surfaces, and test a hypothesis that the Ti nanostructure has the potential to enhance bone–titanium integration. The nanostructure creation effectively provided geometrical undercut and increased the surface area by up to 40% compared with the acid-etched surface with microtopography. Depending on the size control, the nanonodules can be added without smearing the existing micro-texture, creating a nanomicro-hybrid architecture. It was found that (i) titanium implants with 560-nm nanonodules produced 3.1 times greater strength of osseointegration than those with an acid-etched surface in a rat femur model, and (ii) the discovered titanium nano-nodular self-structuring has been proven feasible on biocompatible materials other than titanium, offering new avenues for the development of implant surfaces and other implantable materials for better bone-generative and -regenerative potential. It was further mentioned that the titanium nano-nodular structuring technology based on the self-assembly phenomenon of nanonodules on specifically conditioned micro-roughened titanium surfaces offered new avenues for the development of implant surfaces and other implantable materials for better bone-generative and -regenerative potential [45].

The modification of the surface of low-density polyethylene and PU by means of the pulsed ion-plasma deposition of nanostructural carbon coatings at 20 °C to 60 °C has been studied, and the effect of this low-temperature treatment on the biocompatibility of the low-density polyethylene and PU has been assessed [46]. Optimum technological parameters for the formation of mosaic carbon nanostructures with a thickness of 0.3–15 nm and a cluster lateral size of 10–500 nm are determined. These structures give the polymer surface increased hemocompatible properties. The effect of the UV light of a krypton lamp (λ = 123.6 nm) and white synchrotron radiation on the surface of poly(methyl methacrylate) (PMMA) preliminarily treated in an oxygen-containing RF (radio frequency) discharge plasma has been investigated by varying the duration of exposure (from several minutes to several dozen minutes) and the residual gas pressure (2 and 100 Pa). It was reported that (i) this processing ensures the smoothing of the surface relief on micro- and nanoscale levels, which can improve the biocompatibility of the modified PMMA film surface, and (ii) this technology consists of the chemical pretreatment of the surface for creating a microrelief (2–3 μm roughness), followed by the deposition of a titanium oxide film with controlled composition (TiO_2) and thickness (10–60 nm) [46].

Mehdikhani-Nahrkhalaji et al. [47] conducted the *in vitro* and *in vivo* evaluations of novel bioactive, biodegradable, and antibacterial nanocomposite coating for the improvement of stem cells attachment and antibacterial activity as a candidate for dental implant applications. Poly(lactide-*co*-glycolide)/bioactive glass/hydroxyapatite (PBGHA) nanocomposite coating was prepared via the solvent casting process. The nanoparticle amounts of 10, 15, and 20 wt% were chosen in order to determine the optimum amount of nanoparticles suitable for preparing uniform coatings. Bioactivity and degradation of the coating with an optimum amount of nanoparticles were evaluated by immersing the prepared samples in simulated body fluid (SBF) and phosphate buffer saline (PBS), respectively. The effect of nanocomposite coating on the attachment and viability of human adipose-derived stem cells (hASCs) was investigated. Kirschner wires (K-wires) of stainless steel were coated with the PBGHA nanocomposite coating, and mechanical stability of the coating was studied during intramedullary implantation into rabbit tibiae. The results showed that using 10 wt% nanoparticles (5 wt% HA and 5 wt% BG) in the nanocomposite could provide the desired uniform coating. The study of *in vitro* bioactivity showed rapid formation of bone-like apatite on the PBGHA coating. It was degraded considerably after about 60 days of immersion in PBS. The hASCs showed excellent attachment and viability on the coating. PBGHA coating remained stable on the K-wires with a minimum of 96% of the original coating mass. It was, therefore, concluded that (i) PBGHA nanocomposite coating provides an ideal surface for the stem cells attachment and viability, and (ii) it could induce antibacterial activity, simultaneously [47].

An important aspect of orthopedic implant integration is the enhancement of functional activity of osteoblasts at the tissue–implant interface without any fibrous tissue intervention. Nanostructured implant surfaces are known to enhance osteoblast activity. A simple hydrothermal method for the fabrication of nonperiodic nanostructures (nanoscaffold, nanoleaves, and nanoneedles) on titanium implants exhibited good biocompatibility and a distinct osteoblast response *in vitro* in terms of osteoblast adhesion to the surface [48]. Rani et al. [48] evaluated nanostructures for their detailed *in vitro* cellular response as well as *in vivo* osseointegration. It was reported that (i) a specific surface nanomorphology provided a distinct increase in osteoblast cell proliferation, and (ii) the *in vivo* osseointegration study over 12 weeks on the rat model (Sprague–Dawley) showed early-stage bone formation (60% bone contact by week 2 and ~85% by week 8) in the leaf-like nanopattern, without any inflammatory cytokine production [48].

Ballo et al. [49] developed an implantable model system and investigated the effects of nanoscale surface properties on the osseointegration of titanium implants in rat tibia. Topographical nanostructures with a well-defined shape (semispherical protrusions) and variable size (60 nm, 120 nm, and 220 nm) were produced by colloidal lithography on the machined implants. Furthermore, the implants were sputter-coated with titanium to ensure a uniform surface chemical composition. The histological evaluation of bone around the implants at 7 days and 28 days after implantation was performed on the ground sections using optical and scanning electron microscopy. Differences between groups were found mainly in the new bone formation process in the endosteal and marrow bone compartments after 28 days of implantation. Implant surfaces with 60 nm features demonstrated significantly higher bone-implant contact (BIC, 76%) compared with the 120 nm (45%) and control (57%) surfaces. This effect was correlated to the higher density and curvature of the 60 nm protrusions. It was concluded, within the developed model system, that (i) nanoscale protrusions could be applied and systematically varied in size in the presence of microscale background roughness on complex screw-shaped implants, and (ii) the model can be adapted for the systematic variation of surface nanofeature density and chemistry, which opens up new possibilities for *in vivo* studies of various nanoscale surface–bone interactions [49].

Ti-based alloys are widely used in orthopedic implants because of their excellent mechanical properties and biocompatibility. However, in the complex physiological environment and influenced by other factors like cyclic loading, these implants can lose their natural properties and become incompatible or cytotoxic to the body tissues and cells. Two of the causes are the deteriorated mechanical properties in this dynamic environment and the effects of by-products stemming from corrosion. In serious cases, implant failure results. It was mentioned that nano architectures on the surface of these alloys can improve the *in vivo* and *in vitro* biocompatibility of these alloys [50].

7.3.2. Biomimetic Functionalization

Construction and application of nanostructured surface and interface is an active multi-interdisciplinary research area involving chemistry, physics, material science, and biology. Methods used for the fabrication of nanostructured surfaces are commonly catalogued as "top-down" and "bottom-up," as well as their combination [51]. Uncontrolled interactions between synthetic materials and human tissues are a major concern for implants and tissue engineering. To date, such biofunctonalization techniques have relied on surface immobilization methods that are often applicable only to a limited range of materials and require the presence of specific functional groups, synthetic pathways, or biologically hostile environments. Khatayevich et al. [52], using peptide motifs that have been selected to bind to materials (gold, platinum, glass, and titanium), modified surfaces with poly(ethylene glycol) anti-fouling polymer and the integrin-binding RGD (Arg-Gly-Asp) sequence. The peptides have several advantages over conventional molecular immobilization techniques; they require no biologically hostile environments to bind, are specific to their substrates and could be adapted to carry various active entities. It was reported that (i) cell-resistant properties was successfully imparted to gold and platinum surfaces using gold- and platinum-binding peptides, respectively, in conjunction with poly(ethylene glycol) (PEG), (ii) a several-fold increase in the number and spreading of fibroblast cells was accomplished on glass and titanium surfaces using quartz and titanium-binding peptides in conjunction with the integrin ligand RGD, indicating that control over the extent of cell–material interactions can be achieved by relatively simple and biocompatible surface modification procedures using inorganic binding peptides as linker molecules [52].

Nanotubular titanium oxide (TiO_2) produced by self-ordering processes using electrochemical anodization have been extensively explored in recent years as a new biomaterial for implants, drug delivery systems, cell growth, biosensors, immunoisolations, bioartificial organs, and tissue engineering. Chemical inertness is the main weakness of this material when placed in contact with biological systems and surface modification is a possible solution of this problem. Vasilev et al. [53] developed a flexible and facile method for surface modification of TiO_2 nanotubes to tailor new interfacial properties important in many biomedical applications. TiO_2 nanotubes were prepared by electrochemical anodization of titanium foil using ethylene glycol: NH_4F electrolyte (2% water and 0.3% NH_4F). Plasma surface modification using allylamine (AA) as a precursor has been applied to generate a thin and chemically reactive polymer film rich in amine groups on top of the TiO_2 nanotube surface. This initial polymer film was used for further surface functionalization by attachment of desired molecules. Two modification techniques were used to demonstrate the flexibility for building of new functionalities on titania nanotube surface: electrostatic adsorption of poly(sodium styrenesulfonate) as an example of layer-by-layer assembly (LbL), and covalent coupling of PEG as an example of creating a protein-resistant surface. It was concluded that these approaches for tailoring the surface chemistry and wettability of TiO_2 nanotubes offer considerable prospects for advancing their interfacial properties to improve existing and develop new functional biomaterials for diverse biomedical applications [53]. To be better used as medical implants in orthopedic and dental clinical applications, titanium and titanium-based alloys need to be capable of inducing osteogenesis. Ren et al. [54] introduced a method that allows the facile decoration of titanium surfaces to impart an osteogenesis capacity. A Ti surface was first deposited on a poly(OEGMA-*r*-HEMA) film using surface-initiated atom-transfer radical polymerization (SI-ATRP) with the further step of carboxylation. The modified surfaces were resistant to cell adhesion. Fibronectin (FN) and recombinant human bone morphogenetic protein-2 (rhBMP-2) were further immobilized onto p(OEGMA-*r*-HEMA) matrices. Based on these results, it was demonstrated that the FN- and rhBMP-2-conjugated polymer surfaces could induce the adhesion of MC3T3 cells on Ti surfaces. Moreover, it was reported that (i) the protein-tethered surface exhibited enhanced cell differentiation in terms of alkaline phosphatase activity compared to that of the pristine Ti surface at similar cell proliferation rates, (ii) a simple modification method of Ti surfaces via Ti-thiolate self-assembled monolayers (SAMs) was established, and (iii) a dual-functional Ti surface that combines antifouling and osseointegration promotion was identified [54].

Stable tethering of bioactive peptides like RGD (Arg-Gly-Asp) to surfaces can be achieved via chemical bonding, biotin streptavidin interaction, or photocross-linking. More challenging is the immobilization of proteins, since methods applied to immobilize peptides are either not specific or versatile enough or might even compromise the protein's bioactivity. To overcome this limitation, Sala et al. [55] employed a scheme that by enzymatic (transglutaminase) reaction allows the site-directed and site-specific coupling of growth factors and other molecules to nonfouling poly(L-lysine)-graft-poly(ethylene glycol) (PLL-*g*-PEG) coated surfaces under physiological conditions. It was found that coated surfaces were functionalized directly with peptides and growth factors or precisely position poly(ethylene glycol) (PEG)-like hydrogels for the presentation of growth factors as exemplified with vascular endothelial growth factor (VEGF) [55].

The time required for osseointegration with a metal implant having a smooth surface ranges from 3 to 6 months. Ravichandran et al. [56] hypothesized that biomimetic coating surfaces with poly(lactic-*co*-glycolic acid) (PLGA)/collagen fibers and nanohydroxyapatite (*n*-HA) on the implant would enhance the adhesion of mesenchymal stem cells. Therefore, this surface modification of dental and bone implants might enhance the process of osseointegration. PLGA or PLGA/collagen (50:50 w/w ratio) fiber was coated on Ti disks by modified electrospinning for 5 seconds to 2 minutes, followed by further deposition *n*-HA on the fibers. PLGA fibers of fiber diameter 0.957 ± 0.357 μm had a contact angle of $9.9 \pm 0.3°$ and PLGA/collagen fibers of fiber diameter 0.378 ± 0.068 μm had a contact angle of 0°. Upon *n*-HA incorporation, all the fibers had a contact angle of 0° owing to the hydrophilic nature of *n*-HA biomolecule. The cell attachment efficiency was tested on all the scaffolds for different intervals of time (10, 20, 30, and 60 min). The alkaline phosphatase activity, cell proliferation, and mineralization were analyzed on all the implant surfaces on days 7, 14, and 21. It was reported that (i) results of the cell adhesion study indicated that the cell adhesion was maximum on the implant surface coated with PLGA/collagen fibers deposited with *n*-HA compared to the other scaffolds, (ii) within a short span of 60 minutes, 75% of the cells adhered onto the mineralized PLGA/collagen fibers, (iii) similarly by day 21, the rate of cell proliferation was significantly higher on the mineralized PLGA/collagen fibers owing to enhanced cell adhesion on these fibers, and (iv) this enhanced initial cell adhesion favored higher cell proliferation, differentiation, and mineralization on the implant surface coated with mineralized PLGA/collagen fibers [56]. In order to enhance the cell adhesion and improve the biocompatibility, various types of biomimetic coatings are prepared. HA nanorods are coated with gelatin [57].

Besides the above-mentioned techniques, there should be more methods for biofunctionalization. The polyelectrolyte-mediated electrostatic adsorption of poly-L-lysine was prepared by the LbL self-assembly technique [58]. The collagen/elastin-based biomaterials were further modified by UV-irradiation [59]. The organic/mineral composite coating consisting of gelatin methacrylate hydrogel and HA was prepared [60]. HA was incorporated in collagen gels [61]. A biomimetric composite was prepared with poly(lactic-*co*-glycolic acid)/collagen fibers and nano HA [56]. More complex composite of poly(lactide-*co*-glycolide)/bioactive glass/HA (PBGHA) nanocomposite coating was prepared via the solvent casting process [47]. *N*-carboxyethylchitosan/nano-hydroxyapatite composite films were fabricated [62]. The hybrid 3D porous structure of chitosan-silver nanoparticles was fabricated simply by a one-step method [63].

7.4. New Technologies

There is a variety of high-technology spin-off applications such as the 3D bio-printing. We will review recently developed, yet not well-established, technologies which possess high potential for dental/medical applicability.

7.4.1. Tissue Engineering

Engineering oral tissues as a multidisciplinary approach to build complex structures such as bone, teeth, or soft dental tissues remains a challenging endeavor which will also require significant additional development of materials chemistry before it will be successful. The isolation of stem cell populations from various sources in the oral cavity and advances in utilizing their differentiation potential has been driving the field forward. So far, bioinert materials have mainly been used as carriers and delivery vehicles, relying on the intrinsic cellular competence to form tissues. As this may not be sufficient to induce regeneration, there is a need for novel biomimetic scaffolds capable of providing chemical and mechanical cues to promote multiple specific interactions between cells and matrix. These signals can orchestrate processes such as cell adhesion, migration, differentiation, matrix synthesis, mineralization, and vasculogenesis [64]. Tissue engineering and regenerative medicine strategies have gained increased attention in dental implantology, since dental implantology faces new challenges in clinical dentistry. Whereas conventional implant placement and implant loading protocols under ideal anatomical and biological conditions seem to be clinically solved, engineering and regenerative strategies are aimed at allowing implant placement under compromised conditions (lack of bone or mucosa tissue, impaired regenerative capacity, need for early loading protocols). To understand the new approaches in engineering and regenerative medicine therapies, it is important to recapitulate the history and basics of implant dentistry in order to assess the clinical impact of new approaches [65]. The human body comprises molecules; hence, the availability of molecular nanotechnology will permit dramatic progress to address medical problems and will use molecular knowledge to maintain and improve human health at the molecular scale. Nanomedicine could develop devices that are able to work inside the human body in order to identify the early presence of a disease, and to identify and quantify toxic molecules and tumor cells, for example. Nanodentistry will make possible the maintenance of comprehensive oral health by employing nanomaterials, including tissue engineering and, ultimately, dental nanorobots [39].

7.4.2. Three-Dimensional Printing

The three-dimensional printing process is a solid freedom fabrication (SFF) technique, in which parts are built up in layers from a computer-aided design model. Each layer begins with a thin distribution of powdered metal spread over the surface of a part-build bed. A binder material is deposited via inkjet printing technology to selectively join the metal particles in the shape of the part at that layer. The powder bed and part are lowered by a few thousands of an inch, and a new layer of powder is spread over the previous layer, and selectively joined in the part pattern appropriate for the new layer. This LbL process repeats until the part is completed and removed from the powder bed. The densification method consists of heat-treating processes for debinding, sintering, and infiltration with a second, lower melting temperature metal to near full density. The component may then be finish machined and polished as needed. The final result is a component that is near full density [66,67]. The application of 3D printing technology is versatile, including fabricating customized dental and medical implants [67,68]. The application of 3D printing in medical area is called 3D bioprinting [68].

7.4.3. Laser Technologies

Laser-related technology has been widely used in different ways. The compositionally graded materials of Ti–25V–15Cr–2Al–0.2C and Ti–6Al–4V have been fabricated using direct laser fabrication [69]. By photothermal laser processing, a thin film of anatasetitania nanoparticles with a thickness of about 500 nm was fabricated [70].

Stress-shielding and weak interfacial bond between the tissue and the implant can be eliminated by the use of porous metals. The use of porous materials can effectively reduce the MOE mismatch and provide stable long-term anchorage for biological fixation of the implant due to bone tissue ingrowth through pores. The fabrication of net shape load-bearing implants with complex anatomical shapes to meet desired mechanical and biological performance is still a challenge. Bandyopadhyay et al. [71] discussed applicability of laser engineered net shaping toward load-bearing implants to increase *in vivo* life time.

The interest in NiTi alloys for medical applications has been steadily growing in recent years because of its biocompatibility, superelasticity, and shape memory characteristics. However, the high Ni content in NiTi alloys is still a concern for its long-term applications in the human body. The release of Ni ion into the human body might cause serious problems, as Ni is capable of eliciting toxic and allergic responses. In view of this, surface modification to reduce the surface content of Ni and to improve the corrosion resistance, both of which would reduce Ni release, is an important step in the development of NiTi implants. Ng et al. [72], using laser processing, surface-alloyed NiTi with Nb or Co element. It was reported that (i) the amount of surface elemental Ni was reduced to 10% and 35% for the Nb-alloyed and Co-alloyed layer, respectively, (ii) the corrosion resistance in Hanks' solution (an SBF) was increased as evidenced by a reduced passive current density and a higher pitting potential for both the Nb- and Co-alloyed specimens, (iii) the composition and hardness profiles along the depth of the modified layer were correlated with the distribution of the dendrites, and (iv) the microhardness of the alloyed layers was around 700–800 Hv, which was about four times that of the untreated NiTi specimens [72].

Traini et al. [73] employed the laser sintering of metal powder to fabricate the gradient of porosity, from the inner core to the outer surface case. Surface appearance, microstructure, composition, mechanical properties, and fractography were evaluated. All the specimens were prepared by a selective laser sintering procedure using a Ti–6Al–4V alloy powder with a particle size of 1–10 μm. It was reported that (i) the sintered alloy was composed of 90.08% Ti, 5.67% Al, and 4.25% V, (ii) the MOE of the inner core material was 104 ± 7.7 GPa, while that of the outer porous material was 77 ± 3.5 GPa, and (iii) the fracture face showed a dimpled appearance typical of ductile fracture. Based on these data, it was concluded that the laser metal sintering proved to be an efficient means of construction of dental implants with an FGM which is better adapted to the elastic properties of the bone, suggesting that such implants should minimize stress shielding effects and improve long-term performance [73]. Similarly, Mangano et al. [74] investigated on retrieved laser metal foamed CTi implant. The load-bearing bone implants materials should have sufficient stiffness and large porosity, which are interacted since larger porosity causes lower mechanical properties. Xiao et al. [75] investigated the maximum stiffness architecture with the constraint of specific volume fraction by topology optimization approach, that is, maximum porosity can be achieved with predefined stiffness properties. The different porosities of 41.1%, 50.3%, 60.2%, and 70.7% were fabricated by a selective laser melting process. It was reported that (i) the computational effective elastic modulus of optimized scaffolds was ~13% higher than cubic scaffolds, the experimental stiffness values were reduced by 76% than the conventional ones, and (ii) the combination of topology optimization approach and selective laser melting process would be available for development of titanium implant materials in consideration of both porosity and mechanical stiffness [75].

Due to its good biocompatibility, titanium is widely used for dental and orthopedic implants and for biomedical microsystems. For these applications, Chauvy et al. [76]

applied unique micromachining methods. A new four-step method for electrochemical micromachining of titanium is composed of anodic oxidation, Excimer laser sensitising irradiation, anodic dissolution, and ultrasonic cleaning. The method is applied to the fabrication of two 3D model structures, surface structuring of a cylinder, and machining of a complex two-level architecture. It was reported that the absence of debris and of a heat-affected zone as well as the resulting surface smoothness are the main advantages of the process [76].

7.4.4. Electrospinning

Electrospinning has attracted tremendous interest in the research community as a simple and versatile technique to produce synthetic polymeric ultrafine fibers with diameters ranging from a few micrometres to tens of nanometers [77, 78]. HA fibers were prepared by electrospinning a precursor mixture of $Ca(NO_3)_2{\cdot}4H_2O$ and $(C_2H_5O)_3PO$ with a polymer additive [78]. Tissue engineering and biomedical applications of electrospun polymeric nanifibers are promising [77]. Scaffolds constituted by micro and nanofibers of silk fibroin were obtained by electrospinning [79]. Fibers of fibroin meshes were coated with polypyrrole (pPy) by chemical polymerization; chemical linkages between polymers were observed by SEM and IR spectroscopy. It was reported that (i) mechanical resistance of the meshes was improved by polypyrrole coating, (ii) coated meshes present a high electroactivity allowing anion storage and delivery during oxidation/reduction reactions in aqueous solutions, (iii) uncoated and pPy-coated materials support the adherence and proliferation of adult human mesenchymal stem cells (*ah*MSCs) or human fibroblasts (*h*Fb), and (iv) the bioactivity of fibroin mesh overcomes that of the polypyrrole-coated meshes [79].

Some natural origin polymers have also been successfully electrospun [77]. Owing to their very small diameter, polymeric nanofibers exhibit unusual properties such as high specific surface area, flexibility in surface functionalities, and superior mechanical properties. In addition, electrospun nonwoven meshes could physically mimic the ECM structure of native tissues. These remarkable properties render electrospun nanofibres useful for many applications, particularly those related to the field of biomedical engineering. The prospective tissue engineering/biomedical applications of electrospun polymeric nanofibers should include wound dressings, medical prostheses, drug delivery systems, DNA release, and tissue engineering scaffolds [77].

Electrospinning has been recognized as a versatile method for the fabrication of continuous ultrafine fibers using electrical forces [77,78,80]. Wu et al. [80] prepared HA ($Ca_{10}(PO_4)_6(OH)_2$, HA) fibers by electrospinning a precursor mixture of $Ca(NO_3)_2{\cdot}4H_2O$ and $(C_2H_5O)_3PO$ with a polymer additive, followed by a thermal treatment. The X-ray diffraction (XRD) analysis of the annealed composite fibers revealed that the pure HA phase could be obtained by annealing at 600 °C for 1 hours. It was reported that (i) the SEM analysis showed the surface of as-electrospun composite fibers with an average diameter of 50 μm was smooth due to the amorphous nature of the polymer; however, (ii) the surface of the calcined HA fibers was rough because of the complete removal of the polymer, and (iii) the pure HA fibers obtained by electrospinning were up to 10 mm in length and 10–30 μm in diameter and the HA grain size was ~1 μm in the HA fibers [78].

7.4.5. Atmospheric Plasma Treatment

Atmospheric pressure (or normal pressure) plasma treatment is the key technology for custom surface treatments, including ultrafine cleaning, surface activation, and plasma coating of almost all materials, including plastics, metals, glass, cardboard, textiles, and composite/hybrid materials. Atmospheric pressure plasmas have prominent technical significance because in contrast with low-pressure plasma or high-pressure plasma no reaction vessel is needed to ensure the maintenance of a pressure level differing from atmospheric pressure. Accordingly, depending on the principle of generation, these plasmas can be employed directly in the production line [81–86]. It is possible to coat varied surfaces by means of this technique. Thus, anticorrosive layers and adhesion promoter layers can be applied to many metals without the use of solvents and hence in an environmentally friendly manner [82].

7.4.6. Friction Stir Welding

The friction stir welding (FSW) technique is widely accepted to be one of the most significant welding techniques to emerge in the last 20 years. This application should include Al alloys, Mg alloys, Cu alloys, steels, Ti alloys, and metal matrix composites, focusing particularly on microstructural aspects, including texture formation, and the resulting properties of these joints, and for coating surfaces [87–89].

7.4.7. Near-Net Shape (NNS) Forming

In order to achieve the better condition for fit, for example, the superstructure for implants or denture base for prostheses, the accuracy of the final products is very crucial and need to be improved. Among various manufacturing technologies, NNS forming and nanotechnology are most promising and supportive for these specific aims. New classes of fabrication processes, such as direct-write (DW) technique [90] and SFF [91], have established the capability to produce three-dimensional parts faster, cheaper, and with added functionality. The choice of starting materials and the specific processing technique will produce unique microstructures that impact the final performance, especially of macroscopic structural and electronic parts. Furthermore, the ability to do point-wise deposition of one or more materials provides the opportunity for fabricating structures with novel microstructural and macrostructural features, such as micro-engineered porosity, graded interfaces, and complex multi-material constructions. NNS processing offers cost reduction by minimizing machining, reducing part count, and avoiding part distortion from welding. NSS technologies such as flow-forming (FF), superplastic forming (SPF), casting, forging, powder metallurgy

(P/M) methods, three-dimensional laser deposition, and plasma arc deposition (PAD) have been explored for potential use in tubular geometries and other shapes of varying complexity. It appears that the reduction in cost of a given titanium product will be maximized by achieving improvements in all of the manufacturing steps, from extraction to finishing [92].

7.4.8. Miscellaneous

Ti alloys, such as Ti–6Al–4V or Ti–6Al–7Nb, are currently used in biomedical or dental implant, or both, applications. Ti alloys are used because they are stronger than CpTi due to the presence of alloying elements. However, toxicity of alloying elements (e.g., V element) during long-term use of implants is of concern. Another means of increasing the strength of materials is grain size refinement. Dheda et al. [93] produced ultrafine-grained (grain size: ~250 nm to 1 μm) CpTi by cryomilling followed by spark plasma sintering. Electrochemical impedance spectroscopy (EIS) and cell culture experiments were performed to compare the corrosion and biocompatibility properties of coarse grained Ti and untrafine-grained Ti. It was found that (i) ultrafine- grained Ti exhibited corrosion resistance comparable to coarse grained Ti in Ringers solution, and (ii) ultrafine-grained Ti exhibited a reduced inflammatory response and enhanced cell adhesion compared to coarse-grained Ti [93].

In order to improve the biomedical properties of a titanium alloy surface, Tang et al. [94] employed an electro-spark surface alloying using a graphite electrode in air, in a nitrogen gas atmosphere and in silicone oil. It was reported that (i) alloyed layers, completely covering the substrate surface and about 40 μm thick mainly composed of the TiC phase and with strong metallurgical bonding and adhesion to the substrate, were obtained, indicating markedly improved hardness and wear resistance of the surface layer of the substrate, and (ii) the electron-spark surface strengthened layer treated in silicone oil shows good biocompatibility and biological activity, and can help cell attachment to the substrate surface [94].

When patients have hip, knee, or dental replacement surgery, they run the risk of having their bodies reject the implant. But the smart coating mitigates that risk by fostering bone growth into the implant. The coating creates a crystalline layer next to the implant, and a mostly amorphous outer layer that touches the surrounding bone. The amorphous layer dissolves over time, releasing calcium and phosphate, which encourages bone growth—osseointegration. This bonding also makes the implant more functional, because the bonding helps ensure that the bone and the implant do a better job of sharing the load.

Currently, implant patients are subjected to an intense regimen of antibiotics to prevent infection immediately following surgery. However, the site of the implant will always remain vulnerable to infection. But by incorporating silver into the coating, the silver particles will act as antimicrobial agents as the amorphous layer dissolves. This will not only limit the amount of antibiotics patients will need following surgery, but will provide protection from infection at the implant site for the life of the implant. Moreover, the silver is released more quickly right after surgery, when there is more risk of infection, due to the faster dissolution of the amorphous layer of the coating.

Silver release will slow down while the patient is healing. Furthermore, it is reported that this coating can be the functionally graded HA coatings doped with antibacterial components [95].

Every year, more than a million Americans receive an artificial hip or knee prosthesis. Such implants are designed to last many years, but in about 17% of patients who receive a total joint replacement, the implant eventually loosens and has to be replaced early, which can cause dangerous complications for elderly patients. To help minimize these burdensome operations, a new coating for implants that could help them better adhere to the patient's bone, preventing premature failure was developed [96]. To secure the implant, surgeons use bone cement, a polymer that resembles glass when hardened. In some cases, this cement ends up cracking and the implant detaches from the bone, causing chronic pain and loss of mobility for the patient. The new coating consists of a very thin film, ranging from 100 nm to one micron, composed of layers of materials that help promote rapid bone growth. One of the materials, HA, is a natural component of bone, made of calcium and phosphate. This material attracts mesenchymal stem cells from the bone marrow and provides an interface for the formation of new bone. The other layer releases a growth factor that stimulates mesenchymal stem cells to transform into bone-producing cells called osteoblasts. Once the osteoblasts form, they start producing new bone to fill in the spaces surrounding the implant, securing it to the existing bone and eliminating the need for bone cement. Having healthy tissue in that space creates a stronger bond and greatly reduces the risk of bacterial infection around the implant. It was also reported that the MIT team is now performing animal studies that have shown promising results: (i) the coatings lead to rapid bone formation, locking the implants in place, and (ii) this coating could be used not only for joint replacements, but also for fixation plates and screws used to set bone fractures [96].

Titanium (Ti) foams are attracting increasing interest in bone tissue engineering. The elastic modulus of Ti and its alloys can be reduced through the introduction of a porous structure, thereby addressing the stress shielding problem. Moreover, a porous structure may also provide new bone tissue ingrowth abilities and vascularization. Hsu et al. [97] prepared highly porous Ti scaffolds through a sponge replication method. The results showed that the Ti foam samples sintered in air at 800 °C, 900 °C, or 1000 °C exhibit the presence of rutile TiO_2 on the Ti strut surfaces, which could bioactivate Ti foams. The oxide layers formed on the surface were relatively smooth and the thickness increased with an increase in sintering temperature. Additionally, the total porosities of the Ti foams sintered at three different sintering temperatures are larger than 79%, and open porosity is larger than 74%. The open porosity ratio is in excess of 0.92, suggesting that most pores are interconnected. Moreover, the strength and modulus of the sintered Ti foams conforms to the basic mechanical property requirement of cancellous bones. Hence, it was concluded that the highly porous Ti foams with a bioactive oxide layer were successfully fabricated by single-step sintering in air instead of a conventional vacuum atmosphere [97].

Wettability is an important and complex property of solid surfaces. In recent years there has been much interest in novel wetting behavior and its adaption for use in commercial applications. One area that has attracted significant attention is that of switchable wettability, specifically the controlled and reversible conversion between superhydrophobic and superhydrophilic wetting states. Targeted drug delivery, water-harvesting, and antireflective, water-proofing, and liquid self-transportation coatings are just a few examples where such switchable or smart surfaces are finding applications. For these aims, electrowetting [98] or surface morphological manipulation through the micro-/nano-/micro-nano-binary surface roughness [99] has been developed.

Zirconim films were prepared on titanium by the cathodic arc deposition technique [100]. The surface topography and element composition of the films were characterized by SEM and X-ray photoelectron spectroscopy, respectively. Osteoblast-like MG63 cells were cultured on the surface of the zirconium films *in vitro*, and cell behavior was investigated, with titanium control. The results obtained from SEM and immuno-fluoescence studies showed that the MG63 cells on ZrO_2 films spread better than those on Ti. The CCK8 assay indicated that the zirconia films promoted the proliferation of MG63 cells. The results of alkaline phosphatase (ALP) activity test and the expression of osteogenic marker genes, such as ALP, collagen I, and osteocalcin, demonstrated that the differentiation of MG63 cells might be enhanced by zirconia films. In addition, the zirconia films possibly regulated osteoclastogenic gene expression by stimulating the expression of osteorotegerin. Based on these results, it was suggested that the ZiO_2 film is worth further consideration for orthopedic implant applications [100].

O'Sullivan et al. [101] deposited a series of doped apatites onto titanium substrates using a novel ambient temperature blasting process. The potential of these deposited doped apatites as noncolonizing osteoconductive coatings has been evaluated *in vitro*. XPS, EDX, and gravimetric analysis demonstrated that a high degree of coating incorporation was observed for each material. The modified surfaces were found to produce osteoblast proliferation comparable to, or better than, an HA finish. Promising levels of initial microbial inhibition were observed from the Sr- and Ag-doped surfaces, with the strontium showing prolonged ability to reduce bacteria numbers over a 30-day period. Ion elution profiles have been characterized and linked to the microbial response and based on the results obtained, mechanisms of kill have been suggested. The direct contact of coated substrate surfaces with microbes was observed to be a significant contributing factor to the antimicrobial performance and the anticolonizing activity. It was also reported that the silver substituted apatite was observed to out-perform both the SrA and ZnA in terms of biofilm inhibition [101].

In order to determine whether a newly developed implant material conforms to the requirements of biocompatibility, it must undergo rigorous testing. To correctly interpret the results of studies on implant material osseointegration, it is necessary to have a sound understanding of all the testing methods. The review study was conducted to elucidate the methods that are used for the experimental evaluation of the osseointegration of implant materials [102]. It was found that (i) in recent decades, there has been a constant proliferation of new materials and surface modifications in the field of dental implants; (ii) this continuous development of innovative biomaterials requires a precise and detailed evaluation in terms of biocompatibility and implant healing before clinical use; (iii) the current gold standard is *in vivo* animal testing on well-validated animal models; (iv) however, long-term outcome studies on patients have to follow to finally validate and show patient benefit. Accordingly, it was concluded that no experimental setup can provide answers for all possible research questions. However, a certain transferability of the results to humans might be possible if the experimental setup is carefully chosen for the aspects and questions being investigated. To enhance the implant survival rate in the rising number of patients with chronic diseases which compromise wound healing and osseointegration, it was suggested that dental implant research on compromised animal models will further gain importance in future [102].

Although dental implants exhibit only limited failure rates, their fracture is associated with major modifications of the prosthetic treatment and complex surgery for the removal of the remaining embedded implant part. Michailidis et al. [103] developed stress fields in the bone–implant interface during mastication to assess the failure modes of oral implants. In order to achieve this, an FEM (finite element method) model of an implant as reverse engineered and virtually loaded at the top of the crown for a force spectrum ranging from 75 to 225 N in a vertical, horizontal, and oblique occlusal direction. The calculated stress fields were compared with clinically retrieved fractured implants with identical geometrical characteristics and the fracture modes of both cases were corrected. It was reported that the developing stress patterns, facilitated the interpretation of the implant failure as the maximum stresses, indicated critical values in both, lingual and buccal sides of the implant–bone interface at a certain critical level of bone resorption, in which failure occurs [103].

Jung et al. [104] assessed the literature on accuracy and clinical performance of computer technology applications in surgical implant dentistry. Electronic and manual literature searches were conducted to collect information about (1) the accuracy and (2) clinical performance of computer-assisted implant systems. Meta-regression analysis was performed for summarizing the accuracy studies. Failure/complication rates were analyzed using random-effects Poisson regression models to obtain summary estimates of 12-month proportions. Twenty-nine different image guidance systems were included. From 2,827 articles, 13 clinical and 19 accuracy studies were included in this systematic review. The meta-analysis of the accuracy (19 clinical and preclinical studies) revealed a total mean error of 0.74 mm (maximum of 4.5 mm) at the entry point in the bone and 0.85 mm at the apex (maximum of 7.1 mm). For the five included clinical studies (total of 506 implants) using computer-assisted implant dentistry, the mean failure rate was 3.36% (0%–8.45%) after an observation period of at least 12 months. In 4.6% of the treated cases, intraoperative complications were reported; these included limited interocclusal distances to perform guided implant placement, limited primary implant stability, or need for additional grafting procedures. Differing levels and quantity of evidence were available for computer-assisted implant placement, revealing high implant survival rates after only 12 months of observation in different indications and a reasonable level of accuracy. However, future long-term clinical data are necessary to identify clinical indications and to justify additional radiation doses, effort, and costs associated with computer-assisted implant surgery [104].

Recently, the time-depending aging process of titanium implants has been addressed [105–108]. Suzuki et al. [105] investigated the effect of ultraviolet (UV) light irradiation on rejuvenate aged titanium so that the original bioactivity can be regained. Fresh Ti, aged Ti, and UV-treated Ti were subjected to test. It was reported that proliferation, alkaline phosphatase activity, and calcium deposition of the cells were substantially lower on the aged surfaces than on the fresh surfaces, while those on the UV-treated aged surfaces were higher than on the fresh surfaces, suggesting that the bioactivity of titanium surfaces degrades with time and that UV treatment of the aged surface increases the bioactivity over the level of the freshly prepared surface. It is, therefore, concluded that ultraviolet treatment overcomes time-related degrading bioactivity of titanium [105]. Similar results are reported elsewhere [106, 107].

Despite the substantial contribution of titanium implants in the field of dental and orthopedic constructive therapy, there is a crucial unaddressed question of why bone–implant contact does not reach the ideal 100%. Lee et al. [108] introduced the recently reported time-dependent reduction in osteoconductivity and other biological capabilities of titanium since processing. This phenomenon is defined as the biological aging of titanium and provides insight to significantly advance the understanding of osseointegration and to further improve implant surfaces in the future [108].

References

1. Zivić, F., Babić, M., Grujović, N. and Mitrović, S., 2010, Tribometry of materials for bioengineering applications, *Tribol Industry* 32:25–32.
2. Zivić, F., 2007, Nanotribometer area of application, *Tribol Industry* 29:34–39.
3. Goodman, S.B., Yao, Z., Keeney, M. and Yang, F., 2013, The future of biologic coatings for orthopaedic implants, *Biomaterials* 34:3174–3183. doi: http://dx.doi.org/10.1016/j.biomaterials.2013.01.074.
4. Guarino, V., Gloria, A., Raucci, M. G., De Santis, R. and Ambrosio, É., 2012, Bio-inspired composite and cell instructive platforms for bone regeneration, *Int Mater News* 57:256–275. doi: http://dx.doi.org/ 10.1179/0950660812Z.00000000021.
5. Khaled, S.M., Sui, R., Charpentier, P.A. and Rizkalla, A.S., 2007, Synthesis of TiO_2–PMMA nanocomposite: Using methacrylic acid as a coupling agent, *Langmuir 23:*3988–3995. doi: http://dx.doi.org/10.1021/la062879n.
6. Chae, T., Yang, H., Leung, V., Ko, F. and Troczynski, T., 2013, Novel biomimetic hydroxyapatite/alginate nanocomposite fibrous scaffolds for bone tissue regeneration, *J Mater Sci Mater Med* 24:1885–1894. doi: http://dx.doi.org/10.1007/s10856-013-4957-7.
7. Schuster, M., Turecek, C., Varga, F., Lichtenegger, H., Stampfl, J. and Liska, R., 2007, 3D-shaping of biodegradable photopolymers for hard tissue replacement, *Appl Surf Sci* 254:1131–1134. doi: http://dx.doi.org/10.1016/j.apsusc.2007.07.182.
8. Titanium foams replace injured bones; Research News September 01, 2010.http://www.fraunhofer.de/en/press/research-news/2010/09/titanium-foams-replace-injured-bones.html
9. http://nextbigfuture.com/2010/09/titanium-foams-replace-injured-bones.html
10. Metal Powder Report; Steel foam could replace bones, March 4, 2010. http://www.metal-powder.net/view/7801/steel-foam-could-replace-bones/
11. Bencharit, S., Byrd, W.C., Altarawneh, S., Hosseini, B., Leong, A., Reside, G., Morelli, T. and Offenbacher, S., 2013, Development and applications of porous tantalum trabecular metal-enhanced titanium dental implants, *Clin Implant Dent Relat Res.* doi: http://dx.doi.org/10.1111/cid.12059.
12. Sargeant, T.D., Guler, M.O., Oppenheimer, S.M., Mata, A., Satcher, R.L., Dunand, D.C. and Stupp, S.L., 2008, Hybrid bone implants: Self-assembly of peptide amphiphile nanofibers within porous titanium, *Biomaterials* 29:16–171.
13. Man, H.C., Zhang, S., Cheng, F.T. and Guo, X., 2005, Laser fabrication of porous surface layer on NiTi shape memory alloy, *Mater Sci Eng* 404:173–178. doi: http://dx.doi.org/10.1016/j.msea.2005.05.020.

14. Shishkovsky, I., Morozov, Y. and Smurov, I., 2007, Nanofractal surface structure under laser sintering of titanium and nitinol for bone tissue engineering, *Appl Surf Sci* 254:1145–1149. doi: http://dx.doi.org/10.1016/j.apsusc.2007.09.021.
15. Li, J.P., Habibovic, P., van den Doel, M., Wilson, C.E., de Wijn, J.R., van Blitterswijk, C.A. and Klaas de Groot, K., 2007, Bone ingrowth in porous titanium implants produced by 3D fiber deposition, *Biomaterials* 28: 2810–2820. doi: http://dx.doi.org/10.1016/j.biomaterials.2007.02.020.
16. Wei, W., Macak, J.M., Shrestha, N.K. and Schmuki, P., 2009, Thick self-ordered nanoporous Ta_2O_5 films with long-range lateral order nanostructured materials, carbon nanotubes, and fullerenes, *J Electrochem Soc 156:*K104–K109. doi: http://dx.doi.org/0.1149/1.3116243.
17. Dong, C., Campell, A.S., Eldawud, R., Perhinschi, G., Rojanasakul, Y. and Dinu, C.Z., 2013, Effects of acid treatment on structure, properties and biocompatibility of carbon nanotubes, *Appl Surf Sci* 264:261–268. doi: http://dx.doi.org/10.1016/j.apsusc.2012.09.180.
18. Chen, L., Hu, J., Shen, X. and Tong, H., 2013, Synthesis and characterization of chitosan—multiwalled carbon nanotubes/hydroxyapatite nanocomposites for bone tissue engineering, *J Mater Sci Mater Med* 24:1843–1851. doi: http://dx.doi.org/10.1007/s10856-013-4954-x.
19. Mazare, A., Dilea, M., Ionita, D., Titorencu, I., Trusca, V. and Vasile, E., 2012, Changing bioperformance of TiO_2 amorphous nanotubes as an effect of inducing crystallinity, *Bioelectrochemistry* 87:124–131. doi: http://dx.doi.org/10.1016/j.bioelechem.2012.01.002.
20. Wepasnick, K.A., Smith, B.A., Bitter, J.L. and Fairbrother, D.H., 2010, Chemical and structural characterization of carbon nanotube surfaces, *Anal Bioanal Chem* 396:1003–1014. doi: http://dx.doi.org/10.1007/s00216-009-3332-5.
21. Yang, X.F. and Lu, J., 2013, A new way to synthesize carbon nanofiber film on bulk titanium via hybrid surface mechanical attrition treatment, *Appl Surf Sci* 264:191–196. doi: http://dx.doi.org/10.1016/j.apsusc.2012.09.169.
22. Jiang, Y., Yin, H., Sun, Y., Liu, H., Lei, L., Chen, K. and Wada, Y., 2007, Effects of organic acids on the size-controlled synthesis of rutile TiO_2 nanorods, *Appl Surf Sci* 253:9277–9282. doi: http://dx.doi.org/10.1016/j.apsusc.2007.05.068.
23. Wang, N., Li, H., Lü, W., Li, J., Wang, J., Zhang, Z. and Yiran Liu, Y., 2011, Effects of TiO_2 nanotubes with different diameters on gene expression and osseointegration of implants in minipigs, *Biomaterials* 32: 6900–6911. doi: http://dx.doi.org/10.1016/j.biomaterials.2011.06.023.
24. Hassan, F.M.B., Nanjo, H., Tetsuka, H., Kanakubo, M., Aizawa, T., Nishioka, M., Ebina, T. and Bond, A.M., 2009, Formation of self-ordered TiO_2 nanotubes by electrochemical anodization of titanium in 2-propanol/ NH_4F nanostructured materials, carbon nanotubes, and fullerenes, *J Electrochem Soc 156:*K227–K232. doi: http://dx.doi.org/10.1149/1.3115520.
25. Kowalski, D., Kim, D. and Schmuki, P., 2013, TiO_2nanotubes, nanochannels and mesosponge: Self-organized formation and applications, *Nano Today* 8:235–264. doi: http://dx.doi.org/10.1016/j.nantod.2013.04.010.
26. More, A.M., Gujar, T.P., Gunjakar, J.L., Lokhande, C.D. and Joo, O-S., 2008, Growth of TiO_2 nanorods by chemical bath deposition method, *Appl Surf Sci* 255:2682–2687. doi: http://dx.doi.org/10.1016/j.apsusc.2008.08.003.
27. Lei, L., Yuming, C., Bo, L., Xingfu, Z. and Weiping, D., 2010, Study on the surface erosion route to the fabrication of TiO_2 hollow spheres, *Appl Surf Sci* 256:2596–2601. doi: http://dx.doi.org/10.1016/j.apsusc.2009.11.001.

28. Ma, Y., Zhan, G., Ma, M., Wang, X. and Li, C., 2012, Direct electron transfer of hemoglobin in a biocompatible electrochemical system based on zirconium dioxide nanotubes and ionic liquid, *Bioelectrochemistry* 84:6–10. doi: http://dx.doi.org/10.1016/j.bioelechem.2011.09.003.
29. Choe, H-C., 2011, Nanotubular surface and morphology of Ti-binary and Ti-ternary alloys for biocompatibility, *Thin Solid Films* 519:4652–4657. doi: http://dx.doi.org/10.1016/j.tsf.2011.01.011.
30. Grigorescu, S., Ungureanu, C., Kirchgeorg, R., Schmuki, P. and Demetrescu, I., 2013, Various sized nanotubes on TiZr for antibacterial surfaces, *Appl Surf Sci* 270:190–196. doi: http://dx.doi.org/10.1016/j.apsusc.2012.12.165.
31. Hsu, S-H., Tang, C-M. and Tseng, H-J., 2008, Biostability and biocompatibility of poly(ester urethane)–gold nanocomposites, *Acta Biomater* 4:1797–1808. doi: http://dx.doi.org/10.1016/j.actbio.2008.06.015.
32. Allaker, R.P., 2010, The use of nanoparticles to control oral biofilm formation, *J Dent Res* 89:1175–1186. doi: http://dx.doi.org/10.1177/0022034510377794.
33. Ichikawa, S., Iwamoto, S. and Watanabe, J., 2005, Formation of biocompatible nanoparticles by self-assembly of enzymatic hydrolysates of chitosan and carboxymethyl cellulose, *Biosci Biotechnol Biochem* 69:1637–1642. doi: http://dx.doi.org/10.1271/bbb.69.1637.
34. Das, B., Mandal, M., Upadhyay, A. and Chattopadhyay, P., 2013, Bio-based hyperbranched polyurethane/Fe_3O_4 nanocomposites: Smart antibacterial biomaterials for biomedical devices and implants, *Biomed Mater 8:*035003. doi: http://dx.doi.org/10.1088/1748-6041/8/3/035003.
35. Matsumoto, T.J., An S-H., Ishimoto, T., Nakano, T., Matsumoto, T. and Imazato, S., 2011, Zirconia–hydroxyapatite composite material with micro porous structure, *Dental Materials* 27:e205–e212. doi: http://dx.doi.org/10.1016/j.dental.2011.07.009.
36. Oshida, Y., 2007, *Bioscience and Bioengineering of Titanium Materials*, Elsevier, London, UK, pp.389–390.
37. Lee, B-T., Kim, K-H., Youn, H-C. and Song, H-Y., 2007, Functionally gradient and micro-channeled Al_2O_3–(t-ZrO_2)/HA p composites, *J Am Ceram Soc* 90:629–631. doi: http://dx.doi.org/10.1111/j.1551-2916.2006.01394.x.
38. Lin, D., Li, Q., Li, W. and Swain, M., 2010,Bone remodeling induced by dental implants of functionally graded materials, *J Biomed Mater Res Appl Biomater* 92:430–438. doi: http://dx.doi.org/10.1002/jbm.b.31531.
39. Kanaparthy, R. and Kanaparthy, A., 2011, The changing face of dentistry: Nanotechnology. *Int J Nanomed* 6:2799–2804. doi: http://dx.doi.org/10.2147/IJN.S24353.
40. Drexler, K.E., 2006, *Nanosystems: Molecular Machinery Manufacturing and Computation*. John Wiley and Sons, New York, NY.
41. Tomsia, A.P., Lee, J.S., Wegst, U.G.K. and Saiz, E., 2012, Nanotechnology for dental implants, *Oral Craniofac Tissue Eng* 2:23–34.
42. www.artoss.com/fileadmin/pdf-download/NanoBone-Productbrochure_en.edf
43. Ertorer, O., Topping, T.D., Li, Y., Moss, W. and Lavernia, E.J., 2011, Nanostructured Ti consolidated via spark plasma sintering, *Metallur Mater Trans A*42:964–973. doi: http://dx.doi.org/10.1007/s11661-010-0499-5.
44. Peng, P-W., Ou, K-L., Lin, H-C., Pan, Y-N. and Wang, C-H., 2010, Effect of electrical-discharging on formation of nanoporous biocompatible layer on titanium, *J Alloys Comp* 492:625–630. doi: http://dx.doi.org/10.1016/j.jallcom.2009.11.197.
45. Ogawa, T., Saruwatari, L., Takeuchi, K., Aita, H. and Ohno, N., 2008, Ti Nano-nodular structuring for bone integration and regeneration, *J Dent Res* 87:751–756. doi: http://dx.doi.org/10.1177/154405910808700809.

46. Alekhin, A.P., Boleiko, G.M., Gudkova, S.A., Markeev, A.M., Sigarev, A.A.,Toknova, V.F., Kirilenko, A.G., Lapshin, R.V., Kozlov, E.N. and Tetyukhin, D.V., 2010, Synthesis of biocompatible surfaces by nanotechnology methods, *Nanotechnol Russia*5:696–708. doi: http://dx.doi.org/10.1134/S1995078010090144.
47. Mehdikhani-Nahrkhalaji, M., Fathi, M.H., Mortazavi, V., Mousavi, S.B., Hashemi-Beni, B. and Razavi, S.M.J., 2012, Novel nanocomposite coating for dental implant applications in vitro and in vivo evaluation, *J Mater Sci Mater Med*23:485–495. doi: http://dx.doi.org/10.1007/s10856-011-4507-0.
48. Rani, V.V.D., Vinoth-Kumar, L., Anitha, V.C., Manzoor, K., Deepthy, M. and Shantikumar, V.N., 2012, Osteointegration of titanium implant is sensitive to specific nanostructure morphology, *Acta Biomater* 8:1976–1989. doi: http://dx.doi.org/10.1016/j.actbio.2012.01.021.
49. Ballo, A., Agheli, H., Lausmaa, J., Thomsen, P. and Petronis, S., 2011, Nanostructured model implants for in vivo studies: influence of well-defined nanotechnology on de novo bone formation on titanium implants, *Int J Nanomed* 6:3415–3428. doi: http://dx.doi.org/10.2147/IJN.S25867.
50. Wu, S., Liu, X., Yeung, K.W.K., Guo, H., Li, P., Hu, T., Chung, C.Y. and Chu, P.K., 2013, Surface nano-architectures and their effects on the mechanical properties and corrosion behavior of Ti-based orthopedic implants, *Surf Coat Technol* 233:13–26. doi: http://dx.doi.org/10.1016/j.surfcoat.2012.10.023.
51. Narayan, R.J., Hobbs, L.W., Jin, C. and Rabiei, A., 2006, The use of functionally gradient materials in medicine, *JOM* 58:52–56. doi: http://dx.doi.org/10.1007/s11837-006-0142-5.
52. Khatayevich, D., Gungormus, M., Yazici, H., So, C., Cetinel, S., Ma, H., Jen, A., Tamerler, C. and Sarikaya, M., 2010, Biofunctionalization of materials for implants using engineered peptides. *Acta Biomater* 6:4634–4641. doi: http://dx.doi.org/10.1016/j.actbio.2010.06.004.
53. Vasilev, K., Poh, Z., Kant, K., Chan, J., Michelmore, A. and Losic, D., 2010, Tailoring the surface functionalities of titania nanotube arrays, *Biomaterials* 31:532–540. doi: http://dx.doi.org/10.1016/j.biomaterials.2009.09.074.
54. Ren, X., Wu, Y., Cheng, Y., Ma, H. and Wei, S., 2011, Fibronectin and bone morphogenetic protein-2-decorated poly(OEGMA-*r*-HEMA) brushes promote osseointegration of titanium surfaces, *Langmuir 27:*12069–12073. doi: http://dx.doi.org/10.1021/la202438u.
55. Sala, A., Ehrbar, M., Trentin, D., Schoenmakers, R.G., Vöroös J. and Weber, F.E., 2010, Enzyme mediated site-specific surface modification, *Langmuir 26:*11127–11134. doi: http://dx.doi.org/10.1021/la1008895.
56. Ravichandran, R., Ng, C.C.H., Liao, S., Pliszka, D., Raghunath, M., Ramakrishna, S. and Chan, C.K., 2012, Biomimetic surface modification of titanium surfaces for early cell capture by advanced electrospinning, *Biomed Mater* 7:015001. doi: http://dx.doi.org/10.1088/1748-6041/7/1/015001.
57. Chen, M., Tan, J., Lian, Y. and Liu, D., 2008, Preparation of gelatin coated hydroxyapatite nanorods and the stability of its aqueous colloidal, *Appl Surf Sci* 254:2730–2735. doi: http://dx.doi.org/10.1016/j.apsusc.2007.10.011.
58. Gao, W., Feng, B., Ni, Y., Yang, Y., Lu, X. and Weng, J., 2010, Protein adsorption and biomimetic mineralization behaviors of PLL–DNA multilayered films assembled onto titanium, *Appl Surf Sci 257:* 538–546. doi: http://dx.doi.org/10.1016/j.apsusc.2010.07.029.
59. Skopinska-Wisniewska, J., Sionkowska, A., Kaminska, A., Kaznica, A., Jachimiak, R. and Drewa, T., 2009, Surface characterization of collagen/elastin based biomaterials for tissue regeneration, *Appl Surf Sci* 255:8286–8292. doi: http://dx.doi.org/10.1016/j.apsusc.2009.05.127.

60. Tan, G., Zhou, L., Ning, C., Tan, Y., Ni, G., Liao, J., Yu, P. and Chen, X., 2013, Biomimetically-mineralized composite coatings on titanium functionalized with gelatin methacrylate hydrogels, *Appl Surf Sci* 279:293–299. doi: http://dx.doi.org/10.1016/j.apsusc.2013.04.088.
61. Laydi, F., Rahouadj, R., Vuchois, G., Stoltz, J-F. and de Isla, N., 2013, Hydroxyapatite incorporated into collagen gels for mesenchymal stem cell culture, *Bio-Med Mater Eng* 23:311–315. doi: http://dx.doi.org/10.3233/BME-130755.
62. Lu, Y., Zhu, A., Wang, W. and Shi, H., 2010, New bioactive hybrid material of nano-hydroxyapatite based on *N*-carboxyethylchitosan for bone tissue engineering, *Appl Surf Sci*256:7228–7233. doi: http://dx.doi.org/10.1016/j.apsusc.2010.05.056.
63. Jung, G-B., Kim, J-H., Jin SikBurm, J.S. and Park, H-K., 2013, Fabrication of chitosan-silver nanoparticle hybrid 3D porous structure as a SERS substrate for biomedical applications, *Appl Surf Sci*273:179–183. doi: http://dx.doi.org/10.1016/j.apsusc.2013.02.010.
64. Galler, K.M., D'Souza, R.N. and Hartgerink, J.D., 2010, Biomaterials and their potential applications for dental tissue engineering, *J Mater Chem* 20:8730–8746. doi: http://dx.doi.org/10.1039/C0JM01207F.
65. Joos, U., 2009, Tissue engineering strategies in dental implantology, In: U. Meyer, J. Handschel, H.P. Wiesmann, T. Meyer, ed., *Fundamentals of Tissue Engineering and Regenerative Medicine*, Springer, Berlin/Heidelberg, Germany, pp. 839–854.
66. Lembo, J., 2003, Three-dimensional printing, *Ad Mater Porcess* 161:52–53.
67. Sparrow, N., 2013, How 3-D printing is transforming medical technology, *Eur Med Device Technol* 23:1–3.
68. Banham, R., 2013, Printing a medical revolution, http://individual.troweprice.com/public/Retail/Planning-&-Research/Connections/3D-Printing/Printing-a-Medical-Revolution
69. Wang, F., Mei, J. and Wu, X., 2006, Microstructure study of direct laser fabricated Ti alloys using powder and wire, *Appl Surf Sci* 253:1424–1430. doi: http://dx.doi.org/10.1016/j.apsusc.2006.02.028
70. Schade, L., Franzka, S., Hardt, S., Wiggers, H. and Hartmann, N., 2013, Sintering of thin titanium dioxide nanoparticle films via photothermal processing with ultraviolet continuous-wave lasers, *Appl Surf Sci* 278:336–340. doi: http://dx.doi.org/10.1016/j.apsusc.2012.11.077
71. Bandyopadhyay, A., Krishna, B.V., Xue, W. and Bose, S.J., 2009, Application of laser engineered net shaping (LENS) to manufacture porous and functionally graded structures for load bearing implants, *Mater Sci Mater Med* 20:S29–S34. doi: http://dx.doi.org/10.1007/s10856-008-3478-2
72. Ng, K.W., Man, H.C. and Yue, T.M., 2011, Characterization and corrosion study of NiTi laser surface alloyed with Nb or Co, *Appl Surf Sci* 257:3269–3274. doi: http://dx.doi.org/10.1016/j.apsusc.2010.10.154
73. Traini, T., Mangano, C., Sammons, R.L., Mangano, F., Macchi, A. and Piattelli, A., 2008, Direct laser metal sintering as a new approach to fabrication of an isoelastic functionally graded material for manufacture of porous titanium dental implants, *Dent Mater* 24:1525–1533. doi: http://dx.doi.org/10.1016/j.dental.2008.03.029
74. Mangano, C., Piattelli, A., Mangano, F., Rustichelli, F., Shibli, J.A., Iezzi, G. and Giuliani, A., 2013, Histological and synchrotron radiation-based computed microtomography study of 2 human-retrieved direct laser metal formed titanium implants, *Implant Dent* 22:175–181. doi: http://dx.doi.org/10.1097/ID.0b013e318282817d
75. Xiao, D., Yang, Y., Su, X., Wang, D. and Su, J., 2013, An integrated approach of topology optimized design and selective laser melting process for titanium implants materials, *Bio-Med Mater Eng* 23:433–445.
76. Chauvy, P-F., Hoffmann, P. and Landolt, D., 2003, Applications of laser lithography on oxide film to titanium micromachining, *Appl Surf Sci* 208/209:165–170. doi: http://dx.doi.org/10.1016/S0169-4332(02)01361-2

77. Martins, A., Reis, R.L. and Neves, N.M., 2008, Electrospinning: Processing technique for tissue engineering scaffolding, *Int Mater Rev* 53:257–274. doi: http://dx.doi.org/10.1179/174328008X353547
78. Wu, Y., Hench, L.L., Du, J., Choy, K-L. and Guo, J., 2004, Preparation of hydroxyapatite fibers by electrospinning technique, *J Am Ceram Soc* 87:1988–1991. doi: http://dx.doi.org/10.1111/j.1151-2916.2004.tb06351.x
79. Aznar-Cervantes, S., Roca, M.I., Martinez, J.G., Meseguer-Olmo, L., Cenis, J.L., Moraleda, J.M. and Otero, T.F., 2012, Fabrication of conductive electrospun silk fibroin scaffolds by coating with polypyrrole for biomedical applications, *Bioelectrochem* 85:36–43. doi: http://dx.doi.org/10.1016/j.bioelechem.2011.11.008
80. Supaphol, P., Suwantong, O., Sangsanoh, P., Srinivasan, S., Jayakumar, R. and Nair, S.V., 2012, Electrospinning of biocompatible polymers and their potentials in biomedical applications, *Adv Polym Sci* 246:213–239.
81. Wolf, R.A., 2012, *Atmospheric Pressure Plasma for Surface Modification*, Wiley. doi: http://dx.doi.org/10.1002/9781118547519
82. Noeske, M., Degenhardt, J., Strudhoff, S. and Lommattzsch, U., 2004, Plasma jet treatment of five polymers at atmospheric pressure: Surface modifications and the relevance for adhesion, *Int J Adhes Adhes* 24:171–177. doi: http://dx.doi.org/10.1016/j.ijadhadh.2003.09.006
83. Thomas, M. and Mittal K.L., 2013, *Atmospheric Pressure Plasma Treatments of Polymers: Relevance to Adhesion*, Wiley, Schilevener Publishing. doi: http://dx.doi.org/10.1002/9781118747308
84. Gotoh, K., Yasukawa, A. and Tanuguchi, K., 2012, Water contact angles on poly(ethylene terephthalate) films exposed to atmospheric pressure plasma, *J Adh Sci Technol* 25: 307–322. doi: http://dx.doi.org/10.1163/016942410X511114
85. Kim, J.S., Kim, Y.K. and Lee, K.H., 2004, Effects of atmospheric plasma treatment on the interfacial characteristics of ethylene-vinyl acetate/polyurethane composites, *J Colloid Interface Sci* 271:187–191. doi: http://dx.doi.org/10.1016/j.jcis.2003.10.013
86. Tang, S., Kwon, O.J. and Choi, H.S., 2005, Surface characteristics of AISI 304L stainless steel after an atmospheric pressure plasma treatment, *Surf Coat Technol* 195:298–306. doi: http://dx.doi.org/10.1016/j.surfcoat.2004.07.071
87. Threadgill, P.L., Leonard, A.J, Shercliff, H.R. andWithers, P.J., 2009, Friction stir welding of aluminum alloys, *Int Mater Rev* 54:49–93. doi: http://dx.doi.org/10.1179/174328009X411136
88. Çam, G., 2011, Friction stir welded structural materials: Beyond Al-alloys, *Int Mater Rev* 56:1–48. doi: http://dx.doi.org/10.1179/095066010X12777205875750
89. Li, B.,Shen, Y. and Hu, W., 2013, Surface nitriding on Ti–6Al–4V alloy via friction stir processing method under nitrogen atmosphere, *Appl Surf Sci* 274:356–364. doi: http://dx.doi.org/10.1016/j.apsusc.2013.03.060
90. Ringeisen, B.R., Chrisey, D.B., Piqué, A., Krizman, D., Bronks, M. and Spargo, B., 2001, Direct write technology and a tool to rapidly prototype patterns of biological and electronic systems, *Nanotechnol*1:414–417.
91. Finke, S. and Feenstra, K., 2002, Solid freedom fabrication by extrusion and deposition of semi-solid alloys, *J Mater Sci*37:3101–3106. doi: http://dx.doi.org/10.1023/A:1016137723481
92. Klug, K.L., Ucok, I., Gungor, M.N., Gulu, M., Kramer, L.S., Tack, W.T., Nastac, L., Martin, N.R. and Dong, H., 2004, The near-net-shape manufacturing of affordable titanium components for the M777 lightweight howitzer, *JOM*56:35–42.
93. Dheda,S.S., Kim,Y.K., Melnyk,C., Liu,W. and Mohamed, F.A., 2013, Corrosion and in vitro biocompatibility properties of cryomilled-spark plasma sintered commercially pure

titanium, *J Mater Sci Mater Med* 24:1239–1249. doi: http://dx.doi.org/10.1007/s10856-013-4889-2

94. Tang, C-B., Liu, D-X., Wang, Z. andGao, Y., 2011, Electro-spark alloying using graphite electrode on titanium alloy surface for biomedical applications, *Appl Surf Sci* 257:6364–6371. doi: http://dx.doi.org/10.1016/j.apsusc.2011.01.120
95. ASM, 2010, Smart coating containing silver nanoparticles helps implants bond better. http://asmcommunity.asminternational.org/portal/site/www/NewsItem/?vgnextoid=747ed5f6fb896210VgnVCM100000621e010aRCRD
96. http://web.mit.edu/newsoffice/2012/hip-implants-nanoscale-coating-0419.html
97. Hsu, H-C., Hsu, S-K., Wu, S-C., Wang, P-H. and Ho, W-F., 2013, Design and characterization of highly porous titanium foams with bioactive surface sintering in air, *J Alloys Comp* 575:326–332. doi: http://dx.doi.org/10.1016/j.jallcom.2013.05.186
98. Zhao, Y-P. and Wang, Y., 2013, Fundamentals and applications of electrowetting, *Rev AdhesAdhes* 1:114–174. doi: http://dx.doi.org/10.7569/RAA.2013.097304
99. Zhang, J. and Severtson, S., 2013, Fabrication and application of reversibly switchable surfaces: Super-non-wetting to super-wetting, *Rev Adhes Adhes* 1:248–270. doi: http://dx.doi.org/10.7569/RAA.2013.097306
100. Zhang, S., Sun, J., Xu, Y., Qian, S., Wang, B., Liu, F. and Liu, X., 2013, Adhesion, proliferation and differentiation of osteoblasts on zirconia films prepared by cathodic arc deposition, *Bio-Med Mater Eng* 23:373–385.
101. O'Sullivan, C., O'Hare, P., O'Leary, N.D., Crean, A.M., Ryan, K., Dobson, A.D.W. and O'Neill, L., 2010, Deposition of substituted apatites with anticolonizing properties onto titanium surfaces using a novel blasting process, *J Biomed Mater Res B Appl Biomater* 95:141–149. doi: http://dx.doi.org/10.1002/jbm.b.31694
102. von Wilmowsky, C., Moest, T., Nkenke, E., Stelzle, F. and Schlegel, K.A., 2013, Implants in bone: Part II. Research on implant osseointegration : Material testing, mechanical testing, imaging and histoanalytical methods, *Oral Maxillofac Surg* www.ncbi.nlm.nih.gov/pubmed/23430020
103. Michailidis, N., Karaninas, G., Tsouknidas, A., Maliaris, G., Tsipas, D. and Koidis, P., 2013, A FEM based endosteal implant simulation to determine the effect of peri-implant bone resorption on stress induced implant failure, *Bio-Med Mater Eng* 23:317–327.
104. Jung, R.E., Schneider, D., Ganeles, J., Wismeijer, D., Zwahlen, M., Hämmerle, C.H. and Tahmaseb, A., 2009, Computer technology applications in surgical implant dentistry: a systematic review, *Int J Oral Maxillofac Implants* 24:S92–S109.
105. Suzuki, T., Hori, N., Att, W., Kubo, K., Iwasa, F., Ueno, T., Maeda, H. and Ogawa, T., 2009, Ultraviolet treatment overcomes time-related degrading bioactivity of titanium, *Tissue Eng Part A* 15:3679–3688. doi: http://dx.doi.org/10.1089/ten.tea.2008.0568
106. Att, W., Hori, N., Takeuchi, M., Ouyang, J., Yang, Y., Anpo, M. and Ogawa, T., 2009, Time- dependent degradation of titanium osteoconductivity: An implication of biological aging of implant materials, *Biomaterials* 30:5352–5363. doi: http://dx.doi.org/10.1016/j.biomaterials.2009.06.040
107. Hori, N., Ueno, T., Suzuki, T., Yamada, M., Att, W., Okada, S., Ohno, A., Aita, H., Kimoto, K. and Ogawa, T., 2010, Ultraviolet light treatment for the restoration of age-related degradation of titanium bioactivity, *Int J Oral Maxillofac Implants* 25:49–62.
108. Lee, J.H. and Ogawa, T., 2012, The biological aging of titanium implants, *Implant Dent* 21:415–421. doi: http://dx.doi.org/10.1097/ID.0b013e31826a51f4

Index

CPSIA information can be obtained at www.ICGtesting.com
Printed in the USA
BVOW07*0840070414

349351BV00002B/2/P

9 781606 506271